Evidence-Based Practice in Nursing and Healthcare

Evidence-Based Practice in Nursing and Healthcare

Editor: Byrant Hill

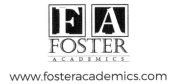

www.fosteracademics.com

www.fosteracademics.com

Cataloging-in-Publication Data

Evidence-based practice in nursing and healthcare / edited by Byrant Hill.
   p. cm.
Includes bibliographical references and index.
ISBN 978-1-63242-585-0
1. Nursing. 2. Nursing--Practice. 3. Medical care. 4. Medicine--Practice. I. Hill, Byrant.
RT42 .E95 2019
610.73--dc23

Foster Academics,
118-35 Queens Blvd., Suite 400,
Forest Hills, NY 11375, USA

ISBN 978-1-63242-585-0 (Hardback)

Contents

Preface

Every book is initially just a concept; it takes months of research and hard work to give it the final shape in which the readers receive it. In its early stages, this book also went through rigorous reviewing. The notable contributions made by experts from across the globe were first molded into patterned chapters and then arranged in a sensibly sequential manner to bring out the best results.

Nursing is concerned with the provision of care to maintain a quality of life for individuals, families or communities. It is extended to individuals across all ages and cultural backgrounds in a manner that takes into consideration the patient's physical, psychological, intellectual, social and emotional needs. Evidence-based nursing refers to the provision of nursing care that is based on an integration of personal clinical expertise and current research. This approach is founded on evidence-based practice. It strives to improve the health and safety of patients in a cost-effective manner. Evidence-based practice is based on the principles of cultivating a spirit of inquiry, asking clinical questions, collecting evidence, appraising the evidence, integrating the evidence, evaluating outcomes and disseminating outcomes. The topics covered in this extensive book deal with the core aspects of nursing and healthcare. It aims to present the researches that have transformed this discipline and aided its advancement. In this book, using case studies and examples, constant effort has been made to make the understanding of this field as easy and informative as possible for the readers.

It has been my immense pleasure to be a part of this project and to contribute my years of learning in such a meaningful form. I would like to take this opportunity to thank all the people who have been associated with the completion of this book at any step.

Editor

Assessment of Factors Affecting Implementation of Nursing Process Among Nurses in Selected Governmental Hospitals, Addis Ababa, Ethiopia; Cross Sectional Study

Mulugeta Aseratie[1], Rajalakshmi Murugan[2] and Mulugeta Molla[*3]

[1]Department of Nursing, College of Health Science, Addis Ababa Science and Technology University, Addis Ababa Ethiopia

[2]School of Nursing, College of Health Science, Addis Ababa University, Addis Ababa, Ethiopia

[3]Department of Nursing, College of Health Science, Mekelle University, Mekelle, Ethiopia

*Corresponding author: Mulugeta Molla, Department of Nursing, College of Health Sciences, Mekelle University, Tigray, Ethiopia, P.O. Box 187, E-mail: muler.warso@gmail.com

Abstract

Background: Nursing Process is a systematic problem-solving approach used to identify, prevent and treat actual or potential health problems and promote wellness. It has five steps- assessment, diagnosis, planning, implementation, and evaluation.

Objective: To assess factors affecting implementation of nursing process among nurses in selected governmental hospitals from February-April, 2011 at Addis Ababa, Ethiopia.

Method: A cross-sectional quantitative study was conducted on selected governmental hospitals in Addis Ababa. Purposive sampling was used for selection of hospitals. Black Lion, St. Paul, Ras Desta Damitew Memorial, and Yekatit 12 hospitals were convenient for the study. The sample size was 202. Data was analyzed using SPSS 16th version.

Result: Nurses working in a stressful working environment were 2.8 (adjusted OR: 0.357, 95%CI: (0.157-0.814)) times less likely to implement nursing process than disorganized working environment adjusting for facility accessibility, knowledge, and sex. Forty eight (25%) of respondents were anxious from high patient flow. Among those 15(31.3%), 22(45.8%), and 11(22.9%) have committed knowledge, executive, and slip/slap error respectively. Highly knowledgeable respondents were 38.913 (Adjusted OR: 38.913, 95%CI: (10.3-147.006) times more likely to implement nursing process than low knowledge group nurses adjusted for working environment, facility, and sex.

Conclusion: The study has identified organizational factors, patient related factors, and level of knowledge and skill were among those factors highly influenced nursing process implementation. This factors cause poor quality of nursing care, disorganized caring system, conflicting role, medication error and readmission with similar problem, dissatisfaction with the care patients have received, and increased mortality.

Keywords: Nursing process; Factors; Ethiopia and hospitals

Introduction

Based on a nursing theory developed by Ida Jean Orlando in the late 1950's as she observed nurses in action, the *Nursing Process* is an essential part of the nursing care plan [1].

The Nursing Process is a systematic problem-solving approach used to identify, prevent and treat actual or potential health problems and promote wellness. It has five steps; Assessment, Diagnosis, planning, implementation and evaluation [2].

Despite their knowledge of the nursing process, certain factors limited the ability of nurses to implement it in their daily practice, including lack of time, high patient volume, and high patient turnover. Despite these hurdles, the daily application of the nursing process is characterized by the scientific background of the professionals involved since it requires knowledge and provides individualized human assistance [3].

However, the existence of failures was shown among the nursing diagnoses in the patients' history, as well as the implementation of nursing prescriptions without recording the evaluation of the expected results [4].

Similar results were also shown in a study published in 2006 during the implementation of the nursing diagnosis, in which the research subjects indicated difficulties in developing the nursing process at all stages, and the need for changes to speed up the work process and optimize the quality of actions in care and education [5]. This research was done in University hospital where students are doing clinical practice. Students who attached in those hospitals learn from patient records but if there is no full implementation of nursing process, they cannot obtain what they should get from patient record. Furthermore, the patient care outcome might be poor which results into poor quality of life. Poor quality of life of an individual is one determinant factor for family disturbance. Family health will be impaired and societal problem become complicated.

It is reasonable to conclude that the nursing process is important for the practice of nursing; however, its use is not an easy task. Therefore, a continuous evaluation of how the nursing process is executed within the health services is required [6].

Nurses comprise the key connective tissue for Ethiopia's health care. They are also the largest cadre of health-care providers in Ethiopia and function in many different roles, from traditional bedside nursing to primary health care in regional health centers. It is common to see nurses working as laboratory personnel, dentists, councilors, and social workers to accommodate the shortages [7].

Nursing process is a multipurpose approach that enables nurses to perform their activities with logical justification. It safeguards the right of both the patient and the nurse. Recently in Ethiopia clients accuse nurses due to their haphazard practice. Clinton foundation is now giving in service training for nurses working in hospitals. Following this, training nurses are trying to practice nursing process and it becomes the focus of Ministry of Health throughout the country.

Nursing process implementation could be highly influenced by different factors that can lead to Poor quality of nursing care, disorganization of the service, conflicting roles, medication error, poor diseases prognosis, readmission, dissatisfaction with the care provided, and increased mortality. These problems are manageable if a nurse can properly implement nursing process. Therefore, the main aim of this study was to assess factors affecting implementation of nursing process among nurse in selected governmental hospitals of Addis Ababa. The finding will provide pragmatic evidence for educators, clinicians, program planner, decision makers to design a new and/or strengthen the existing nursing process and it will also serve as a baseline for future researchers.

Materials and Methods

Study area

The study was conducted in Addis Ababa, the capital city of Ethiopia and seat of African Union & United Nations World Economic Commission for Africa. Addis Ababa has a population size of over 3 million. Its average elevation is 2,500 m above sea level, and hence has a fairly favorable climate and moderate weather conditions. There were 12 governmental hospitals, among these Black Lion, St. Paul, Ras Desta Damitew Memorial, and Yekatit provides multi-dimensional aspects of care to clients. The data was collected in those areas only because the rest were giving a specialized care for homogeneous groups and it would be difficult to analyze with the findings of those 4 hospitals.

Study design

Institution based quantitative cross sectional study was conducted in four selected governmental hospitals in Addis Ababa.

Study period

The study was conducted from February-April, 2011.

Sample size determination

The overall minimum sample size was determined using single population proportion formula by considering; Z=standard normal distribution (Z=1.96) with confidence interval of 95% and =0.05, p=0.5, d=0.05. And By assuming this the final sample size was calculated as:

$$n^i = \frac{z_{a/2}^2 (p(1-p))}{d^2}$$

Where n= minimum sample size required for the study

P=prevalence/ population proportion (p=0.5); since we didn't get other p-value we took p_0.5.

d=is a tolerable margin of error (d=0.05)

= 1.96(1.96) (0.5(1-0.5))/0.05(0.05) = 384.16 => n^i=384

Since the total population is less than 10,000 we used correction formula. The exact sample size therefore was calculated as follows.

$f \frac{n_i x N}{n_i + N}$ Where n^i= calculated sample size n^f= exact sample size

N= sample population

= (384x354)/ (384+354) =135,936/738=184.19=184

= 184+10% none response rate = 184+18.4 =202.4

=202

Sampling procedure and technique

According to the data obtained from the selected hospitals there were 126, 100, 59, and 69 BScN nurses in BLH (Black lion Hospital), SPH (St. Paul), RDDMH (Ras Deasta Damtew Memorial Hospital), and Yekatit 12 hospital respectively. There were a total of 354 BScN nurses.

For the hospitals to proportionate the number of study subject using nf/N x n, is allocated a proportionate sample to their size.

BLH = (202x126)/354=71.89=72

SPH = (202x100)/354=57.06=57

RDDMH = (202x59)/354= 33.66=34

Yekatit 12 = (202x69)/354=39.3=39

Among those participants, Simple random sampling method has been used to select the participants from each Hospital.

Data collection and quality control

For data collection structured questionnaire was used. Structured English version questionnaire was developed from different literatures. And it was collected by self-administered questionnaire. The data collection process was supervised by the principal investigator from February-April/2011. Before the actual data collection, data collectors have obtained half day training about the aim of the study and the content of the instrument.

Study variables

The outcome variable was the Implementation of nursing process and the independent variable includes: Year of experience, Knowledge of nurses, Nurse to patient ratio, Nurse demographics, Hospital organizational structure, Patient turn over and Skill.

Eligibility criteria

Inclusion criteria:

- All BSc nurses with more than 6 months of working experience.
- Nurses who were willing to participate in the study.

Exclusion criteria:

- Diploma clinical nurse
- Nurses who are giving free service, absent during data collection time

Statistical analysis

Data first was cleared, coded and entered into computer using Epi-info and exported into SPSS16th version for analysis. The Uni-variate analysis such as percentage and frequency distribution of different characteristics of the questionnaire were analyzed. Bivariate analysis was used to see the association of independent with the dependent variable. Logistic regression model was employed to control confounding variables, variables included in the model were restricted to those significantly related to implementation of nursing process at the bivariate level and some of the statistical test like, odds' ratio (crude & adjusted) was used to measure their association and some of the results were compared with results of other studies available.

Ethical considerations

Ethical clearance was obtained from institutional review board of Addis Ababa University and selected hospital officials was communicated using support letter from school of nursing. No personal identification was registered and confidentiality was also maintained. No raw data was given to other parties

Result

In this study the response rate was 95%. Among the total respondents 102(53.1%) were females and 90(46.9%) were males. Ninety two (47.9%) of the respondents were in the age range of below 24 years, 81(42.2%) were in 25-44 years. one hundred fifty seven (81.8%) of the respondents were worked overtime. Only 9(5.7%) of the respondents were satisfied with the overtime payment whereas 148 (94.3%) were not satisfied with the payment (Table 1).

Characteristics		Frequency	Percentage
sex	Female	102	53.1
	Male	90	46.9
age	below24	92	47.9
	25-44	81	42.2
	45-54	17	8.9
	55-64	2	1
marital status	Single	135	70.3
	Married	52	27.1
	Widowed	3	1.6
	Divorced	2	1
year of graduation	<2yrs	130	67.7
	2-5yrs	57	29.7
	5-10yrs	3	1.6
	>10yrs	2	1
work experience	< 5 years	144	75
	5-10years	23	12
	10-15 years	7	3.65
	15-20 years	9	4.69
	20-25 years	5	2.6
	>25 years	4	2.1

Table 1: Socio-demographic characteristics of nurses in governmental hospitals of Addis Ababa, Ethiopia, 2011.

Vis-à-vis on method of making work of nurses visible one hundred sixteen (60.4%), 100(52.1%), 33(17.2%), and 68(35.4%) of the respondents have used recording, nursing process, reporting to higher officials, and only working on the patient's problem to make their work visible respectively. Nine (4.7%) of the respondents have used nothing to make their work visible. From the total respondents 116(60.4%) of them were always record their activities while 4(2.1%) never recorded their activities.

In this study forty eight (25%) of respondents were anxious from high patient flow. Among those 15(31.3%), 22(45.8%), and 11(22.9%) have committed knowledge, executive, and slip/slap error respectively.

From the total respondents 104(54.2%) of them said the dissatisfying aspect of their job was caring for so many patients followed by rules being made up without staff or residents in mind 79(41.1%); useless paper work 40 (20.8%) and new reporting system 31(16.1%). From those dissatisfied with any reason stated above 95(49.5%) of the total respondents were dissatisfied due to their profession (Table 2).

Character		Frequency		Percentage
Working hours/day	<8hrs	11		5.7
	8hrs	148	77.1	

Category	Subcategory	Response	Count	Percentage
		12hrs	19	9.9
		>12hrs	14	7.3
Distribution of patient flow		<8pts	14	7.3
		5-10pts	51	26.6
		10-15pts	49	25.5
		>15pts	78	40.6
Overtime work		Yes — With payment	134	69.8
		Yes — Without payment	23	12
		No	35	18.2
Satisfied with payment		Yes	9	5.7
		No	125	94.3
Dissatisfying aspect of nursing	Caring for so many patients	Yes	104	54.2
		No	88	45.8
	New reporting system	Yes	31	16.1
		No	161	83.9
	Rules made without considering staff	Yes	79	41.1
		No	113	59.9
	Useless paper work	Yes	40	20.8
		No	152	79.2
Work place	Stressful		140	72.9
	Negligent at a time		21	10.9
	Disorganized		31	16.2
Effect of staff turnover	Decreasing productivity	Yes	68	35.4
		No	124	64.6
	Disorganized service delivery	Yes	134	69.8
		No	58	30.2
	Decrease spread of organizational knowledge	Yes	46	24
		No	146	76
Cause of employee turnover	Job and employee skill mismatch	Yes	88	45.8
		No	104	54.2
	Inferior facility	Yes	40	20.8
		No	152	79.2
	Less recognition	Yes	68	35.4
		No	124	64.6
	Less/ no appreciation	Yes	55	28.6
		No	137	71.4

	Less growth opportunity	Yes	68	35.4	
		No	124	64.6	
	Poor training	Yes	41	21.4	
		No	151	78.6	
	Poor supervision	Yes	28	14.6	
		No	164	85.4	

Table 2: Organizational factors affecting implementation of nursing process among Nurses in governmental hospitals of Addis Ababa, Ethiopia, 2011

Regarding working hour distribution (Table 2) seventy eight (40.6%) of nurses have cared for more than 15 patients per day and 49(22.5%) were cared for 10-15 patients per day while 51(26.6%) have cared for 5-10 patients per day and only 11(5.7%) were cared for less than 8 patients per day. 148(77.1%) of respondents have worked eight hours per day whereas 14(7.3%) have worked more than 12 hours per day.

Seventy eight (40.6%) of respondents were challenged to provide their nursing care due to early discharge of patients before completing the planned intervention. Seventy five (39.1%) of respondents believed that patients discharged before completing their treatment and came back to their institution with a complicated problem which was difficult to manage.

Regarding the knowledge assessment of nurses (Table 3) majority of respondents 175(91.1%) have answered the correct answer, which is evidence based practice is not among the five components of nursing process while the remaining 16(8.9%) have chosen the incorrect answer one among the components of nursing process.

Characteristics	Correct Answer No (%)	Incorrect Answer No (%)	Total No (%)
One is not among the component of nursing process	175(91.1%)	17(8.9%)	192(100%)
A nurse should do one at the first step of nursing process	156(81.2%)	36(19.8%)	192(100%)
The Gordon approach is directly targeted at-----	102(53.1%)	90(46.9%)	192(100%)
Which nursing diagnosis is better to solve a patient's problem with diabetes mellitus chronic complication in the future?	136(70.8%)	56(29.2%)	192(100%)
What makes nursing process different from medical approach?	137(71.4%)	55(28.6%)	192(100%)
Among the individuals in a hospital one is not mandatory for the better accomplishment of nursing process.	101(52.6%)	91(47.4%)	192(100%)
One is not included under the activities to be performed in the planning phase of nursing process.	64(33.3%)	128(66.7%)	192(100%)
In implementation step of nursing process a nurse is expected to perform------	108(56.2%)	84(43.8%)	192(100%)
One could not be a guide for evaluation of nurses performance in nursing process	112(58.3%)	80(41.7%)	192(100%)
Disturbed sleeping pattern related to unresolved fears and anxieties as evidenced by difficulty in falling /remain asleep. Identify the problem, etiology and sign/symptom of the above nursing diagnosis	92(47.9%)	100(52.1%)	192(100%)
Write one full actual nursing diagnosis	39(20.3%)	153(79.7%)	192(100%)

Table 3: Nurses' knowledge about nursing process among nurses in selected governmental hospitals of Addis Ababa, Ethiopia, 2011.

Regarding factors affecting of implementation of nursing process (Table 4) sixty one (32.8%) of female and 39(20.3%) of male respondents were implemented nursing process. Out of one hundred respondents who were implemented nursing process 80(41.6%) were working in a stressful working environment, 10(5.2%) were worked in a neglecting environment, and 10(5.2%) were worked in a disorganized environment. Seventy three (38%) were implemented nursing process without facility shortage while 27(14%) were implemented with an inferior facility. Among those implemented nursing process only four nurses were highly knowledgeable and equal number of respondents 48(25%) were moderately and poorly knowledgeable.

Characteristics		Implementation of nursing process		Crude P-value	COR	AOR(95%CI)
		Yes	No	(95%CI)		
		No (%)	No (%)			
Sex	Female	61(32.8%)	41(21.4%)	0.023	0.514(0.289-0.913)	0.712(0.361-1.407)*
	Male	39(20.3%)	51(26.6%)			
Work place	Stress full	80(41.6%)	60(31.3%)	0.014	0.357(0.157-0.814)	0.180(0.065-0.501)
	Negligent	10(5.2%)	11(5.7%)	0.266		
	Disorganized	10(5.2%)	21(10.9%)			
Facility	Accessible	73(38%)	79(41.1%)	0.031	2.248(1.079-4.684)	3.109(1.277-7.570)
	Inferior	27(14%)	13(6.8%)			
Knowledge	Highly knowledgeable	4(2.1%)	27(6.8%)	0	27(7.924-91.994)	38.913(10.3-147.006)
	Moderately knowledgeable	48(25%)	53(27.6%)	0	4.417(2.1-9.289)	4.913(2.178-11.084)
	Low knowledgeable	48(25%)	12(41.1%)			

Table 4: Factors Affecting implementation of nursing process among nurses in selected governmental hospitals of Addis Ababa, Ethiopia, 2011.

From binary logistic regression analysis (Table 4) being a female were significantly associated with implementation of nursing process than male (COR: 0.514, 95%CI :(0.284-0.913), p: 0.023).

Working in a hospital with high facility were 2.248 times significantly and more likely to implement nursing process than those working in an inferior facility (COR: 2.248, 95%CI: (1.079-4.684), P: 0.030).

Highly knowledgeable nurses were 27 times more likely and significantly associated with implementation of nursing process than low knowledge group nurses (COR: 27, 95%CI: (7.924-91.994), P: <0.001). Moderately knowledgeable nurses were positively and significantly associated with implementation of nursing process (COR: 4.417, 95%CI: (2.1-9.289), P: <0.001).

In a multivariate analysis (multivariate logistic regression) (Table 4) nurses working in a stressful working environment were 0.357(AOR: 0.357, (0.157-0.814)) times less likely to implement nursing process than disorganized working environment adjusting for facility accessibility, knowledge, and sex. Accessibility of facilities needed for nursing care were 2.248(AOR: 2.248, (1.079-4.684) times more likely to implement nursing process than nurses working in an inferior facility controlling for working environment, knowledge, and sex. Highly knowledgeable and highly skillful, moderately skillful, and poorly skillful accounting 19,11, and 1 respectively were 38.913(AOR: 38.913, (10.3-147.006) times more likely to implement nursing process than low knowledge group nurses adjusted for working environment, facility, and sex. Moderately knowledgeable were 4.913 (AOR: 4.913, (2.178-11.407)) times more likely to implement nursing process than low knowledge group nurses adjusted for work place, facility, and sex.

Discussion

The study tried to assess factors affecting implementation of nursing process among nurses working in selected government hospitals of Addis Ababa. One hundred (52.1%) nurses were implemented nursing process while 92(47.9%) of them were not implemented nursing process. From those implemented nursing process 61(61%) were female and 39(39%) were male.

From the total respondents 104 (54.2%) of them said the dissatisfying aspect of their job was caring for so many patients. In a research conducted about nurse to physician communication, nursing workload definitely affects the time that a nurse can allot to various tasks. Under a heavy workload, nurses may not have sufficient time to perform tasks that can have a direct effect on patient safety. A heavy nursing workload can influence the care provider's decision to perform various procedures [8]. This similarity might be due to the nature of the profession and when nurses become dissatisfied about their job the nursing care to be provided will not have systematic approach or nursing process may not be implemented in a hospital with high patient flow beyond the capacity of nurses.

The average nurse-to-population ratio in high-income countries is almost eight times greater than in low-income countries. Factors contributing to the nursing shortage vary in different parts of the world [9]. As registered nurse-to-patient ratios decrease from 1:4 to 1:10, the number of post-op surgical patient deaths climbs dramatically [10]. In this study seventy eight (40.6%) of nurses have cared for more than 15 patients per day and 49(22.5%). This significant difference might be due to a difference in socio-economic status of those countries.

One hundred thirty four (69.8%) of respondents in this study had believe that staff turn over from a specific public health institution obligates the organization to provide a disorganized service. Sixty eight (35.4%) of respondents had believe that staff turnover can cause decrease in productivity whereas 46(24%) had believed that staff turnover can cause decreased spread of organizational knowledge. In line with this research, several studies have shown the relationship between nurses' working conditions, such as high workload, and job dissatisfaction [11]. Job dissatisfaction of nurses can lead to low morale, absenteeism, turnover, and poor job performance, and potentially threaten patient care quality and organizational effectiveness [12]. Thus, workload leads to staff turnover that could be a burdensome for implementation of nursing process.

According to the report released from Cambridge UK workload can be a factor contributing to errors [13]. In this study forty eight (25%) of respondents were anxious from high patient flow. Among those 15(31.3%), 22(45.8%), and 11(22.9%) have committed knowledge, executive, and slip/slap error respectively.

There was a study conducted in the United Kingdom to assess whether data obtained from nursing records could be reliably used to identify interventions for patients who had suffered acute myocardial infarction or a fracture of the head of the femur, showed that the analyzed nursing records did not provide an adequate picture of patients' needs for nursing interventions [14]. Similarly in this study ninety two (47.9%) of respondents were able to identify the problem, etiology and sign and symptoms of a given actual nursing diagnosis. Only 39(20.3%) of respondents were able to write a full actual nursing diagnosis that have consisted of problem, etiology, and manifestations of the problem. This tells us the inability of nurses to identify the components of nursing diagnoses and recording it in a well-organized manner that could be understandable by other staff members. This may be due to the difficulty of nurses to write nursing diagnosis than other nursing process components.

An investigation conducted in Brazil on the steps of nursing process actually implemented in the routine of a university hospital showed that all phases were performed. However, problems were identified in the nursing diagnosis process, involving recording the history and implementing nursing prescriptions. The evolution of expected results, in particular, was not adequately recorded [15]. From 100(52.1%) respondents who have implemented nursing process 61, 22, 8, 7, and 2 were recorded their activities always, sometimes, every once in a while, rarely and never respectively. The part of nursing process which was not written is not separately identified in this study. But we can conclude that nurses could not fully document what they have performed cognizant of the fact that they have implemented nursing process.

High workload is a key job stressor of nurses in a variety of care settings, such as ICUs. A heavy nursing workload can lead to distress (e.g., cynicism, anger, and emotional exhaustion) and burnout. Nurses experiencing stress and burnout may not be able to perform efficiently and effectively because their physical and cognitive resources may be reduced; this suboptimal performance may affect patient care and its safety. In this study from the characteristics work place, nurses who were working in a stressful environment were 0.357 times significantly and less likely to implement nursing process than those worked in a disorganized environment (COR: 0357, 95%CI (0.157-0.814), P: 0.014). Neglecting working environment had no significant association with implementation of nursing process. Hence nursing process implementation needs a safe and encouraging working environment.

Conclusion

From this study 100(52.1%) of the respondents were implementing nursing process. Among the factors which affect the nursing process were high patient flow 48(25%), patient load 78(40.6%) of nurses cared for more than 15 patients per day, early discharge 78(40.6%). Nurses who were working in a stressful environment were 0.357 times less likely to implement nursing process than those worked in a disorganized environment.

Highly knowledgeable nurses were 27% times more likely to implement nursing process than low knowledge group nurses.

Strength and Limitation of the Study:

Strength of the study

This study was probably the first/ among the pioneers research related to nursing process in Ethiopia. It will be helpful as baseline information for other researchers.

Limitations of the study

Since this was quantitative study it may not explore all the associated factors and it is advisable to use both quantitative and qualitative methods as well.

Since the study subjects were recruited from selected governmental hospitals of Addis Ababa. The study didn't included nurses working in other hospitals. Thus the study may not be generalized to all nurses in Addis Ababa because nurses out of selected hospitals may have different experience and opinion.

Acronyms and Abbreviations

AAU: Addis Ababa University

BLH: Black Lion Hospital

Dx:Diagnosis

ICU: Intensive Care Unit

NANDA: North American Nursing Diagnosis Association

NCP: Nursing Care Plan

NP: Nursing Process

RDDMH: Ras Desta Damitew Memorial Hospital

SPH: St. Paul Hospital

USA: United States of America

Competing interest

We don't have any competing interest.

Acknowledgement

Above all we would like to express our gratitude to my Lord- Jesus Christ and His mother the Virgin St. Marry who carries all my burdens and shepherded us healthy.

We are pleased to thank AtoFekadu Aga (MSN), AtoYosephTsgie (MSN), Addis Ababa University) , AtoAbdurahman Mohamed(MPH), Dr.Mulusew A and his wife Etalemahu M. for their professional, moral and material support. Our gratitude also goes to our friends for their direct or indirect contribution to the development of this study.

The last but not the least we would like to extend our gratitude to data collectors, Addis Ababa University, staff of Black Lion, St. Paul, RasDestaDamitew, and Yekatit12 hospitals for their cooperation in the realization of the study.

References

1. CGS (2010) Nurse Practice Act

2. S Carlson (2010) Nursing Process

3. De Freitas MC, Queiroz TA, de Souza JA (2007) [The nursing process according to the view of nurses from a maternity]. Rev Bras Enferm 60: 207-212.

4. Lima AF, Kurcgant P (2006) [The nursing diagnosis implementation process at the University Hospital of the University of São Paulo]. Rev Esc Enferm USP 40: 111-116.

5. Lima AF, Kurcgant P (2006) Meanings of the nursing diagnosis implementation process for nurses at a university hospital. Rev Lat Am Enfermagem 14: 666-673.

6. J Schaefer (2010) Nursing process and its determinant factors.

7. Global health council (2010) Building a Winning Nursing Work Force for HIV-Care in Ethiopia.

8. Griffith CH 3rd, Wilson JF, Desai NS, Rich EC (1999) Housestaff workload and procedure frequency in the neonatal intensive care unit. Crit Care Med 27: 815-820.

9. WHO (2006) The World Health Report 2006

10. Darvas JA, Hawkins LG (2002) What makes a good intensive care unit: a nursing perspective. Aust Crit Care 15: 77-82.

11. Cavanagh SJ (1992) Job satisfaction of nursing staff working in hospitals. J Adv Nurs 17: 704-711.

12. Reason J (1990) Human error. Cambridge, UK: Cambridge University Press.

13. Hale CA, Thomas LH, Bond S, Todd C (1997) The nursing record as a research tool to identify nursing interventions. J Clin Nurs 6: 207-214.

14. Reppetto MA, de Souza MF (2005) [Evaluation of nursing care systematization through the phases of nursing process performance and registration in a teaching hospital]. Rev Bras Enferm 58: 325-329.

15. Oates RK, Oates P (1995) Stress and mental health in neonatal intensive care units. Arch Dis Child Fetal Neonatal Ed 72: F107-110.

Big Data Analytics in Heart Attack Prediction

Cheryl Ann Alexander[1] and Lidong Wang[2*]

[1]*Department of Nursing, University of Phoenix, USA*

[2]*Department of Engineering Technology, Mississippi Valley State University, USA*

[*]**Corresponding author:** Lidong Wang, Department of Engineering Technology, Mississippi Valley State University, USA; E-mail: lwang22@students.tntech.edu

Abstract

Introduction: Acute myocardial infarction (heart attack) is one of the deadliest diseases patients face. The key to cardiovascular disease management is to evaluate large scores of datasets, compare and mine for information that can be used to predict, prevent, manage and treat chronic diseases such as heart attacks. Big Data analytics, known in the corporate world for its valuable use in controlling, contrasting and managing large datasets can be applied with much success to the prediction, prevention, management and treatment of cardiovascular disease. Data mining, visualization and Hadoop are technologies or tools of big data in mining the voluminous datasets for information.

Aim: The aim of this literature review was to identify usage of Big Data analytics in heart attack prediction and prevention, the use of technologies applicable to big data, privacy concerns for the patient, and challenges and future trends as well as suggestions for further use of these technologies.

Methods: The national and international databases were examined to identify studies conducted about big data analytics in healthcare, heart attack prediction and prevention, technologies used in big data, and privacy concerns. A total of 31 studies that fit these criteria were assessed.

Results: Per the studies analyzed, Big Data analytics is useful in predicting heart attack, and the technologies used in Big Data are extremely vital to the management and tailoring of treatment for cardiovascular disease. And as the use of Big Data in healthcare increases, more useful personalized medicine will be available to individual patients.

Conclusion: This review offers the latest information on Big Data analytics in healthcare, predicting heart attack, and tailoring medical treatment to the individual. The results will guide providers, healthcare organizations, nurses, and other treatment providers in using Big Data technologies to predict and manage heart attack as well as what privacy concerns face the use of Big Data analytics in healthcare. Effective and tailored medical treatment can be developed using these technologies.

Keywords: Big data; Big Data analytics; Heart attack; Nursing; Health care; Personalized patient care; Privacy; Data mining; Machine learning; Internet of things (IoT); Telecardiology

Introduction

Acute Myocardial infarction (AMI), commonly referred to as a heart attack, is among one of the deadliest of cardiovascular diseases. AMI happens as circulation or blood flow to heart muscle is interrupted, causing the heart muscle to damage or die (become necrotic) [1]. The primary reason for most heart attacks is a blockage which causes blood flow to one of the coronary arteries, vital channels through which blood travels to the heart muscle, to become reduced or obstructed. When blood flow is obstructed or reduced, the heart muscle is rapidly deprived of red blood cells which carry the necessary oxygen essential for sustaining life and consciousness in the human body. It takes as few as six to eight minutes without oxygen to cause the heart muscle to arrest, leading to the individual's death [2]. The cause of most heart attacks is plaque, a hard substance which builds up over time in the coronary arteries. Plaque, a substance made up of numerous cells and cholesterol (fat), draws platelets, which increase over time, causing a blockage large enough to diminish or block blood flow to heart muscle. Some individuals have a build-up of plaque in the arteries over many years and this is known as atherosclerosis. Examining the cause and etiology of atherosclerosis, it can be described as a chronic inflammation. And when examining AMI, it also could be described as acute inflammation. White blood cell production in the bone marrow is increased due to signaling via the sympathetic nervous system after the AMI as well as in the spleen. This increase in white blood cell production migrate to the heart and vessel wall and can be recruited into other atherosclerotic plaques, causing more inflammation and likely subsequent ischemic events such as reinfarction or stroke [3].

There are generally two phases of wound healing when it comes to monocytes and macrophages. Initially there is an early inflammatory phase and afterwards, a reparative phase begins. However, both phases are necessary for proper wound healing; but if either of these phases is stalled or if the inflammation continues too long, resolution of the inflammation never happens and it leads to heart failure [3]. On the other hand, a more unusual type of heart attack strikes when there is an acute spasm or constriction of one of the coronary arteries. The spasm then cuts off blood flow to the heart causing oxygen deprivation. These spasms can appear in coronary arteries without any signs of atherosclerosis. As far as symptoms, men are significantly more likely to experience chest pain than women. Furthermore, women are far more likely to experience a heart attack if their pain lasts more than one hour, while men are more like to experience pain durations of less than one hour when having a heart attack [2]. AMI occurs within the entire physiological system; it does not just happen to the heart, but changes happen everywhere, including remote organs such as the spleen and bone marrow [3].

The old way of handling data included small and expensive methods. Input data from clinical trials were too small and too costly; data was limited so the modelling effort was small. However, in today's market, the electronic health record (EHR) has revolutionized data management. Data has become cheaper, larger, and there is a broader patient population to be included. Data has become noisy, heterogeneous, diverse in scale and longitudinal in the EHR. In addition, Medicare now penalizes hospitals with high rates of readmissions amid patients with Heart failure, Heart attack, and Pneumonia [4]. Care plans and outcomes-based discharge measures have been established by Medicare so that hospitals must conform to Medicare admission and discharge regulations for these diseases for reimbursement. Outcomes measures have become the primary mode of evaluating patients for discharge and reimbursement since the establishment of the Health Insurance Portability and Accountability Act of 1996. Some examples of different outcome in health care include: binary outcomes (death or adverse events), continuous outcomes (length of stay or visual analogue score), ordinal outcomes (quality of life, grade of tumor, number of heart attacks), survival outcomes (cancer survival or clinical trials) [4]. Big data, a concept now several years old, is becoming the primary method to harness data as more and more health care organizations discover opportunities to better understand and predict customer behaviors and interests. Big data is the data that exceeds the processing capacity of conventional database systems. The data is too big, moves too fast, or doesn't fit the strictures of conventional database architectures [5]. Big data characteristics can be described by "6Vs". They are: Volume, Velocity, Variety, Value, Variability and Veracity [5-14].

Volume: It means data size such as terabytes (TB: approximately 10^{12} bytes), petabytes (PB: approximately 10^{15} bytes) and zettabytes (ZB: approximately ^{21} bytes), etc.

Velocity: Data is generated at a high speed.

Variety: Data can be structured, semi-structured, or unstructured.

Value: It refers to the value that the data adds to creating knowledge.

Variability: It refers to data changes during processing and lifecycle.

Veracity: It includes two aspects: data consistency (or certainty) and data trustworthiness.

Big data fosters newer opportunities to predict and/or more rapidly respond to critical clinical events, generating better health outcomes and more efficient cost management. Oracle, an international technology firm, proposes that big data often has low value density if data is received in its original form. Intelligent electronic devices - used by some individuals while both at home and while traveling about their day - now capture and transmit data for analysis in the management of chronic diseases and conditions providing more frequent data about the heart, the breathing process, blood sugar or blood pressure - as the patient goes about daily life - and significantly increases a provider's ability to make appropriate clinical decisions. A cardiologist can receive data daily about each ambulatory - roughly one hundred times more often than possible with quarterly office visits - thereby occasionally giving the provider an early warning of problems, which could prevent a heart attack. Data compiled by these medical devices is quite frequently voluminous and rapidly increasing; this necessitates intensive and complex analysis to both augment clinical decisions and guide research on improved practices, thus improving outcomes [15].

But big data is not only about size, there is also the insight it derives from complex, noisy, heterogeneous, longitudinal, and voluminous data. Challenges, however, include capturing, storing, searching, sharing and analyzing. And social communication in varied digital forms is on the increase [16]. Already established as a novel field, data mining is now a primary method for discovering knowledge in buried patterns among the big datasets. In the health care industry, this uncharted knowledge can be utilized in different application domains, for example heart attack prediction. Data mining techniques and machine learning can be used to develop new software to assist providers and others in the health care industry to make decisions about heart attacks in the early stages [17,18]. Big Data is created by a growing plurality of resources, including Internet clicks, mobile transactions, user-generated content, and social media, and currently, genomics data, as well as purposefully generated content through sensor networks or corporate transactions. Currently, the most vital advances include the use of genomic data in drug discovery, the sharing of clinical-trial data, the use of EHRs, and the growing availability of data from mHealth applications such as telemedicine, patient registries, and social media [19]. Medication data vary in EHR systems and can be in both structured and unstructured formats. The availability and completeness of medication data vary while inpatient medication data may be complete, but outpatient medication data may not be. Prescription records may be incomplete as data is usually only stored as prescriptions but we cannot be sure whether patients filled those prescriptions. Clinical notes also hold rich and various sources of information, most of which is unstructured [16]. The new generation of information about the efficacy of treatments and the prediction of outcomes are the most fundamental applications of big health care data. Big Data varies from traditional decision support tools as it fosters collection and analysis of real-time patient data [19]. It is extremely vital to patient care and reducing both mortality and morbidity associated with heart attacks that providers can utilize big data applications to improve or establish a heart attack prediction program. Predicting heart attacks will not only save numerous lives but will assist providers in establishing personalized medicine, one of the many applications of big data in health care currently available..

Aim

The aim of this comprehensive literature review is to examine current standards, methods, and uses for big data to develop a heart attack prediction system to assist providers in establishing higher standards of care and a more personalized medical care plan for the patient.

Literature Review Questions

- What is Big Data Analytics and how is it used in health care?

- Can using Big Data Analytics be used to predict heart attacks?
- What is the role of nursing in the application of Big Data?
- What are some of the challenges of using Big Data Analytics in health care?
- What are the future trends associated with Big Data, heart attack prediction and personalized medicine?
- Will society punish violations before they occur based solely on investigative predictions of future behaviors?

Methods

Search strategy

A systematic review of the literature concerning Big Data Analytics in Health Care, Big Data Analytics, Big Data in Heart Attack Prediction, Big Data and telemedicine, visualization, and The Internet of Things in all countries was conducted in December of 2016. Studies published between 2011 and 2016 were examined using the following search engines per the search criteria: Google Scholar, EBSCOhost Online Research Databases, Medline/PubMed, Mississippi State University Library Database, and the University of Phoenix e-campus library databases. The search strategy included all English language peer reviewed articles and all types of trials and studies. The selected titles were from appropriate articles also hand-searched to detect further relevant papers.

Search terms

Specific search terms were utilized in this study. Some of the search terms applied to the selected databases include: Big Data Analytics, Big Data Analytics in Health Care, Heart Attack Prediction, Heart Attack Prevention, Visualization and Big Data, Telecardiology, Sensors and Big Data applications. All the search terms were applied in English only. Each keyword was combined using "or" then combining it with "and."

Review procedure

Most of these studies were conducted either in the US, United Kingdom or Australia, using different definitions, various methods to collect the data, and both qualitative and quantitative study types. We did not however, try to analyze this data statistically, but results were summarized through Big Data Analytics in Health Care, Big Data and Heart Attack Prediction, The Internet of Things, Visualization and Telecardiology. Challenges and future trends as well as the conclusion are original research.

Article selection criteria

Inclusion/exclusion criteria

This article encompasses various types of studies, for example, randomized controlled trials, non-randomized controlled trials, longitudinal studies, cohort or case-control studies and descriptive and qualitative studies. Full-text peer reviewed articles that included Big Data in Health Care, Big Data and Heart Attack Prediction, The Internet of Things, Visualization, and Telecardiology were selected to comprise a sample group. However, studies related to Big Data Analytics in other fields, general studies on heart attack, and studies conducted unrelated to heart attack and Big Data were excluded from

the sample. Conference papers, reports, and Power Point presentation material was considered when relevant to the primary sample.

Results

Features of the studies

A total of 1,224 studies were screened per title and 568 titles were excluded because the topic was not related to our research, or that they were editorials or letters. That left 142 peer reviewed article abstracts to be judged and after the title evaluation, 67 articles were examined for full text fitness and 36 articles were excluded due to the relevancy to our topic. Considering the evaluation, only 31 articles were deemed appropriate for this paper based on topic and relevancy.

Big data analytics in health care

The general process of data analytics can be comprised of two phases which are illustrated in Figure 1 [20]. Big Data analytics is changing the way we experience, provide, and receive health care. Providers are using big data more frequently than ever before to achieve a more personalized approach to their health care. As more and more data becomes available, through the EHR, medication refill records, insurance reports, genomics, telemedicine, and more currently, sensor data, we assume that innovators will design even more exciting ideas for using big data—nearly all of which that would help considerably diminish the soaring cost of health care in the US. The health care system must make a significant transformation for stakeholders to take full advantage of big data. The old levers for capturing value—chiefly cost-reduction efforts, most notably unit price discounts dependent upon contracting and negotiating power, or the rejection of redundant treatments—do not take full advantage of the insights that big data provides and therefore need to be enhanced or substituted for other methods linked to the new value pathways created by big data. Finally, traditional fee-for-service payment structures must be exchanged for a new system that bases reimbursement on gainful insights offered by big data [21].

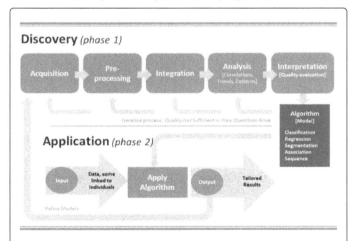

Figure 1: The general process of data analytics.

Structured data, for example, tables of numbers, do not reveal everything understood about a medication or biological process and most of the current knowledge about living organisms exists in unstructured formats [16]. Primary data pools are at the heart of the big-data revolution in healthcare. Integration of data pools is required for major opportunities. Table 1 [16] explains the primary data pools:

Primary Data Pools	Description
Clinical data	· Owners: providers
	· Example datasets: medical images, electronic medical records (EMR)
Activity (claims) and cost data	· Owners: providers, payors
	· Example datasets: utilization of care, cost estimates
Pharmaceutical R&D data	· Owner: academia, pharmaceutical companies
	· Example datasets: clinical trials, high-throughput-screening libraries
Patient behavior and sentiment data	· Owners: consumers and stakeholders outside health care (e.g., apparel, retail)
	· Example datasets: retail purchase history, patient behaviors and preferences, exercise data captured in running shoes

Table 1: Primary data pools of the big-data revolution in health care.

Biomedicalization denotes the on-going expansion of medicalization into new territory due to relatively fresh technology and scientific changes. Health care organizations, insurance agencies, pharmaceutical companies, and providers are now struggling to form new techno scientific innovations and organizational methods to meet their ever-growing needs. There has been a tremendous growth of the techno scientific nature of biomedicine in recent years, primarily due to three overlapping areas: computerization and data banking; molecularization and genericization of biomedicine and drug design; and medical technology, design, development and distribution [22]. Numerous medical characteristics combined with big data analysis based on the medical diagnostics of multiple fields rather than just by an individual provider relying on each patient's medical information [23]. Big data now plays a critical role in health care operations as data from large EHR systems, refill profiles, insurance information, genomic data and currently sensor data from both wearable and stationary nodes. Providers can utilize the data to manage many disease processes, personalize treatment to the individual, and improve outcomes through researching the database. Nursing care can also now be tailored to the individual's specific needs.

Smart Healthcare, now a current trend in health care contributing to the sources big data supports, has used multiple products such as home health care, wearable healthcare, and bio-transplant health care. For patients needing monitoring at home, home health care systems are sensors installed in the home that help manage the individual's health along with individual users and their smartphones. In the case of wearable health care, sensors are worn on the human body, providing personalized service through the measurement, transmission, and analysis of the bio-signal of the user's body in real time [23]. Sensors provide invaluable real time data to the provider.

Precise analysis in big data can lead to more certain decision-making. Apache Hadoop, an influential aspect in big data was developed by Yahoo, is an open-source software framework written in Java and is primarily for distributed processing and distributed storage of enormous datasets on computer clusters. Enormous data storage and faster processing are supported by Hadoop. Hadoop Distributed File System (HDFS) makes numerous copies of each data block and distributes them on systems to a cluster for reliable access. HDFS

supports cloud computing using Hadoop, a distributed data processing platform. A distributed column oriented database—Hbase—is built on top of HDFS. It can be used when we need random access to very large datasets. HDFS provides reliable and scalable data storage. The central core of Apache Hadoop consists of a storage part—HDFS—and a processing segment, Map Reduce. Apache Mahout executes distributed or scalable machine learning and data mining algorithms [17,24]. Proposed system architecture is described in Figure 2 [17].

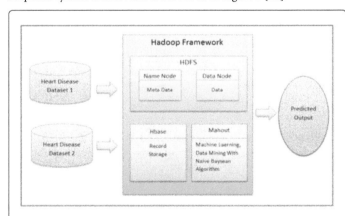

Figure 2: A system architecture dealing with big data.

This system is primarily concerned with two datasets—the original big dataset and the updated dataset. There are also two nodes: the Name Node which keeps a record of all files in the file system, and tracks the site of each file in a cluster; there is also the Data Node which warehouses data in the Hadoop File System. Any efficient file system is comprised of more than one Data Node, with data replication. Hbase is used when an engineer needs random; real time read or writes access to Big Data. The goal of Hbase is to accommodate especially large tables [17]. The Hadoop framework fractures big data into smaller parts stored on clusters of commodity hardware. Hadoop concurrently processes huge quantities of data utilizing various low cost computers for speedy results. HBase is a column-based database management system running above HDFS. It is well suited for scant datasets common in numerous big data use cases. HBase applications use a Java programming language like typical MapReduce applications. An HBase system is comprised of sets of tables. Each table holds columns and rows like a traditional database. An HBase column characterizes an attribute of each item. HBase permits several characteristics to be grouped together into column families, so that each of the elements of a column family is stored together. In HBase you must first predefine the table schema and clarify the column families. New columns can be added to families virtually any time, making the schema highly flexible. Hadoop manages huge amounts of structured as well as unstructured data much more efficiently than the traditional enterprise data warehouse. Since Hadoop is an open source framework and can run on commodity hardware, initial cost cuts are dramatic. Hadoop has a vigorous Apache community behind it which continues to subsidize its advancement. HDFS, a Java oriented file system, delivers reliable and scalable data storage [18].

Patient-customized health care and big data

Ciccone et al. conducted a feasibility study of incorporating care managers (specially trained nurses) into the healthcare system to support general practitioners (GPs) and specialists in the management of patients with cardiovascular disease (CVD), diabetes, heart failure or CVD risk. Care managers worked directly with individual patients, assisting them in making lifestyle changes, monitoring their conditions and providing the necessary information and advice to promote patient empowerment, and enhance self-management skills. This resulted in a tangible improvement in the clinical service and patients achieved better control of their disease. Ultimately, the care manager role has a positive influence on patient health and self-management, and their outcomes can be attributed to the solid "partnership" between the care manager and the patient and the collaboration between the provider and the care manager [25]. Specially trained nurses are now at the forefront of the new data revolution in healthcare. Not only do nurses provide care at the bedside, in the data-driven society we live in currently, nurses must shift their roles to assist their patients in becoming more empowered, changing their lifestyles, and improving their overall health based on the data. Never before in history has this system of personalized medicine been at the threshold of revolutionary evidence-based patient care.

Recently, a Patient-customized Healthcare System based on Hadoop with Text Mining (PHSHT) was developed as a method to efficiently manage diseases and the health care system. Subsequently, the PHSHT not only supplements the glitches within the existing decision-making algorithm, which ignores the relationship among attributes, but it also produces precise disease rules. Also, the patient's status is revealed to the individual so preventing any unexpected accidents since the patient can then take immediate action. The Text Mining based Hadoop platform determines an individual's disease, predicts the disease process, and creates more precise information about any diseases by converting the patient's unstructured generated data to structured data. There are four modules in PHSHT: (a) MDCM stores big data such as a patient's health information in the Hbase, which happens within a hospital or a portable health care system. Afterward, the collected big data is separated into structured data like patient information, family history, and medical prescriptions, as well as unstructured data like clinical notes, EHR, and PACs data; (b) TMHM analyzes the amassed unstructured data with Text Mining based Hadoop and transforms it to structured data. TMHM also distributes and stores structured data in the Hbase then merges the stored structured data and stores it in Hbase again with a MapReduce Framework; (c) DRCM generates

disease rules by using the disease information stored in the Hbase and CPST algorithm and stores them again in the Hbase; (d) DMPM notifies a patient or the provider of a risk index as the result of disease prediction after analyzing the patient's risk with the patient's collected information or by predicting a disease by relating the disease rules generated by DRCM with collected information [26]. The modules and flowchart of the PHSHT is illustrated in Figure 3 [26].

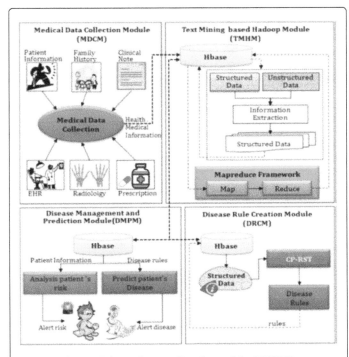

Figure 3: The modules and entire flowchart of the PHSHT.

Troponin and implanted sensors

Following medical advice about controlling risk factors plays a key role in reducing the severity and relapse, prevention, and health promotion of cardiovascular diseases. Cardiac patients who may be undergoing CABG could be the main determinant of compliance with health advice treatment outcomes and the quality of life in patients after surgery. On the other hand, the disease negatively affects their psychological well-being; usually cardiac patients have lower psychological well-being than patients without heart disease [27]. There is also solid evidence that a higher incidence of anxiety and depression follows a heart attack. Young age, heart murmur, history of implantable cardioverter defibrillator (ICD) shock and generalized anxiety all point to greater anxiety after cardiac arrest and may well be predictive for people who have had a heart attack without arrest. Problems arise not only from the onset of depression and anxiety for cardiac patients but also predict poorer recovery and a higher long term risk for complications [22]. Factors other than chest pain can predict a heart attack before it occurs. Some chemicals that the body produces in response to an AMI can be detected hours prior to the actual heart attack. An electrocardiogram (ECG) can also be a reliable method to predict heart attacks and refer patient to the hospital for rapid treatment and prevention of the disabling effects of heart attacks. It is vital to utilize every tool available to predict, manage, and treat heart disease.

Troponin levels, a chemical produced by the heart in response to ischemia, usually increase in the blood some hours before a heart attack occurs. Measuring this chemical can lead to preventive or immediate treatment for a heart attack. Measurement of troponin must be done by detecting it inside the body. Very recently, there have been some developments in various institutes to develop a mechanism to detect troponinT/I and transmit this data via a smart phone. In effect, this would be an early heart attack detection system where an implanted troponin detection sensor is attached trans receiver to a real-time monitoring center. Reports from the real-time monitoring system, individualized to the user are analyzed and the patient alarmed to the condition. Troponin I (cTnI) is more reliable test specificity than troponin T (cTnT). An electrochemical biosensor as well as a microprocessor can be utilized for the recognition of troponin levels. The biosensor is surgically implanted inside the skin of a patient so that it can be exposed to blood flow, preferably an artery. Data is received from the sensor in analogue form then it is necessary to amplify the magnitude and convert it to digital form. It is then that the processed data transmitted by the Wireless Body Network Controller (BNC) attached RF device is sent to the medical monitoring system. The EHR database, updated in real-time, is equipped with a monitoring and administration zone and fault tolerant base alarm system. Troponin levels from various users are provisioned and updated in the EHR database in real-time. The implanted sensor sends troponin related data through Bluetooth and other access networks for the monitoring center to analyze in real-time or a short periodic manner [1].

The internet of things and disease prediction

The Internet of Things (IoT) is an advanced technology which exploits several specialties such as sensor development, data acquisition, management and processing, and communication and networking where subjects (e.g. objects, people) with unique characteristics can link to a remote server and form local networks. Since the connectivity in IoT-based systems permits objects to trade and fuse data to gain more comprehensive knowledge about their functionality and qualities of the neighboring environments, it offers superior, intelligent, and well-organized services. IoT technologies offer an improved quality of life for individuals through continuous (i.e., 24/7) remote monitoring systems which is one of the primary features of this technology. Although several efforts exist to use IoT-based systems for monitoring and care of the elderly, most only target specific conditions from a too limited standpoint (e.g. health monitoring, safety monitoring, etc.). Deliberating on the importance of remote monitoring of the elderly and the complete variety of possible services available with such a system, it is difficult not to realize that the technology still lacks a user-centered study. For example, a user-centered design would use numerous resources to present a system which focuses on the proficiencies, conditions, and abilities of the users. Various literature has focused on IoT-based elderly care which provides a comprehensive review of monitoring services; that is, essentials of user-centered system design for monitoring the elderly and the development of a multipurpose system which monitors a large group of users to detect (or predict) patterns or health-related situations that may happen to elderly patients such as heart attack, stroke, or diabetes. Remote health monitoring becomes even more important in the care of elderly patients due to the increased frailty and susceptibility to various diseases (e.g. acute and chronic diseases) of old age. Not only does remote health monitoring improve the quality of life of elderly patients, detects and notifies caregivers and

providers of emergencies, reduces nursing care needs and hospital stays (e.g. health care cost reduction), it can predict and track disease processes such as heart attacks [28].

Wireless detection of a heart attack

Smartphones and sensors can detect and transmit varied health data. A wrist watch has been designed as Heart Attack Detection equipment used daily to indicate heart condition, detect heart attack and to call for emergency help. Designed especially for patients with heart disease, it can not only decrease morbidity and mortality but disability as well.

The ECG is extremely valuable as a tool for detecting a heart attack. The ECG is an electrical recording of heart activity and can be utilized in the investigation of heart disease. Electrical impulses initiate heart muscle contraction, which results in the heartbeat. Notice that the spacing between each pulse measure a heart's rhythm and the height of the pulse is an indicator of pumping strength. The wrist watch contains an ECG circuitry unit which captures abnormal heart beat signals from the patient. The microcontroller on the watch then runs a heart attack algorithm and the Bluetooth emergency calling system dials medical help during the time of heart attack. There are two biosensors worn on the patient's wrist which sends the ECG signal to the analog ECG circuitry. Then the amplified and filtered analog output of the circuitry is translated from an analog to digital signal and then transmitted to the unit on the walking watch. The ECG circuitry unit, the A/D converter and the transmitter are worn on one of the patient's wrists. This watch is wireless, giving the user more freedom to move by avoiding wires between the watch and the wrist. The patient wearing the watch receives a digital ECG signal, and the microcontroller runs a heart attack algorithm to detect potential heart attack symptoms. If any symptom of a heart attack is detected, the risk level rises. Once a patient's risk level reaches the emergency mode, the Bluetooth module activates the user's mobile phone to call 911 for medical help. The latest mobile phones include a GPS function [29].

Telecardiology in heart attack prediction

Telecardiology can be defined as the monitoring or diagnosis of cardiac activities at a distance via telecommunication technology. ECG and imaging-based echocardiography (ECHO) are tools most often applied in cardiology. ECHO has become a widely-used tool in telecardiology due to its ability to physically evaluate cardiac and vascular anatomical structures and physiological functions, which can affect intervention strategies. The strongest advantage of telecardiology is that it allows timely remote diagnosis by cardiologists and for the provider to evaluate effective therapeutic strategies, especially for rurally located patients where professional cardiologists are not as accessible. Telecardiology lowers the mortality rate for patients with heart attack and can reduce the cost of transportation from the home to the emergency setting or unnecessary transfers between hospitals [30].

A critical tool for telecardiology applications is wireless telecommunication, which delivers pervasive services with less interruption errors when compared to traditional telephone lines. Therefore, thanks to this technology, individuals residing in rural areas or disparate health care areas around the world will benefit from remote. However, it is possible to achieve ECG monitoring in a home environment without Internet connections using only traditional telephone lines by recording ECG signals as audio input which is then transmitted to a hospital via a fixed phone line or mobile phone [30].

Tele-ICU, a hospital-based form of telecardiology is only conducted by qualified and experienced nurses and cardiologists, who are responsible for the 24 h continuous remote monitoring of vital signs. A second significant feature of tele-ICU technology is the real-time tele-communication and tele-consultation among the bedside paramedics, off-site professionals and ICU patients via surveillance and the 24-hour alert system [30].

Data mining in big data processing and heart attack prediction

Currently, data mining can help health care insurance organizations to detect hypocrites and misuse, health care institutions to make decisions of customer relationship management, providers to identify effective treatments and best practices and patients now receive enhanced and more economical health care services. This predictive analysis is widely used in health care. Classification is one of the data mining methods used to predict and classify the predetermined data for the specific class. There are diverse classifications procedures proposed by researchers. Different data mining techniques have been applied to predict heart disease. The accuracy of each algorithm has been verified and stated as Naïve Bayes, Decision Tree and ANN. The three-different data mining algorithms, ANN, C4.5 and Decision Trees are utilized to investigate heart related diseases using ECG signals. The analysis results clearly show the Decision Tree algorithm performs best and provides better accuracy than the C4.5 or Naïve Bayes algorithm. It requires less space when the volume of data is increased; it has a lower error rate, and minimizes the predictive error. C5.0 algorithm is the most potentially suitable algorithm for any kind of medical diagnoses. In cases of the C5.0 algorithm performs faster and provides the best accuracy with lower memory consumption [24].

Data mining techniques can be utilized for pre-processing and machine learning algorithms can be utilized for implementation; cloud computing is used for deployment. Currently, popular machine learning algorithms have already become useful in determining the heart disease risk level and in helping the doctors correctly predict it. Data Mining is a process of extracting valuable and significant knowledge from huge datasets. Data Pre-processing is an important process in data mining and machine learning. Thus, dimensionality reduction is a valuable tool for downsizing data. The most key procedures for dimensionality reduction are feature selection and feature extraction. Feature selection is the method of choosing a subset of applicable features. Feature selection techniques are a subset of the more universal field of feature extraction [31].

Technology and its tools can be utilized for visualization and investigation, to automate the progression of detecting promising ideas to foster more efficient discovery of content, and to provide the facility to track its influence after the presentation of hopeful ideas into the discourse community. There are varied types of discourse analysis, including automated content analysis, which uses natural language processing and machine learning techniques. Running the discourse through I2A using KBDeX for visualization, it was possible to classify discourse units (DUs) and their corresponding contents into distinctive idea types. First, I2A was used to detect ideas, followed by the determination of pertinent and promising ideas, then by conducting an analysis of discourse belonging to different idea types for validation purposes [32].

With Naïve Bayes' assumption, all the attributes are autonomous, significantly reducing the calculations later developed. Using Naïve Bayes assumption, the probability can be divided into a continuous product of class conditional probabilities. Each patient has the risk intensity for which the posterior probability is extreme. Using a normal distribution accounting for age, cholesterol and thalach provides an approximately excellent assumption. The general idea of the algorithm is to use a weighted average calculation for all heart disease symptoms. Providers may sometimes be unsuccessful in correctly diagnosing the severity of the disease. Inside Mapper, the function of each line from the input file is used as input to map the phase and is then fed to different map-tasks in parallel, considering a multi-node cluster. Each node follows the same procedure in parallel [31].

The issue of privacy in big data

Faulty results and seriously compromised privacy are only two concerns when algorithms and data whose quality is suspicious, yield faulty results although used appropriately. Even when the algorithms and data are appropriate for their intended purpose, privacy concerns are paramount and may seriously compromise individual rights. Big Data analytics support automated processes which arrive at decisions about an individual, health care organization, or disease, and raise important questions about self-determination, personal autonomy and fairness. Results may also yield predictions about patients which may be conceived as invasive or against patient choice. Policymakers, users of data, and data protection authorities must carefully consider how principles are honestly and effectually harnessed by analytics. Although there are risks associated with the use of big data analytics, as a society, if we fail to utilize its benefits to solve old problems in health care, research, education, and development, we deprive individuals, patients, and society of the potential benefits. Preferably, there will be thoughtful guidance which studies the realities of big data and the nature of analytic processing and will empower organizations to utilize analytics in a vigorous and accountable style to reach long-sought out solutions [20].

Challenges and future trends in big data analytics

Big data in health care has many challenges including but not limited to: deducing knowledge from complex heterogeneous patient sources; leveraging the patient/data correlations in longitudinal records; understanding unstructured clinical notes in the appropriate context; competently managing huge volumes of medical imaging data and mining potentially beneficial information and biomarkers; analyzing genomic data, a computationally rigorous task and merging it with standard clinical data to increase layers of complexity; capturing the behavioral data through multiple sensors with their various social interactions and communications. Big data does have some goals, which include: taking advantage of massive amounts of information and providing the right intervention to the right patient at the right time; personalized care for the patient; potentially utilize all components of the health care system, that is, provider, payer, patient, and management. Sources and techniques for big data in health care can be structured EHR data, unstructured clinical notes or PACS data, genetic data, or research data. The biggest challenge for handling the data include ungrammatical phrases, grammar mistakes, short phrases, abbreviations, misspellings, semi-structured information which is copy-paste from other sources such as lab results and vital signs [16].

Other challenges for big data use include the structured template of some clinical notes (SOAP notes), text mining information such as extraction of the name, entity recognition, information retrieval, clinical text versus biomedical text, and medical literature (well-written medical text. Clinical text is that which is written by clinical staff in the clinical setting [16]. Other challenges of include analysis, capture, data collection, search, sharing, storage, transfer, visualization and information privacy. The term big data simply denotes the use of predictive analysis or other specific advanced methods to mine valuable information from data, and often refers to the size of dataset [17]. The size and heterogeneity of data being gathered is a significant challenge. The high volume, velocity and variety of available data collection methods is likely to drive this data-driven society to a point where sampling will not be required because the entire background of a population is available [19].

The future scope of our health care system is aimed at offering a big data infrastructure for our designed risk calculation tools, to design more sophisticated prediction models and feature extraction techniques and extend our proposed system to predict other clinical risks [17]. Some other future possibilities are for the discovery of ground-breaking pharmaceuticals, the development of more effective treatment protocols and for the development of personalized medicine [19].

Summarization of main findings

The following Table 2 is a summarization of our results based on the literature research. Each section is denoted and a summary of findings associated with the results is indicated. The results of this review were conclusive in one sense: personalized medicine is the key to the future of medicine and nurses play a key role in helping patients navigate the data-driven healthcare society that was once driven by the provider.

Sections	Main Findings
Big Data analytics in health care	Big Data analytics is a novel method of handling the numerous amounts of healthcare data that is streamed daily. It includes technologies and tools adept at navigating the massive amounts of data in any given healthcare system and mining useful information to treat patients
Patient-customized health care and big data	Big Data tools are now able to predict, prevent, and suggest the best evidence-based treatment plans for the patient based on the data from a variety of sources. Care managers, specially trained registered nurses trained to work with providers to empower and assist patients to make lifestyle changes, are essential in the data-driven society to personalize medicine.
Troponin and implanted sensors	Implanted sensors are now available to detect troponin levels in the blood prior to some heart attack and potentially alert emergency personnel to the problem and prevent mortality and morbidity associated with heart attacks.
The Internet of Things (IoT) and disease prediction	The IoT can be used to predict diseases based on monitoring of the elderly, sensors, and the data which can then be processed using Big Data analytics.
Wireless detection of a heart attack	Smartphones, wristwatches, and other human-based sensors can be used in predicting and preventing heart attacks prior to occurrence by reading the EKG which may show changes prior to heart attack and alert key personnel immediately.
Telecardiology in heart attack prediction	Telemedicine is in a key position to monitor and indicate when a person is having a heart attack in healthcare systems where cardiologists may not be available immediately. The data relayed in these eICU and eER settings are key to preventing morbidity and mortality in small rural healthcare area.
Data mining in big data processing and heart attack prediction	Data mining is a key tool of Big Data used to predict, prevent, and suggest the best treatment plan for heart attacks.
The issue of privacy in big data	Privacy is a key issue in today's data-driven healthcare society as most information is de-identified; however, it can be re-identified under certain circumstances. With the onset of Big Data uses in healthcare, it is imperative that privacy against hackers, identity theft, and the illegal uses of healthcare data is prevented.

Table 2: Gathering the main findings.

Conclusion

The analysis of voluminous, structured and unstructured data, as well as disorganized data has produced substantial discoveries. The absence of cross-border direction and technology integration demands standards to enable interoperability amid the elements of the big data value chain. Big data proposes vast promises for detecting interactions and nonlinearities in relationships among variables. Mobile devices, such as smart phones and tablets, and sensors, will continue to be the most indispensable tools available to deliver heart attack prediction and telecardiology services over wireless networks to reduce cardiovascular disease morbidity and mortality. The deployment of cloud computing has inexpensively facilitated the collaborative application of telecardiology between hospitals and has expanded services from regional to global. The most important factor, however, in the development and application of big data, telecardiology, sensor use, mobile phone or tablet use and landline use is patient privacy and to safeguard the patient's ability to direct and discover the use of his or her health care information. Care managers, specially trained nurses who are revolutionizing healthcare by empowering patients directly to change their lifestyle and habits based on evidentiary research and data are needed to assist patients in this new data-driven healthcare scene. Nurses have always been on the forefront of revolutionary medicine and in today's data-driven healthcare system, nurses are critical in assisting their patients to navigate the data landmines and empower them to change unhealthy habits and reach a more improved health status.

References

1. Al Mamoon I, Sani AS, Islam AM, Yee OC, Kobayashi F, Komaki S (2013) A proposal of body implementable early heart attack detection system, 1-4.

2. Morley SR (2013). Heart attack experiences described in weblogs: An analysis of sex differences. CMC Senior Theses.

3. Patterson K (2016) Matthias Nahrendorf. Circ Res 119: 790-793.

4. Sun J, Reddy CK (2013) Big data analytics for healthcare. In Proceedings of the 19th ACM SIGKDD international conference on Knowledge discovery and data mining, pp: 1525-1525.

5. Dumbill E (2013) Making sense of big data. Big Data 1: 1-2.

6. Russom P (2011) Big data analytics. TDWI best practices report, fourth quarter, pp: 1-35.

7. Eaton C, Deroos D, Deutsch T, Lapis G, Zikopoulos P (2012) Understanding big data. Analytics for Enterprise class Hadoop and Streaming Data. McGraw-Hill Companies.

8. Dumbill E (2012) Planning for big data. O'Reilly Media, Inc.

9. Zikopoulos P, Eaton C (2011) Understanding big data: Analytics for enterprise class hadoop and streaming data, McGraw-Hill Osborne Media.

10. Bellini P, Di Claudio MARIANO, Nesi P, Rauch N (2013) Tassonomy and review of big data solutions navigation. Big Data Computing, pp: 57–101.

11. Demchenko Y, Grosso P, De Laat C, Membrey P (2013) Addressing big data issues in scientific data infrastructure. In Collaboration Technologies and Systems (CTS) 2013 International Conference on IEEE, pp: 48-55.

12. Megahed FM, Jones-Farmer LA (2013) A Statistical Process Monitoring Perspective on "Big Data", Frontiers in Statistical Quality Control, Springer, New York, pp: 1-21.

13. Minelli M, Chambers M, Dhiraj A (2012) Big data, big analytics: emerging business intelligence and analytic trends for today's businesses, John Wiley and Sons.

14. Rajpathak T, Narsingpurkar A (2013) Managing knowledge from Big Data analytics in product development. White Paper, Tata Consultancy Services, Software AG, pp: 1-8.

15. Winter R (2011) Big Data: Business Opportunities, Requirements and Oracle's Approach. Executive Report, Winter Corporation, 2.

16. Sun J, Reddy CK (2013) Big data analytics for healthcare. Tutorial presentation at the SIAM International Conference on Data Mining, Austin, TX.

17. Ghadge P, Girme V, Kokane K, Deshmukh P (2015) Intelligent heart attack prediction system using big data. International Journal of Recent Research in Mathematics Computer Science and Information Technology 2: 73-77.

18. Wanaskar UH, Ghadge P, Girmev V, Deshmukh P, Kokane K (2016) Intelligent Heart attack prediction system using big data. International Journal of Advanced Research in Computer and Communication Engineering 5: 723-725.

19. European Commission, Directorate-General for Health and Consumers, Unit D3 eHealth and Health Technology Assessment (2014) The Use of Big Data in Public Health Policy and Research: Background information document. Brussels, pp: 1-17.

20. Center for Information Policy Leadership, Hunton and Williams LLP (2013) Big Data and Analytics: Seeking Foundations for Effective Privacy Guidance. A Discussion Document, pp: 1-16.

21. Groves P, Kayyali B, Knott D, Kuiken SV (2016) The big data revolution in healthcare: Accelerating value and innovation. Center for US Health System Reform Business Technology Office, Copyright © McKinsey and Company, pp: 1-19.

22. Langdridge D (2016) Recovery from Heart Attack, Biomedicalization, and the Production of a Contingent Health Citizenship. Qualitative Health Research.

23. Lee SH, Kim M, Chung H, Yang S (2016) Designing of efficient technique blocking abnormal packets through correlation analysis in the healthcare environment. Indian J Sci Technol 9.

24. Ebenezer JGA and Durga S (2015) Big data analytics in healthcare: A survey. Arpn Journal of Engineering and Applied Sciences 10: 3645-3650.

25. Ciccone MM, Aquilino A, Cortese F, Scicchitano P, Sassara M, et al. (2010) Feasibility and effectiveness of a disease and care management model in the primary health care system for patients with heart failure and diabetes (Project Leonardo). Vasc Health Risk Manag 6: 297-305.

26. Lee B, Jeong E (2014) A design of a patient-customized healthcare system based on the hadoop with text mining (PHSHT) for an efficient disease management and prediction. International Journal of Software Engineering and Its Applications 8: 131-150.

27. Fard AD, Mojtabaei M (2016) The effect of cognitive behavioral stress management and psychological well-being and adherence to treatment in patients with coronary heart disease (Chd). IJHCS 1: 271-284.

28. Azimi I, Rahmani AM, Liljeberg P, Tenhunen H (2016) Internet of things for remote elderly monitoring: A study from user-centered perspective. J Ambient Intell Humaniz Comput, pp: 1-17.

29. Kumar KG, Arvind R, Keerthan PB, Kumar SA, Dass PA (2014) Wireless methodology of heart attack detection. International Journal for Scientific Research and Development 2: 673-676.

30. Hsieh JC, Li AH, Yang CC (2013) Mobile, cloud, and big data computing: Contributions, challenges and new directions in telecardiology. Int J Environ Res Public Health 10: 6131-6153.

31. Prerana THM, Shivaprakash NC, Swetha N (2015) Prediction of heart disease using machine learning algorithms- Naïve Bayes, Introduction to PAC Algorithm, Comparison of Algorithms and HDPS. International Journal of Science and Engineering 3: 90-99.

32. Lee VYA, Tan SC, Chee JKK (2016) Idea identification and analysis (I2A): A search for sustainable promising ideas within knowledge-building discourse. In: CK Looi, J Polman, U Cress, P Reimann (eds.,), Transforming learning, empowering learners: The International Conference of the Learning Sciences (ICLS), International Society of the Learning Sciences, Singapore.

3

Assessment of Knowledge and Attitude of Nurses towards Ionizing Radiation during Theatre/Ward Radiography

Geofery Luntsi[1*], Aishatu Babagana Ajikolo[1], Nkubli Bobuin Flaviuos[1], Lola Nelson[2], Chigozie Nwobi[1], Jamila Muhammed Hassan[1] and Fati Adamu Malgwi[1]

[1]Department of Medical Radiography, College of Medical Sciences, University of Maiduguri, Borno State, Nigeria

[2]Department of Nursing Sciences, College of Medical Sciences, University of Maiduguri. Borno State, Nigeria

*Corresponding author: Geofery Luntsi, Department of Medical Radiography, College of Medical Sciences, University of Maiduguri, Borno State, Nigeria, E-mail: geostuffy@unimaid.edu.ng

Abstract

Title: Assessment of Knowledge and Attitude of Nurses towards Ionizing Radiation during Theatre/Ward Radiography

Objective: To assess the knowledge and attitude of nurses towards radiation protection In Maiduguri metropolis.

Methods: A descriptive cross-sectional survey design was used. A quota sampling technique was used to draw a total of 188 registered nurses from three tertiary hospitals in Maiduguri metropolis; University of Maiduguri Teaching Hospital (UMTH), Federal Neuro-Psychiatric Hospital Maiduguri (FNPH), and State Specialist Hospital Maiduguri (SSH) participated in the study. Data was obtained using a 14- item self completion questionnaire that was administered to nursing staff of these hospitals. The questionnaire was divided into 2 sections. Section A; on demographic data and Section B; on knowledge and attitude. Data obtained were analyzed using SPSS version 18.0 and descriptive statistics was used for the analysis.

Results: There were more female than male participants with a ratio of 1.09:1. Majority of the nurses (74%) were below the age of forty (40). Most of the nurses 68 (36.2%) had diploma as their highest qualification followed by 61 (32.4%) certificate holders. The level of knowledge on radiation was found to be good and positive attitude towards radiation during ward/theater radiography.

Conclusion: Findings of this study revealed that nurses within Maiduguri metropolis had good knowledge of ionizing radiation, although their attitude towards radiation protection during ward/theater radiography is still less than required.

Keywords: Knowledge; Attitude; Radiation; Nurses; Ward; Theater; Radiography

Introduction

Radiation has always been present in our environment; however, mankind was not directly aware of its existence until the end of the 19th century, when flurries of scientific discoveries were made [1]. The risk of radiation awareness among the people by the media is aggressive and exaggerated which creates several misconception, confusion and erroneous beliefs that exist with regard to in-hospital radiation hazards. Studies have documented that most people overestimate the risk of industrial radiation and underestimate the risk of medial radiation application [2].

Ionizing radiation in medical imaging is one of the powerful diagnostic tools in medicine [3], several studies have revealed that many doctors have reported that to complete their diagnosis they always sent their patients for a radiologic examination [4]. Although all medical interventions have potential benefits, but it's potential risks should not be ignored [3].

The potential risks of radiation comprises of stochastic effect of which probability increases with dose and deterministic effect of which

severity increases with dose [5]. Cancer induction and genetic effects are stochastic effects while cataracts, blood dyscrasias and impaired fertility are examples of deterministic effects [5]. Therefore, before undertaking any radiological examination, it is important that the physician, radiologist and radiographer all understand the potential risks of radiation and also its advantages or benefits to the patients [5].

Reduction of exposure time, increasing distance from source, and shielding of patients and occupational workers have proven to be of great importance in protecting patients, personnel, and members of the public from the potential risks of radiation [5]. These three radiation protection actions of "time-distance-shielding" are the triad of radiation protection. Radiation protection is a general term applied to the profession or science related to protecting man and the environment from radiation hazards.

Nurses posted to the radiology department and those in the wards and theatre where radiography procedures are done, offers professional care to patients before, during and after radiologic procedures. They help to book reassure and prepare patients for special radiologic procedures and as well provide after care to patients after the procedures. Nurses also help to support the patient during the procedure and also prepare the equipment and instruments needed during the examination. Nurses working in departments, units or wards where ionizing radiation take place need to be knowledgeable about radiation and radiation protection practices so as to be able to give the patient the rightful information and protect themselves as well as the patients and the general public from unnecessary radiation exposure.

The researchers observed that during radiographic examinations on the ward, some nurses are extremely afraid to stay within the vicinity during radiation exposures, or just move some distance away but on sitting the radiographer with the mobile X-ray machine on the ward, they leave you with the patient and do not even want to come closer and help in lifting the patient even while no exposure is going on, and despite the reassurance and radiation protection measures employed by the radiographer. These reactions of some nurses towards ionizing radiation and the need to understand why they behave differently prompted the researchers' interest to find out the level of knowledge on ionizing radiation and their attitude towards radiation protection. This study aimed to assess the knowledge and attitude of nurses towards radiation protection during ward and theatre radiography.

Materials and Methods

Descriptive survey design was used for the study. The study was conducted in three tertiary hospitals in Maiduguri Borno State, Northeastern Nigeria, and the target population was all nurses working in the departments, units or wards where radiographers may sometimes be requested to carry out certain radiographic examinations on patients who are critically ill and who may not be able to be moved to the radiology department for their examination, like patients in the intensive care unit (ICU), orthopedic ward, accident and emergency unit among others. With the use of quota sampling technique, 95 Nurses were drawn from University of Maiduguri Teaching Hospital (UMTH), 55 from Federal Neuropsychiatric Hospital (FNPH), and 38 from State Specialist Hospital (SSH) making a total of 188 Nurses. A structured close ended 14- items questionnaire was used to collect data. The questionnaire was divided into 2 sections.

Section A consisted of demographic data and Section B consisted of items on knowledge and attitude towards radiation protection during radiography. Data was collected for a period of one month and analyzed using statistical package for social sciences (SPSS), version 18.0 and presented using frequency distribution tables and percentages. Ethical clearance was obtained from research and ethical committee of UMTH to conduct the study. This was done by submitting a letter together with the research proposal to the research and ethical committee of UMTH for permission to conduct the research. After two weeks of submission, approval was granted signed by the chairman of the committee to conduct the study. The approval letter was presented to the heads nursing in each of the hospital for permission to administer the questionnaire. Informed consent was sought from all the participants and acceptance to participate in the study was considered as consent. Confidentiality of the data collected was maintained as no name of any nurse was mentioned in the research.

Results

A total of 230 questionnaires were distributed and 188 were filled and returned within a period of one month giving a response rate of 82%. The study found that female respondents were 98 (52%) while male were 90 (48%).The respondents age ranged from 21 to 46 years and above with a mean age of 26.5 years. Respondents with the age group of 26 -30 years had the highest while those within the age group of 46 and above had the least frequency. Most of the nurses 68 (36%) had diploma as their highest level of qualification followed by certificate holders who were 61 (32%). Only one nurse (1%) had a PhD and two of them (2%) had MSc while 56 (30%) had BSc. In years of experience, 84 (44.7%) had practiced for 0-5 years while 23 (12.2%) had practiced for 16-20 years. University of Maiduguri Teaching Hospital had 95 (50.5%) of the participants while 55 (29.3%) were from FNPH and 38 (20.2%) from SSH (Table 1).

Demographic data		Total			
		UMTH	FNPH	SSH	TOTAL
		N	N	N	N
Sex	Male	49 (52%)	30 (55%)	11 (29%)	90 (48%)
	Female	46 (48%)	25 (45%)	27 (71%)	98 (52%)
Age group	21-25	6 (6%)	14 (25%)	10 (26%)	30 (16%)
	26-30	26 (27%)	20 (36%)	6 (15%)	52 (27.7%)
	31-35	18 (19%)	11 (20%)	2 (5%)	31 (16.5%)
	36-40	18 (19%)	1 (2%)	7 (18%)	26 (13.8%)
	41-45	19 (20%)	3 (5%)	7 (18%)	29 (15.4%)
	46 and above	8 (8%)	6 (11%)	6 (16%)	20 (10.6%)
Level of education	Certificate	22 (23%)	17 (31%)	22 (58%)	61 (32%)
	Diploma	34 (36%)	24 (44%)	10 (18%)	68 (36%)
	BSc	36 (38%)	14 (25%)	6 (11%)	56 (30%)

	MSc	2 (2%)	0 (0%)	0 (0%)	2 (1%)
	PhD	1 (1%)	0 (0%)	0 (0%)	1 (1%)
Years of professional practice	0-5	29 (30.5%)	37 (67.3%)	18 (47.4%)	84 (44.7%)
	10-Jun	16 (16.8%)	7 (12.7%)	4 (10.5%)	27 (14.4%)
	15-Nov	24 (25.2%)	1 (1.8%)	4 (10.5%)	29 (15.4%)
	16-20	15 (15.8%)	4 (7.2%)	4 (10.5%)	23 (12.2%)
	Above 20	11 (11.6%)	69 (10.9%)	8 (21.1%)	25 (13.3%)

Table 1: Demographic characteristics of respondents.

Table 2 shows that, 150 (79.7%) agreed radiation used in medical imaging can possibly cause harmful effects while 30 (16.5%) disagreed to it, and 8 (4.3%) do not know. Majority, 149 (79.3%) of the nurses agreed that X-ray used in medical imaging has more benefit than harm. The remaining 31 (16.5%) answered yes and only 8 (4.3%) of the population admitted that they don't know. Majority of the nurses, 80 (42.6%) wrongly assumed that objects in the room emit radiation after an X-ray exposure. Only 56 making (29.8%) answered no while 51 (27.1%) don't know.

Items	Yes	No	Don't know	Total
Radiation can cause harmful effects	150 (79.7%)	30 (16.5%)	8 (4.3%)	188 (100%)
X-rays used in medical imaging cause more harm than benefit	31 (16.5%)	149 (79.3%)	8 (4.3%)	188 (100%)
Radiation that is used in wards and theatres are more dangerous than those in the radiology department	49 (26.1%)	106 (56.4%)	33 (17.6%)	188 (100%)
Radiation is used for boosting the immune system	26 (13.8%)	141 (75%)	21 (11.2%)	188 (100%)
Generally we receive radiation in our everyday life	137 (72.9%)	45 (23.9%)	5 (2.7%)	187 (100%)
The lifespan of radiology workers are less compared to other health workers	92 (48.9%)	54 (28.7%)	42 (22.3%)	188 (100%)
Objects in the room emit radiation after an x-ray exposure	80 (42.6%)	56 (29.8%)	51 (27.1%)	187 (100%)

Table 2: Nurses knowledge on radiation.

In Table 3, 142 (75.5%) of the respondents keep away from patients during radiographic exposure. Only 5 (2.7%) don't know and 41 (21.8%) do not.

Items	Yes	No	Don't know	Total
Staying away from patient during exposure.	142 (75.5%)	41 (21.8)	5 (2.7%)	188 (100%)
Use lead apron during radiographic exposure.	159 (84.5%)	16 (8.5%)	13 (6.9%)	188 (100%)
Coming to the vicinity after x-ray exposure.	78 (41.5%)	93 (49.5%)	16 (8.5%)	187 (100%)

Table 3: Attitude of nurses towards radiation.

About 159 (84.5%) use lead apron to protect themselves during radiographic exposures, 13 (6.9%) don't know and 16 (8.5%) do not. About 93 (49.5%) come to the vicinity after radiographic exposure while 78 (41.5%) do not and 16 (8.5%) don't know.

On cross tabulating educational qualification and attitude, towards radiation protection, it was found that participants with MSc. and above have good radiation protection practice. This is followed by BSc and the least was among certificate holders.

The study also found that positive attitude increase with increase in years of professional practice. Those with a working experience of 16-20 years and 20 years and above had good positive attitude to radiation protection and least was those with practice experience of 0-5 years (Tables 4 and 5).

Items	Educational level					
	Certificate	Diploma	BSc	MSc	PhD	TOTAL
Staying away from patient during exposure	42 (68.6%)	51 (75%)	46 (82.1%)	200%)	1 (100%)	142 (75.5%)
Use of lead apron	49 (80.3%)	58 (85.3%)	48 (70.6%)	2 (100%)	1 (100%)	159 (84.6%)
Come to vicinity after exposure.	29 (47.5%)	33 (48.5%)	28 (50%)	2 (100%))	1 (100%)	93 (49.5%)
AVERAGE	40 (65.6%)	47 (69.6%)	40 (72.6%)	2 (100%)	1 (100%)	131 (69%)

Table 4: Crosstabulating educational level against attitude toward radiation.

Items	Years of practice					
	0-5	10-Jun	15-Nov	16-20	20 and above	TOTAL
Staying away from patient during exposure	57 (67.9%)	20 (74.1%)	23 (79.3%)	20 (87%)	22 (88%)	142 (75.5%)
Use of lead apron	71 (84.5%)	21 (77.8%)	23 (79.3%)	21 (91.3%)	23 (92%)	159 (84.6%)
Coming to vicinity after exposure.	32 (38.1%)	14 (51.9%)	21 (72.4%)	13 (56.5%)	13 (52%)	93 (49.5%)
AVERAGE	53 (63.5%)	18 (67.9%)	22 (77%)	18 (78.3%)	19 (77.3%)	131 (69%)

Table 5: Cross tabulating years of practice against attitude toward radiation.

Discussion

A total of 230 questionnaires were distributed, 188 were filled and returned within a period of one month giving a response rate of 81.7%. Males were 90 (48%) while 98 (52%) were female with age range from 21-46 years and above and a mean age of 26.5 years. The higher number of female participants could perhaps be because the nursing profession is viewed as a female profession and dominated by them. This is in agreement with a study by Alotaibe and Saeed [6] and Maliro [7] who also found higher frequency of female.

The study found majority of the participants 129 (68%) to be certificates and diploma holders, followed by bachelors of nursing science degree (BNSc) holders with 5 (30%) while masters of science degree (MSc) and doctor of philosophy degree (Ph.D) were the least with 2 (1%) and 1 (0.5%) respectively. These findings were similar to that of Alotaibe and Saeed6 who found that most of the nurses had diploma as their highest qualification. This could be because there are more certificates and diploma awarding nursing institutions than those awarding bachelors of nursing sciences degree (BNSc), master's degree (MSc) and doctor of philosophy degree (Ph.D) as obtainable within the study locality and developing nations like Nigeria. UMTH had the highest number of BSc nurses with 36 (37.9%) followed by FNPH 14 (25%) and SSH with the least having a frequency of 6 (11%).

Working experience shows that, 84 (44.7%) of the respondents had working experience of five years and below signifying that most of the respondents were still young in professional practice.

The participants had good knowledge of ionizing radiation and about 60.4% knew the source, benefit and the potential harm of ionizing radiation. This is probably due to general knowledge about radiation and its associated hazards. These findings are in agreement with that of Rassin et al. [4], who found that majority (70%) of the nurses had average knowledge on radiation. However studies conducted by Alotaibe and Saeed [6] and Maliro [7] revealed that nurses lack knowledge on radiation sources and radiation protection methods.

The study also found that the respondents had positive (good) attitude towards ionizing radiation during theatre and ward radiography, whereas 132 (70%) of them practice good radiation protection by shielding (use of lead apron) and keeping distance from patients during radiographic exposures. This is perhaps because of the fear of radiation motivating them either ignorantly or intentionally to adopt good radiation protection practices. This findings are different from that of Rassin et al. [4] who found that though there was an average knowledge on radiation, most of the participants do not follow radiation safety methods.

The study found that the level of education attained by the participants in this study, impacted positively on their attitude towards radiation protection because good radiation protection practice increased as the participants' level of education increased as seen in this study. This might be as a result of the increased information due to higher level of exposures that might come as a result of increased level of education. This finding are not similar to that of Alotaibe and Saeed [6], Maliro [7], and Urushizaka [8] who found that there is no influence of level of education on attitude of nurses towards radiation protection.

This study also revealed that as participants' years of practice increased, their attitude towards radiation also got better. This might be because of the abated fear and misconceptions about ionizing radiation that may accrue over the length of years of practice. This is not in agreement with to the findings of Alotaibe and Saeed [6] and Maliro [7], who found that years of professional practice did not affect the attitude towards radiation. However, geographical location, place and nature of practice should not be ignored as this could also impact on their attitude towards ionizing radiation.

Conclusion

Findings from this study showed that participants had good knowledge and attitude towards ionizing radiation during theatre and ward radiography and this was influenced by the level of education attained and years of professional practice, however, more needs to be done to improve on the curriculum content on ionizing radiation in the nursing institutions and nurses should also be encouraged to pursue further studies to meet up with the current trend of evidence based practice.

We recommend seminars and symposium on a regular basis within the hospitals to educate all the staff on radiation protection.

References

1. Bushberg, JT, Seibert JA, Edwin ML and Boone MJ (2002) Essential physics of medical imaging, 2nd ed., Lippincott Williams and Wilkins. Philadelphia.

2. Mubeen SM, Abbas Q, Nisar N (2008) Knowledge About Ionizing And Non-Ionizing Radiation Among Medical Students. Ayub Medical College, Abbotabad, Karachi, Pakistan 20: 118-20.

3. Mojiri M, Moghimbeigi A (2008) Awareness and attitude of radiographers towards radiation protection, Journal of Paramedical Sciences 2: 4-5.

4. Rassin M, Granat P, Berger M, and Silner E (2005) Attitude And Knowledge Of Physicians and Nurses About Ionizing Radiation, Journal Of Radiology Nursing 24: 26-30.

5. Grover SB, Kumar J, Gupta A, Hanna L (2002) Protection against radiation hazards: regulatory bodies, safety norms, dose limits and protection devices, Indian journal of radiology and imaging. 12: 157-67.

6. Alotaibe M, Saeed R (2006) Radiology Nurses Awareness of Radiation, Journal of Radiology Nursing l25: 7-12.

7. Maliro FMJ (2011) Ionizing Radiation Protection Awareness among Nurses Working At Queen Elizabeth Central Hospital Malawi, PhD, Department of Health Sciences, University of Johannesburg.

8. Urushizaka M, Noto Y, Ogura N, kitajima M, Nishizawa Y, et al. (2013) Changes in Nurses Impression of Radiation after attending Educational Seminars on Radiation, Radiation Emergency Medicine 2: 35-42.

4

Clinical Supervision as an Integral Part in Training for Bridging Course Learners at Selected Hospitals of Vhembe District, Limpopo Province, South Africa

Mafumo JL*, Netshandama VO and Netshikweta L

Department of Advanced Nursing Science, University of Venda, South Africa

*Corresponding author: JL Mafumo, Department of Advanced Nursing Science, University of Venda, University Road, Thohoyandou, Limpopo 0950, South Africa. E-mail: julia.mafumo@univen.ac.za

Abstract

Purpose: The purpose of this study was to explore and describe the significance of clinical supervision amongst Bridging course learners at the selected hospitals in Vhembe district, Limpopo province.

Methods: A qualitative, exploratory, contextual and descriptive design was used and this approach was regarded as the most appropriate for this study. The population of this study consisted of the learner nurses in the Bridging Course Programme (R683) leading to registration as a General Nurse. Purposive, non-probability sampling method was used to select the participants.

Data collection: Data was collected by means of focus group discussion interviews during which participants were able to describe their experiences of the clinical placement in the real life setting and the support received from the professional nurses, data were collected until data saturation was reached.

Data analysis: The researcher used the process of bracketing and remained neutral, setting aside previous knowledge and beliefs about the phenomenon under investigation. The researcher listened to the audiotapes used for data collection several times until the researcher completely satisfied with the interpretation of the verbatim data.

Ethical consideration: The researcher sought for approval to collect data from the appropriate authority at the University of Venda, the Provincial Department of Health and the bridging students in each institution.

Keywords: Learner nurses; Clinical Supervision; Clinical environment; Nurse educators; Professional nurses

Introduction

Clinical Supervision for learner nurses is viewed as a process for improving clinical practice and reducing the emotional burden of those who are still on training and getting the feet in the profession. It assists in problem identification and provides solutions to problems. It also improves clinical practice, and increase understanding for learner nurses. It is significant in nursing as it can improve patient care. Clinical supervision is important in student nurse training as it socialises them into their future professional role and identity [1].

It also helps learners to be confident and competent during clinical practice. Learner depends on the quality of clinical supervision and experience obtained for their competency when they are placed in the clinical environment. This will influence their practice when they are in the clinical practice. The nurse educators, clinicians, professional nurses and nurse managers have the responsibility to ensure that the clinical supervision of learner nurses is done. They need to guide the learners so that they become the best nurse practitioners we expect them to be.

Background to the Study

Clinical supervision is defined as a formal, systemic and continuous process of professional support and learning for practicing nurses in which nurses are assisted in developing their practice through regular discussion with experienced colleagues with whom they share clinical experience [2]. Globally the training of learner nurses is seen as the basis of nursing practice. Learner nurses need to be supported and guided so that they can become responsible, accountable and independent professionals who are able to function within the precepts of the profession. In nursing we always talk about integration of theory and practice and this can only be achieved if those responsible for teaching theory supervise if the learners are performing as expected in the clinical area. In order to facilitate optimal learning for the student nurse, the student must be presented with a range of real life work experiences that are presented in a supportive environment [3]. Clinical supervision does not only provide learners with an opportunity to work on their own and grow professionally, it also allows them to have self-confidence in performance of nursing skills and functioning independently [4].

Clinical supervision aims to help learner nurses increase both their competence and confidence through exchanges with experienced professionals and the use of reflective skills. Clinical supervision covers all the aspects in nursing practice. A supportive environment and team work in the clinical setting lead to reduction in the workload when it comes to patient care [5]. The students are taught communication skills and interaction with patients.

The student is supervised until such time that he/she is confident and competent in performing the skill then the supervisory role will be reduced bit by bit and not totally taken away. For clinical supervision to be effective, nurse educators and professional nurses in the units need to have a sound knowledge of the learning needs of students as they are supervising them in the clinical setting [6]. Supervision also provides support on increasing students' own responsibility to nurse patients independently.

Problem Statement

Custodians of nursing education have often expressed their different views regarding clinical supervision for learner nurses in hospitals of Vhembe district in Limpopo Province learners. Clinical supervision is a serious concern to learner nurses as nursing is a practice – based profession. Even if the learner preforms exceptionally well in theory she still has to be very competent in clinical skills.

The concern was that learner nurses were not able to integrate theory, practice and skills and would not be able to function independently on completion of their training. From the discussions that were held with stake holders the researcher felt that there is a need to investigate the views of expressed by leaner nurses regarding clinical supervision. The researcher also wanted to investigate if the learners are satisfied with the clinical supervision that they are receiving.

Purpose of the Study

The purpose of the study was to explore and describe views of learner nurses regarding clinical supervision at sampled hospitals of Vhembe district in Limpopo Province, South Africa.

Research Objectives

- To explore learner nurses' views regarding clinical supervision at the sampled hospitals of Vhembe district in Limpopo Province.
- To describe learner nurses' views regarding clinical supervision at the sampled hospitals of Vhembe district in Limpopo Province.

Significance of the Study

Significance to the learners, nurse educators and professional nurses

The study results can contribute enable nurse educators and professional nurses to assist to ensure high quality nursing education, produce competent nurses and promote the charm of the nursing profession. Nurse educators and professional nurses will be able to detect areas of concern which needs improvement and engage the parties involved on how improvements can be made in order to have an efficient and effective system of learner supervision.

Significance of the research

The findings of this study would contribute to nursing research because clinical supervision is such an essential and indispensable field of study in the nursing profession.

Research Methodology and Research Design

Research design aims at providing a plan for answering the research question. The researcher used the qualitative, exploratory, descriptive and contextual research approach, because the study focused on the views of learner nurses. The researcher used interviews to gain the knowledge that will make it possible to describe the learners' views in an effort to obtain complete and accurate information for use in this study.

Research Setting

The study was conducted at sampled hospitals in Vhembe District of Limpopo Province where learners doing Bridging Course are allocated for clinical exposure.

Population

According to Burns and Grove [8]; Polit and Beck [9] population refers to the entire group of persons or objects that is of interest to the researcher that meets the criteria that the researcher is interested in studying. The population was learner nurses doing Bridging Course for enrolled nurses leading to registration as a General Nurse, as stated in Regulation 683 of 14 April 1989. The sampled population was learners who were doing second year of study in Bridging course at sampled hospitals of Vhembe district of Limpopo Province. Purposive, non-probability sampling method was used to sample participants. The study involved a total of twenty-eight (28) participants.

Data Collection

For this study, the researcher conducted unstructured focus group interviews. The unstructured in-depth focus group interviews lasted for approximately 60 to 90 min each and no new information was obtained after completion of the interviews. FGDs were used, rather than in-depth individual interviews, based on the need to identify the experiences, views and perceptions of the participants. The selections of FGD members require careful decision to optimise the usefulness of the focus group. For most purposes, the group of 6 to 10 members are optimal. The researcher stimulates exchange of ideas and encourages debates.

The FGD methodology provides in-depth information, but it does not produce quantifiable data and the findings cannot be generalised to a larger population.

Ethical Considerations

Protecting the rights of the participants

- Non-discrimination

The researcher avoided discrimination against the Bridging course learners on the basis of sex, race, ethnicity or other factors that were deemed to jeopardise the trustworthiness of the study results.

- Beneficence

According to Polit and Beck beneficence is the most fundamental principle in research. To adhere to this principle, the well-being (physical, emotional, social of financial) of the respondent must be protected from discomfort and harm [10]. In this study the researcher did not harm and refrain from exploiting participants, and promoted both individual and societal benefits that are directly related to participation in this research

- Right to be informed

The participants have the right to know what the research entails, how it will influence them, the risks and the benefits and that they may refuse to participate in the study should they choose to do so [11].

- Justice

The principle of justice means that participants need to be treated fairly [12]. The researcher respected the rights of the learners to privacy and the right to fair treatment in the context of research participation

Protecting the rights of the institutions

- Legality

Before research can be commenced, permission needs to be obtained from the authority of the institutions where research will be conducted. The ethical principles that are applicable to participants also apply to the institutions. The researcher understood and obeyed relevant laws and institutional and governmental policies regarding research, protection of human subjects, and any other ethical consideration relevant to the study.

Data Analysis

Tesch's steps of data analysis were followed as stated in Creswell [13]. During the process of analysing, the researcher identified the essence of the phenomenon under investigation based on the data collected and how that data was presented. In a case of describing, the researcher describes critically, in written communication, the meaning of the phenomenon as it has been given by the participants. This step of describing is applied after all data have been analysed, and themes have emerged from the grouped categories and sub-categories. Data belonging to each category was assembled in one place and preliminary analysis was done. The data was sorted. During this process, main ideas were formed and information sorted into themes, categories and subcategories.

Trustworthiness of the Study

Findings were discussed between the researcher and the participants. Accuracy was maintained throughout the study by making use of member checks and allowing the participants who provided the information to check both the data and the interpretation.

Dependability

The researcher enhanced the dependability of this study by involving an expert in qualitative research to assist with data analysis and the interpretation of data. The researcher kept all records of all stages of the research process for the purpose of audits done by experts.

Transferability

The researcher enhanced transferability by providing an in-depth discussion and interpretation of data and by using focus group discussions.

Confirmability

The researcher maintained the confirmability of this study by taking comprehensive notes throughout the research. The researcher also ensured that data is accurately interpreted, and reflected the information that was obtained from the participants. Thus the findings were shared with participants to confirm the information they gave. Information was discussed with the supervisor and the qualitative research expert to prevent any form of bias.

Findings

The study found out the experiences of Bridging course learners as not satisfactory regarding clinical supervision received in the clinical areas. According to the study the findings were that:

Clinical supervision is not adequately done in the clinical environment due to but not limited to the following factors:

- Attitude of trained staff and learners

Attitude of both professional nurses and learners was indicated as another barrier to proper clinical supervision. It was indicated that professional nurse see learners as extra work or burden when they have to supervise them. On the other hand, learners were seen as being arrogant and dodge form the unit most of the time. This worsens the relationship between learners and professional nurses. Another issue that emerged from the discussion was that often learners are less interested and are not inquisitive to ask more about what is happening in the clinical area, they only do routine just like any other staff member without asking anything.

- Shortage of equipment

Shortage of equipment was another barrier to proper clinical supervision. Procedures had to be flawed because there are on equipment. In this instance proper clinical supervision cannot be done as procedures are compromised due to unavailability of equipment are.

- Learners used as part of working force

Another issue was the fact that these learners because they are enrolled nurses, they were used as a work force to patch the shortage in the units. Learners in Bridging course have been trained for certificate courses before therefore they are assumed as "knowing it all". Whenever off-duties are written, they are used to balance the trained staff. Whenever there is shortage of trained staff learners are asked to work overtime. Because of that learners tend to focus on the ward routine than their learning needs.

- Insufficient learning opportunities

The issue of a small and poorly equipped simulation laboratory was raised where learners indicated that they can't practice as much as they would want to in the simulation lab as they are overcrowded during procedure simulations. Learners also indicated that the professional nurses in the units keep them busy with ward routine hence there is not much time to practice their skills.

Generally, learners indicated that they feel that they are not adequately supervised in the clinical area. The learners indicated some dissatisfaction and frustration because they say that they are not properly supervised.

- Shortage of trained staff

Students indicated that the wards are short staffed of professional nurses therefore they concentrate on ward activities and patient care. Students were left to be doing procedures alone without the supervision of the professional nurses.

Discussion

The study results indicated that the majority students were not satisfied with the clinical supervision in the units though few had a different perspective. Students cited many factors that were experienced which lead to clinical supervision not properly done. The study indicated that material and human resources challenges contributed to poor clinical supervision. In the material resources there was shortage of equipment s which compromised the performance of procedures. Professional nurses would flaw some procedures because there is no equipment to perform such procedures.

There were also insufficient learning opportunities created for students to go and practice clinical skills in the laboratories. In human resources the study found that there is shortage of professional nurses leading to the professional nurses concentrating on patient care and ward activities and not patient supervision. The study also revealed that the professional nurses and the student had a negative attitude towards clinical supervision leading to compromising clinical supervision.

During the study students indicated that at times they even forget that they were students as most of the time they were treated as employees of the institution and not students. They were involved in ward activities than in their learning expectations.

Recommendations

Recommendations regarding inadequate clinical supervision

It is recommended that clinical supervision of nursing learners should be prioritised by nurse educators and professional nurses in all the training institutions.

Having clinical supervisors or clinicians made available for the clinical supervision of learner nurses;

Professional nurses to be more supportive towards the training of learner nurses.

Recommendations regarding the need for clinical training specialists and preceptors

It is recommended that the appointment of clinician and preceptors in the training institutions could provide the opportunity to oversee the education and training of learner nurses of different categories.

The clinicians and preceptors should be offered courses on coaching, mentoring and preceptor development.

They could also receive compensation so that they do not see supervision as extra responsibility.

Recommendations regarding the availability of a structured plan or programme

It is recommended nurse educators should provide professional nurses in the clinical setting with a structured clinical supervision programme.

A detailed schedule or programme should be in place in all the units to guide both the learner and supervisor concerning their training needs.

Learners should also have their clinical learning outcomes.

The roles and responsibilities of both supervisor and the student should be clearly defined in the contract, and the contract should clearly define the goals to be achieved through clinical supervision.

Recommendations regarding the use of learners as workforce

Nurse educators need to have good relationship and communication with the professional nurses in the units so that they treat learners as what they are and not a working force.

Learners should not be used to patch the shortage that is in the wars/units at the expense of their training.

They should be allowed the opportunity to be learners and be guided in the clinical placement.

They should work under direct or indirect supervision of the professional nurse allocated to them.

Learners should maintain their supernumerary status of being "learners" not workers.

Recommendations regarding the incorrect guidance and supervisory procedures

Learners should be supervised all the time whenever they are in the clinical placement. They should be under direct or indirect supervision of the professional nurse.

Professional nurses in the unit should take education and teaching of learner nurses seriously. Procedures should be done properly without any compromise in order to allow leaners to see the correct things being.

Recommendations regarding insufficient learning opportunities

The recommendations were:

Simulation laboratory should be well equipped and special attention given to the number of learners taken in for training in the so that overcrowding is avoided.

During simulation learners should be taken in groups of ten in order to prevent overcrowding in the simulation laboratory.

Recommendations regarding learner nurse-professional nurse ration

Allocation of learners in the units should be in such a manner that there is no learner overcrowding in a particular unit.

Learners should be fairly distributed because when there is overcrowding, it is not easy to supervise those learners.

The training of the learners must be considered a high and important priority and every effort should be made to give learners the best clinical experience possible.

Institutions of higher learning using the same clinical environment should work together to ensure fair distribution of learners.

Limitations of the Study

Limitations regarding the target population

This study only focused on learners following the Bridging Course for enrolled nurses that lead to registration as a General Nurse according to Regulation 683 of 14 April 1989, in their second year of study, maybe learners in their first year of study or learner following another training programme could have had different view.

Conclusion

Clinical supervision is regarded as the foundation for nursing practice therefore people who are tasked with training learner nurses should ensure that this is the priority in student learning. The positive outcome of clinical experience for learner nurses depends on joint actions by the nurse educators and professional nurses in the unit. They need to equip learner nurses with knowledge and skills so that they practice competently. The quality of patient care depends on the quality of training provided to the care giver.

References

1. Higgs J (2012) Practice-based education pedagogy: situated, capability-development, relationship practice(s) In: Higgs J, Barnett S, Hutchings M, T Rede f (eds.,) Practice based education: Perspective and Strategies. Sense Publishers, Rotterdam, pp: 71-81.

2. Dimitradou M, Papastravrou E, Efstathiou G, Theudorou M (2015) Baccalaureate student's perception of learning and supervision in the clinical environment. Nurs Health Sci 17: 236-242.

3. Henderson A, Tyler S (2011) Facilitating learning in clinical practice: Evaluation of a trial of a supervisor of clinical education role. Nurse Education in Practice 11: 288-292.

4. Jiang R, Chou C, Tsai P (2012) Preceptor–guided practica and the learning experiences of nursing students. J Nurs Resh 16: 152-157.

5. Carlson E, Pilhammar E, Wann-Hansson C (2010) Time to precept: supportive and limiting conditions for precepting nurses. J Adv Nurs 66: 432-441.

6. Mochaki NW (2009) Clinical teaching by registered nurses. Published master's thesis, University of South-Africa, Pretoria, South Africa.

7. Waldock J (2010) Facilitating student learning in clinical practice. Kai Tiaki Nursing New Zealand 16: 14-16.

8. Burns K, Grove S (2011) The practice of nursing research: Conduct, critique and utilization. St Louis, Saunders, Missouri.

9. Polit DF, Beck CT (2008) Nursing research: Generating and assessing evidence for nursing practise. Philadelphia Lippincott.

10. Brink H, Van Der Walt C, Van Rensburg G (2008) Fundamentals of research methodology for health care professionals. Juta and Company, Cape Town.

11. Jooste K (2009) Supervision in social work. Columbia University Press, New York.

12. Botma Y, Greef M, Mulaudzi FM, Wright SCD (2010) Research in health sciences. Heinemann, Cape Town.

13. Creswell JW (1994) Research designs: Qualitative and quantitative approaches. Thousand Oaks, Sage, CA.

5

Communication Skills of Novice Nurses at Psychiatric Hospital in Saudi Arabia

Zakaria A Mani* and Mohammed Abutaleb

Ministry of Health, Nursing Education, Saudi Arabia

*Corresponding author: Mani ZA, Nursing Instructor, Ministry of Health, Nursing Education, Gizan, Abu Arish 45911, Saudi Arabia, E-mail: mani_zakaria@yahoo.com

Abstract

Objective: The objective of this study is to describe the novice nurses' perceptions of communication skills in Saudi Arabia.

Method: A questionnaire developed by Moss that examined nurses' communication with psychiatric patients was used. The questionnaires were collected during the month of December, 2016.

Results: A total of 59 questionnaires were obtained from 89 participants, representing a 66.29% response rate. Findings revealed that novice psychiatric nurses faced challenges in communicating with psychiatric patients. Education and training from either nursing college or hospital orientation program were lacking.

Conclusion: Nurses who have been in work for more than 12 months were confident in their communications with psychiatric patients. Nursing and hospital orientation program should be improved and empowered to prepare novice nurses for the psychiatric setting.

Keywords: Novice nurse; Psychiatric patient; Hospital; Communication

Background

The transition process of graduated nurse to the clinical environment is a critical phase in the professional life [1]. Factors linked with transition process include insufficiency of practical training, lack of confidence, poor conflict management skills, unrealistic expectations, stress, lack of supervision or support and burnout [2,3].

Providing care for hostile patients in inpatient psychiatric units was considered as stressful situations. That is because there were several patients with complex mental illnesses in the inpatient area [4], where nurses exposed to conflict or unpredictable violence [5]. Violence and unpredicted aggressive reaction indicates unsecure environment for both nurse and other patients [4,6]. Such environment is considered stressful for psychiatric nurses, which made them passive to a level to perceive their mental patients as "dangerous, immature, harmful, and pessimistic" [7].

In preparation for such professional environment, emphasis on communication skills during hospital orientation programs or nursing education colleges could be considered the cornerstone of the care for psychiatric patients [8]. Effective communication has been shown as difficult even for the experienced psychiatric nurse [9]. Lack of the communication skills for new psychiatric nurses represents a challenge in delivering a good care especially with the complexity of psychiatric diseases in inpatients area. Findings of literature search about this topic in Saudi Arabia were limited. Therefore this study could contribute to describe the current practice and help to develop the quality of hospital's orientation programs.

Aim

The aim of this study was to evaluate perceptions of novice nurse-patient relationship and to describe the extent of communication skills of those novice nurses who were placed to work in a secondary care hospital specialized for mental disorders in Jazan, a southwest region in Saudi Arabia. Knowing such perceptions could help to get both hospital and regional nursing leaderships aware of novice psychiatric nurses' use of communication techniques with psychiatric patients.

Method

The study was based on a survey questionnaire validated and previously been used. The main advantage of the questionnaire is that it is an efficient and effective method of collecting self-reported data from the participants [10]. The primary version of instrument which developed by Georgaki et al. [11] examined nurses' truthful communication with cancer patients. This was modified, validated and used by Moss [12] in psychiatric patient. The modified version was adapted in this study and further demographic questions were added in accordance to Saudi's context. It consists of seven demographic questions and 17 items focused on novice nurses communication with psychiatric patients. The 17 items were in the form of Likert scales ranging from one to five, where one means strongly agree, second means agree, third means disagree, fourth means strongly disagree and fifth means not sure. The last question was an open-ended question that ask participant to note any concerns related communications with psychiatric patients and how to improve it.

An interpretation to Arabic language was made by an accredited translation office. The researchers reviewed the validation of the translation and compare it with original questionnaire and then a very little revision was made. The pilot study was conducted in both languages Arabic and English. The pilot test was focused on how nurses find instructions and questions? Is it understandable and clear or they suggesting any modification? Five nurses who conducted the pilot test suggested a very little clarification in the Arabic form. The clarifications were then made and reviewed by both researchers.

An ethical approval for conducting this study was obtained from ethical committee of Health Care Services in Jazan region. An anonymous self-reporting, questionnaire and participation was made by consenting voluntary participants. Participants were encouraged to read the explanatory statement before deciding to participate in this study. The explanatory statement clarified that returning a completed questionnaire would be considered as implied consent.

Only novice nurses who have a work experience in the psychiatric hospital for less than 24 months were considered for this study. Therefore, a convenience sampling was proposed to recruit participants. This sampling approach is considered appropriate for small exploratory quantitative studies [13]. The questionnaires were collected during the month of December, 2016.

Questionnaires were checked for completeness and legibility. All questionnaire items, except for the open-ended responses, were converted to numeric codes, to enable data entry into Microsoft Excel and SPSS Version 20 for analysis. Data entry was considered an error-prone process [14], therefore one researcher (ZM) enter the data carefully and then 10% was checked at random by the other researcher (MA) to ensure the accuracy of data entry. A unique identifier in the form of an identity (ID) number was assigned to each questionnaire and this identifier was utilized to indicate authentic citations. The use of authentic citations increases the trustworthiness of the data and demonstrates how the themes were developed [15].

For data analysis, descriptive statistics were used to describe and summarize the demographic data, including age, sex and years of nursing experiences. Measures of central tendency and reliability statistics were calculated describe the rest of the survey items. Open-ended responses were thematically described.

Results

Approximately eighty-nine nurses were identified as novice in the psychiatric hospital; therefore the questionnaire was distributed to all of them. Only 59 returned the questionnaire. This represented 66.3% of the response rate. Four questionnaires were excluded because they were uncompleted. Consequently, 55 questionnaires were considered for the statistical analysis.

Participants demographic

Majority of the novice nurses were Saudi nationality (76.4%) and male (62.8%). The average years of professional experience were 3.05.

The experiences in the psychiatric hospital were 27.3% have less than 12 months experience, 61.8% have 12-18 months and only 10.9%, their experiences ranges from 19 to 24 months. Other demographics data are shown in Table 1.

Participant demographics		
Characteristics	N	%
Gender		
Male	34	61.80%
Female	21	38.20%
Age		
25 or under	8	14.50%
26 to 40	47	85.50%
Nationality		
Saudi	42	76.40%
Non-Saudi	13	23.60%
Education		
Diploma	16	29.60%
Associate degree	15	27.80%
Bachelor degree	22	40,7%
Master degree	1	1.90%
Departments		
Acute Unit	22	40%
Chronic Unit	9	16.40%
Addiction Unit	7	12.70%
Emergency Department	6	10.90%
Female Unit	11	20%

Table 1: Participant demographics.

Items evaluating the perception of the novice nurses regarding their communication competencies of their work in mental hospital is described in Table 2.

Communication competencies findings							
Items	Strongly agree	Agree	Disagree	Strongly disagree	Not sure	Mean	SD
Feel uncomfortable during emotionally charged situations with psychiatric patients	3.60%	23.60%	49.10%	14.50%	9.10%	2.98	0.952
Feel hesitant to approach psychiatric patients who exhibit aggressive behavior	1.80%	12.70%	52.70%	29.10%	3.60%	2.8	0.779

Have difficulty in communicating with patients with mental illness	3.70%	11.10%	50%	27.80%	7.40%	2.76	0.889
Had sufficient knowledge in communicating about mental illness before being hired in a psychiatric nurse position	1.80%	10.90%	43.60%	34.50%	9.10%	2.62	0.871
The information provided during hospital orientation was sufficient to communicate or interact with the aggressive psychiatric patient	1.80%	10.90%	23.60%	47.30%	16.40%	2.35	0.947
Nurse preceptors provided continuous feedback on your interactions and communication skills with psychiatric patients on the unit	11.10%	7.40%	13%	42.60%	25.90%	2.35	1.261
Able to communicate with a patient who may be aggressive	9.10%	0%	18.20%	54.50%	18.20%	2.27	1.062
The hospital orientation was well organized for a novice psychiatric nurse	5.60%	7.40%	11.10%	57.40%	18.50%	2.24	1.027
The communication skills that were learned in nursing school helped to assess patients with mental illness during the hospital and unit-based orientation	5.60%	5.60%	11.10%	57.40%	20.40%	2.19	1.011
During the unit-based orientation, you were able to describe signs of aggressive behavior in psychiatric terms to staff	10.90%	3.60%	7.30%	49.10%	29.10%	2.18	1.219
You are able to articulate to staff the patient's behavior in psychiatric terminology	5.50%	0%	10.90%	50.90%	32.70%	1.95	0.97
The unit-based orientation provided sufficient time for a novice psychiatric nurse to adapt	5.50%	1.80%	5.50%	50.90%	36.40%	1.89	0.994
You are able to detect the mood of a patient just by observation	0%	0%	18.50%	51.90%	29.60%	1.89	0.691
You maintain a calm disposition when a patient is raising their voice	3.60%	1.80%	9.10%	50.90%	34.50%	1.89	0.916
You avoid discussing sensitive topics with your patients	1.90%	0%	9.40%	54.70%	34%	1.81	0.761
When talking to your patients, you pay close attention to their body language	5.50%	0%	1.90%	50%	42.60%	1.76	0.95
Speak Arabic language fluently	5.60%	0%	13%	24.10%	57.40%	1.72	1.071

Table 2: Communication competencies findings.

Table 3 shows the effect of experience in mental hospital with regard to the competency of the novice nurses in communicating with aggressive patients. As you can depict from the Table 3 that only 6 out of 15 nurses who work in psychiatric hospital for less than 12 months perceived able to communicate with aggressive psychiatric patients while 34 out of 40 nurses who work more than 12 months were able to communicate so.

		Experience in psychiatric hospital			Total
		Less than 12 months	From 12 to 18 months	From 19 to 24 months	
You are able to communicate with a patient who may be aggressive	Strongly agree	0	8	2	10
	Agree	6	20	4	30
	Do not agree	5	5	0	10
	Not sure	4	1	0	5

Total		15	34	6	55

Table 3: Cross tabulation between communication with aggressive patient and experiences in psychiatric hospital.

Table 4 also shows the effect of experience in mental hospital with regard to feeling of difficulty of communication with patients with mental illness. As you can depict from the Table 4 that 13 out of 15 nurses who work in psychiatric hospital less than 12 months have difficulty communicating with patients with mental illness, where only 31 out of 39 who had experience more than 12 months did not have difficulty in their communication.

		Psyc Experience			Total
		Less than 12 months	From 12 to 18 months	From 19 to 24 months	
You have difficulty communicating with patients with mental illness	Strongly agree	1	2	1	4
	Agree	12	2	1	15
	Do not agree	2	24	1	27
	Strongly do not agree	0	4	2	6
	Not sure	0	2	0	2
Total		15	34	5	54

Table 4: Cross tabulation between difficult communications vs. psychiatric hospital experience.

Comments regarding communication with psychiatric patients

Additional comments related the concerns of communications with psychiatric patients and how to improve emerged the following findings.

One nurse stated that nursing college was prepared student in general nursing and psychiatric nursing knowledge was lacking. Many nurses claimed that more education and training for novice psychiatric nurses were needed. Particularly education of both how to communicate with psychiatric patient based on their diagnosis and psychiatric medications. Another nurse recommended further education for how to communicate appropriately, be patience, provide emotional support and build a good relationship with psychiatric patients.

Further comment indicated that psychological and social awareness should be considered by nurses when approaching communication with anyone. One nurse suggested that dealing with psychiatric patients kindly, meet their needs and do not let them be alone should be considered as well.

One nurse suggested that psychiatric patients might not treat appropriately from their families or friends and this might worsen the patient's conditions. Therefore they need quality of care from a well prepared and qualified psychiatric staff. One comment indicated that psychiatric patients needed more attention from the all staff. One nurse claimed that the availability of social worker and social psychologist 24 h daily were important to meet the patients' needs.

One comment indicated that patients continuously requested nurses that they wanted call their families and limited access of call could trouble both patients and nurses. On the other hand nurses claimed a requirement to establish entertainment activities, exercises and games for psychiatric patients.

One comment stated that scarcity of security could effect on psychiatric patients relationship and trust in the treatment that given by nurses particularly when nurses provided security roles, restrain or seclusion.

Discussion

The findings of this study revealed that nurses who worked more than 12 months in psychiatric setting were confident to communicate with psychiatric patients. Nurses who worked less than 12 months had experienced difficulty communicating with psychiatric patients. Duchscher [8] recommended that focus on communication is the cornerstone of the care for psychiatric patients. Thus it is important to improve the novice nurse's communication skills in the beginning of their working period.

One comment suggested that psychiatric nursing knowledge was lacking in nursing college. This comment may request further education and training should be implanted in the nursing college. Moreover, more education and training for novice psychiatric nurses at the hospital should be enabled to improve their communicate skills and how to deal with psychiatric patients competently.

Another comment stated that nurses provided security roles, restrain and seclusion. This can disturb the relationship between nurses and psychiatric patients. They may not trust nurse's treatment anymore. The scarcity of security could become a big challenge for psychiatric nurses to build a relationship with psychiatric patients.

Conclusion

Novice psychiatric nurses have difficulty in communicating with psychiatric patients. Nurses who worked for more than 12 months were confident in their communications with psychiatric patients. Nursing college should develop the psychiatric nursing knowledge in the bachelor nursing curriculum. Furthermore, the hospital orientation program should be improved and expanded to prepare novice nurses for the psychiatric setting.

Limitation

This study was conducted in only one setting with small sample size and therefore this study can't be generalized.

Acknowledgement

Many thanks to statistician Layla shaabi from King Fahad Central Hospital at Gizan for her supports and advices.

References

1. Benner P (1982) From novice to expert. AJN 82: 402-407.

2. Jewell A (2013) Supporting the novice nurse to fly: A literature review. Nurse Educ Pract 13: 323-327.

3. Morrow S (2009) New graduate transitions: Leaving the nest, joining the flight. J Nurs Manag 17: 278-287.

4. Ward L (2013) Ready, aim fire! Mental health nurses under siege in acute inpatient facilities. Issues Ment Health Nurs 34: 281-287.

5. Anderson A, West SG (2011) Violence against mental health professionals: When the treater becomes the victim. Innov Clin Neurosci 8: 34-39.

6. Jones J, Nolan P, Bowers L, Simpson A, Whittington R, et al. (2010) Psychiatric wards: Places of safety? J Psychiatr Ment Health Nurs 17: 131-140.

7. Hamdan-Mansour AM, Wardam LA (2009) Attitudes of Jordanian mental health nurses toward mental illness and patients with mental illness. Issues Ment Health Nurs 30: 705-711.

8. Duchscher JB (2008) A process of becoming: The stages of new nursing graduate professional role transition. J Contin Educ Nurs 39: 441-452.

9. Sharac J, McCrone P, Sabes-Figuera R, Csipke E, Wood A, et al. (2010) Nurse and patient activities and interaction on psychiatric inpatients wards: A literature review. Int J Nurs Stud 47: 909-917.

10. Jirojwong S, Johnson M, Welch A (2011) Research methods in nursing and midwifery: Pathways to evidence-based practice, Oxford University Press, South Melbourne.

11. Georgaki S, Kalaidopoulou O, Liarmakopoulou I, Mystakidou K (2002) Nurses' attitudes toward truthful communication with patients with cancer: A Greek study. Cancer Nurs 25: 436-441.

12. Moss R (2015) Communication skills of novice psychiatric nurses with aggressive psychiatric patients. Walden Dissertations and Doctoral Studies.

13. Schneider Z, Whitehead D, LoBiondo-Wood G, Haber J (2013) Nursing and midwifery research: Methods and appraisal for evidence-based practice, Mosby Elsevier, Sydney: NSW.

14. Polit DF, Beck CT (2012) Nursing research: Generating and assessing evidence for nursing practice, Lippincott Williams and Wilkins, Philadelphia.

15. Elo S, Kyngas H (2008) The qualitative content analysis process. J Adv Nurs 62: 107-115.

6

Connecting Leisure-Time Physical Activity and Quality of Sleep to Nurse Health: Data from the e-Cohort Study of Nurses and Midwives

Tim Henwood[1]*, Anthony Tuckett[2], Nadja E –Bagadi[3] and John Oliffe[4]

[1]The University of Queensland, University of Queensland/ Blue Care Research and Practice Development Centre, School of Nursing, Midwifery and Social Work, Brisbane, Australia

[2]The University of Queensland, School of Nursing, Midwifery and Social Work, Brisbane, Australia

[3]School of Nursing and Midwifery, Freiburg University, Freiburg, Germany

[4]School of Nursing, University of British Columbia, Vancouver, Canada

*Corresponding author: Tim Henwood, The University of Queensland/ Blue Care Research and Practice Development Centre, 56 Sylvan Rd, Toowong, Brisbane, QLD, 4066, Australia; E-mail: t.henwood@uq.edu.au

Abstract

Background: Professional nurses are prone to fatigue and poor health. Getting sufficient physical activity and sleep have reported benefits. However, the benefit of ample sleep and physical activity to nurse health is understudied.

Objective: The goal of the current article is to report nurse general and workplace health, productivity and wellbeing by comparing those professionals with recommended levels of physical activity and sleep to those with reduced profiles.

Design: Data were generated from the 2006-08 delivery of the e-Cohort survey of nurses and midwives.

Methods: The primary analysis (n=3967) was based on the physical activity and sleep categories: (LS1) Meeting the recommended guidelines or above for both leisure physical time activity and sleep; (LS2) Meeting the recommended guidelines or above for leisure time activity but not sleep; (LS3) Meeting the recommended guidelines or above for sleep but not leisure time activity; and (LS4) Not meeting the recommended guidelines for both leisure time activity and sleep.

Results: LS1 were significantly younger, had a lower body mass index than any other group and were the least likely to report in-work difficulty, emotional barriers to workplace productivity and restriction in basic daily tasks. LS4 were more likely to have osteoarthritis, depression and high blood pressure.

Conclusion: The study findings confirm health benefits from achieving recommended levels of physical activity and sleep. Adherence to beneficial lifestyle behaviours has important implications for the self-health of nurses. Workforce administrators should consider this when designing programs to reduce nurse workplace burnout and aid workforce retention.

Keywords Guideline adherence; Nurse health; Physical activity; Sleep; Workplace fatigue; Workplace productivity; Workforce planners

Introduction

Nurses are often reported less than healthy and engaged in health risk behaviours such as poor dietary habits, lack of exercise and physical activity, and smoking [1-3]. The combination of shift work and workplace stress is known to compromise nurse wellbeing, and is a common precursors to poor sleeping quality [4]. As a result, nurses often spiral into fatigue, drowsiness and burnout, which culminate in reduced patient care and staff turnover [5,6]. For those nurses engaged in healthy lifestyle behaviours, measurable positive physical and workplace wellbeing benefits are reported [7-9]. Yet it would appear the translation of this evidence to nurse practice is below expectation. While it could be assumed that nurses might have improved knowledge of habits proven to combat stress and fatigue, such as regular physical activity, research consistently highlights nursing as a profession with poor physical and cognitive health [1,2,7]. Recent work by Blake et al. [1] reported that poor health was endemic among nurses with the majority not adhering to national guidelines or recommendations. Given the growing need for competent and invested nurse professionals, the existence of poor self-health that compounds workplace fatigue and burnout is a valid concern that requires more detailed investigation [10].

In 2010, the World Health Organization named physical inactivity as the fourth leading risk factor for global mortality [11]. Associated with physical inactivity are increased risks of disease and all-cause mortality [12]. In contrast, being physically active and/or involved in regular exercise has a plethora of benefits including reduced risk of disease and improved vitality among other health outcomes [11]. Sleeping patterns are also recognized as a determinant of health.

Relationships exist between sleeping disorders and declining wellbeing, increased morbidity and mortality, as well as reduced productivity and memory performance [13,14]. In addition, sleeping disorders are linked to obesity, back pain, anxiety and depression [15,16], and are predictive of workplace burnout [4]. In contrast, improved sleep benefits function, mood, reaction time and reduced daytime sleepiness [17]. Investigations of improved sleep quality and quantity consistently show improved performance, alertness and mood, with results appearing most beneficial to those who work shift or night-time [17-19], and extended to reduced post-shift motor vehicle incidents and fatalities [20].

Recent work confirms that nurses involved in regular leisure time physical activity and improved lifestyle choices report an improved health and workplace productivity profile [8,21]. However, the benefit of physical activity and sleep recommendation adherence for nurses is poorly understood. From this evidence, it could be hypothesized that beyond health and wellbeing, nurses achieving the recommended levels will experience reduced workplace stress and burnout, and deliver advance patient care [8,9]. The goal of this article is to report nurse general and workplace health, productivity and wellbeing by comparing those professionals with recommended levels of physical activity and sleep to those with reduced profiles. In addition to the potential to improve nurses' self-health, this work can guide the health promotion, recruitment and retention efforts of workplace administrators.

Methods

Study design

Employing survey data captured by the Australian and New Zealand Nurses and Midwifes e-Cohort study, this cross-sectional investigation used a group categorization design to analyse the hierarchal impact of an increased sleep and physical activity profile to individuals reporting reduced profiles, in relation to general and workplace health, productivity and wellbeing.

Data were drawn from the large, self-reported survey of practicing nurses and midwives across multiple working environments. The sample, recruitment and survey structure have been described in detail previously [22-24]. In brief, employing Australia and New Zealand academic network support, nursing and midwifery councils were approached to seek permission to recruit nurses for survey. Recruitment commenced in April 2006 and concluded in March 2008. Of the 290 000 Australian and 44 400 New Zealand registered and enrolled nurses and midwives eligible for inclusion, 8247 participated in the survey [22], and 3967 nurses with sleep and physical activity data were included in this analysis.

Research ethics

Ethics approval was provided by the University of Queensland Human Research Ethics Committee.

Data collection

To all eligible members, a personalized email was sent with a study introduction and invitation to participate. Within the email, a URL link directed participants to the study website. The 108 question e-Cohort survey took approximately 40 minutes to complete and

population-based information were collected around two central themes:

- **Work/Life Balance:** Describing and quantifying the factors associated with the retention of the existing workforce and patterns of employment; and
- **Staying Healthy:** Measuring the prevalence, incidence and associated risk factors of physical, mental and health behaviours, including musculoskeletal disorders and work-place injuries in the cohort.

These themes where submerged among a composite of validated and widely used questionnaires (e.g., International Physical Activity Questionnaire, SF-36) and the direct assessments of markers of workforce involvement and health (e.g., years of shift work, BMI).

Data categorization

In this study, total leisure time physical activity in MET (Metabolic equivalent of task) minutes per week and sleeping time per night were categorized, then merged into four distinct groups. Total leisure time physical activity was a combined measure of self-reported low, moderate and vigorous activity undertaken across a seven day continuum, and reported in METs. Data were generated from the International Physical Activity Questionnaire (IPAQ) [25]. The questions used were:

- 'Not counting any walking you have already mentioned, during the last seven days, on how many days did you walk for at least 10 minutes at a time in your leisure?'
- 'During the last seven days, on how many days did you do moderate physical activities [>10 minutes] like bicycling at a regular pace, swimming at a regular pace and doubles tennis in your leisure time?' and
- 'During the last seven days, on how many days did you do vigorous physical activities [>10 minutes] like aerobic running, or fast swimming in your leisure time?'

Participants reported the number of 'Days per Week' and 'Minutes per Day' they undertook physical activity. Data were then converted to MET minutes/week, and the three levels of leisure time activity were summed to give total leisure time physical activity. Participants were categorized as: Low - below the recommendations for weekly physical activity; Moderate - at the weekly recommendation range; or High - above the weekly recommendations. Categories were based on the American College of Sports Medicine guidelines for developing and maintaining health in adults, with those who reported total leisure time activity less than 630 MET minutes/week categorized low and those reporting greater than 1240 MET minutes/week categorized as high leisure time activity [26].

Sleeping time was categorized in accordance with the National Sleep Foundation guidelines that optimal sleep for adults is 7 - 9 hours per night, and the established evidence that less than optimal sleep has detrimental health and productivity implications [27]. Sleep data were generated from the following question:

- 'How many hours of actual sleep do you usually get in a 24 hour period?'

Those who reported sleeping for less than 7 hours a night were categorized as poor sleepers, and those who reported > 9 hours were categorized as above optimal (7-9 hours/night).

To analyse the impacts of *leisure time activity* and *sleep* on health and vitality, four groups were created. These where: (LS1) Meeting the recommended guidelines or above for both leisure time activity (moderate and high physical activity) and sleep (7-9 hours or above); (LS2) Meeting the recommended guidelines or above for leisure time activity but not sleep; (LS3) Meeting the recommended guidelines or above for sleep but not leisure time activity; and (LS4) Not meeting the recommended guidelines for both leisure time activity and sleep. Group comparisons were then undertaken against questions reflecting self-reported health status, vitality, disease and capacity in activities of daily living.

Data analysis

All data were processed in SPSS version 22.0 (SPSS Inc., Chicago, IL, USA). Data were extensively reviewed and outliers eliminated by case using the parameters described above. Descriptive and frequency analysis were undertaken dependent on the variables status, continuous or categorical. For between group analyses, Pearson's Chi Squared test (χ^2) was conducted for categorical data and where appropriate a logistic regression analysis was undertaken to represent the strength of difference. For continuous data, analysis of variance (ANOVA) was conducted and Bonferroni post-hoc procedure used to identify the source of difference. An alpha level of 0.05 was required for significance. Data are presented as mean ± standard deviation.

Results

Prior to group classification, the cohort age was 42.9 ± 10.2 years (n=3967) and reported 673.9 ± 1069.8 MET minute/week of total leisure activity. They were predominantly female (91.4%), with 86.7% of the cohort achieving 7–9 hours' sleep per night, but greater than 65% not meeting the recommended guidelines for leisure time physical activity per day.

Workplace wellbeing

Those who had the best activity and sleep profile (LS1) were younger and had lower BMI's than all other groups (p < .001) (Table 1). LS1 were most likely to report having difficulty in performing their work "None of the time" (χ^2=88.532, d.f.=12, p < .001). Similarly, LS1 were most likely to report that due to emotional issues (depression, anxiety) they had cut down on time at work (χ^2=46.567, d.f.=12, p < .001), accomplished less at work (χ^2=52.503, d.f.=12, p < .001) or had not demonstrated care in work place tasks (χ^2=30.419, d.f.=12, p=.002) "None of the time". In addition, LS1 were most likely to report feeling full of life "Most of the time" (χ^2=162.493, d.f.=12, p < .001), nervous "None of the time" (χ^2=49.495, d.f.=12, p < .001) and down hearted and depressed "None of the time" (χ^2=91.734, d.f.=12, p < .001).

Table 1: Between group differences for age, BMI, sitting time and days off sick.

	Group				P*	Post-hoc**
	1	2	3	4		
Age (yrs)	41.44 ± 10.15	42.79 ± 10.07	42.80 ± 10.09	44.66 ± 10.23	<.001	4 > 3 > 2, 1
Number†	790	392	1482	880		
BMI (kg/m2)	25.92 ± 4.92	26.71 ± 5.42	27.84 ± 6.02	28.60 ± 6.38	<.001	4 > 3 > 2, 1
Number (%)‡	779 (98.6)	389 (99.2)	1456 (98.2)	872 (99.1)		
Sitting Time Week days (m/d)	1045.39 ± 959.35	845.87 ± 713.14	1121.16 ± 1437.33	988.16 ± 1086.83	0.003	3 > 2
Number (%)‡	605(76.6)	300 (76.5)	1077 (72.7)	626 (71.1)		
Sitting Time Weekends (m/d)	341.47 ± 296.35	347.97 ± 352.33	386.02 ± 385.28	378.21 ± 392.78	0.034	3 > 1
Number (%)‡	730 (92.4)	368 (93.9)	1308 (88.3)	792 (90.0)		
Days off sick	8.41 ± 26.78	6.76 ± 14.90	9.99 ± 48.16	5.91 ± 12.59	0.357	
Number (%)‡	214 (27.1)	150 (38.3)	480 (32.4)	350 (39.8)		

Data are mean ± standard deviation Groups: (1) Meeting the recommended guidelines or above for both leisure time activity and sleep; (2) Meeting the recommended guidelines or above for leisure time activity but with poor sleep; (3) Meeting the recommended guidelines or above for sleep but not leisure time activity; and (3) Not meeting the recommended guidelines for both leisure time activity and sleep. yrs – years, BMI – body mass index, kg/m2 – kilograms per metre squared, m/d minutes per day
* Between group ANOVA   ** Between-group Bonferroni post hoc comparison   † Total number of individual allocated to each group
‡ Total number of responders per group per variable (% of total possible sample)

General health and energy

When asked about levels of energy, LS1 were most likely to have sufficient energy "Most of the time" (39.8%) (χ^2=198.635, d.f.=12, p < .001). In relation to happiness, LS1 were most likely to report feeling happy "All of the time" ($\chi2$=93.241, d.f.=12, p < .001), while LS4 most likely to report feeling tired "All of the time" ($\chi2$=136.012, d.f.=12, p < .001). When asked about General Health, LS1 were most likely to report "Excellent" or "Very Good" (46.1%) health, and LS4 most likely to report "Fair" (18.7%) health (χ^2=244.619, d.f.=12, p < .001). LS4 were least likely and LS1 the most likely to respond "Definitely false" to their health getting worse (χ^2=71.326, d.f.=12, p < .001). These data are presented in more detail in (Table 2).

Table 2: Group differences for self-reported wellbeing and general health by Pearson's chi squared test (χ^2), Omitted responses given in brackets

Group	1		2		3		4		Total		
	n	%	n	%	n	%	n	%	n	%	P*
Difficulty performing work (Most of the time/A little of the time)											
All of the time	8	1	11	2.8	30	2	20	2.3	69	2	<.001
Some of the time	133	17	98	25.3	292	19.8	249	28.4	772	21.9	
None of the time	403	51.4	157	40.6	665	45.1	283	32.3	1508	42.8	
Emotional problem causing:											
Cut down on work (Most of/A little of the time)											
All of the time	7	0.9	7	1.8	13	0.9	12	1.4	39	1.1	< .001
Some of the time	104	13.3	63	16.2	222	15	157	17.9	546	15.5	
None of the time	521	66.5	240	61.5	919	62.2	473	53.8	2153	61	
Accomplish less (Most of/A little of the time)											
All of the time	6	0.8	13	3.3	33	2.2	22	2.5	74	2.1	< .001
Some of the time	148	18.8	86	21.9	291	19.7	217	24.7	742	21	
None of the time	394	50.1	162	41.3	689	46.7	327	37.2	1572	44.5	
Be less careful (Most of/A little of the time)											
All of the time	5	0.6	5	1.3	8	0.5	8	0.9	26	0.7	< .001
Some of the time	102	13	66	17	222	15.1	154	17.6	544	15.5	
None of the time	475	60.4	220	56.6	839	57.1	430	49.1	1964	55.8	
Felt full of Life (Most of/A little of the time)											
All of the time	55	7	11	2.8	39	2.6	16	1.8	121	3.4	< .001
Some of the time	247	31.4	155	39.5	556	37.5	345	39.3	1303	36.8	
None of the time	10	1.3	14	3.6	55	3.7	60	6.8	139	3.9	
Felt nervous (Most of/A little of the time)											
All of the time	3	0.4	5	1.3	6	0.4	11	1.3	25	0.7	< .001
Some of the time	192	24.4	103	26.3	337	22.8	263	30.1	895	25.4	
None of the time	312	39.7	121	30.9	547	37	248	28.4	1228	34.8	
Felt down in the dumps (Most of/A little of the time)											
All of the time	2	0.3	4	1	9	0.6	13	1.5	28	0.8	< .001
Some of the time	104	13.2	80	20.5	208	14	202	23	594	16.8	
None of the time	472	60.1	185	47.4	812	54.9	346	39.4	1815	51.3	
Felt calm and peaceful (Most of/A little of the time)											
All of the time	19	2.4	6	1.5	31	2.1	16	1.8	72	2	< .001
Some of the time	303	38.5	155	39.7	583	39.5	329	37.6	1370	38.8	

	n	%	n	%	n	%	n	%	n	%	p
None of the time	19	2.4	20	5.1	58	3.9	57	6.2	151	4.3	
Had lots of energy (Most of/A little of the time)											
All of the time	33	4.2	10	2.6	19	1.3	21	2.4	83	2.3	< .001
Some of the time	300	38	176	44.9	597	40.3	323	36.9	1396	39.5	
None of the time	30	3.8	16	4.1	116	7.8	106	12.1	268	7.6	
Felt downhearted and depressed (Most of/A little of the time)											
All of the time	2	0.3	7	1.8	12	0.8	13	1.5	34	1	< .001
Some of the time	144	18.3	90	23.1	310	20.9	241	27.4	785	22.2	
None of the time	327	41.6	113	29	503	34	216	24.6	1159	32.8	
Felt worn out (Most of/A little of the time)											
All of the time	19	2.4	22	5.6	61	4.1	56	6.4	158	4.5	< .001
Some of the time	301	38.2	155	39.6	552	37.2	338	38.5	1346	38	
None of the time	91	11.5	25	6.4	115	7.8	37	4.2	268	7.6	
Been happy (Most of/A little of the time)											
All of the time	79	10.1	24	6.2	105	7.1	41	4.7	249	7	< .001
Some of the time	177	22.5	121	31	434	29.3	303	34.5	1035	29.3	
None of the time	3	0.4	4	1	12	0.8	8	0.8	27	0.8	
Felt tired (Most of/A little of the time)											
All of the time	44	5.6	45	11.5	125	8.5	117	13.4	331	9.4	< .001
Some of the time	346	44	156	40	635	42.9	304	34.7	1441	40.8	
None of the time	15	1.9	4	1	25	1.7	12	1.4	56	1.6	
General health (Very good/Fair)											
Excellent	179	22.7	66	16.8	165	11.1	63	7.2	473	13.4	< .001
Good	198	25.1	139	35.4	596	40.2	397	45.2	1330	37.5	
Poor	7	0.9	1	0.3	16	1.18		0.9	32	0.9	
Expect health to get worse (Mostly true/false)											
Definitely true	16	2	10	2.6	27	1.8	30	3.4	83	2.3	< .001
Don't know	181	22.9	108	27.6	425	28.7	261	29.7	975	27.6	
Definitely false	327	41.4	123	31.4	439	29.7	215	24.5	1104	31.2	

Groups: (1) Meeting the recommended guidelines or above for both leisure time activity and sleep; (2) Meeting the recommended guidelines or above for leisure time activity but with poor sleep; (3) Meeting the recommended guidelines or above for sleep but not leisure time activity; and (3) Not meeting the recommended guidelines for both leisure time activity and sleep. n - number, % - percentage of total group. *Pearson's Chi-squared test 2-sided significance.

Physical capacity

Supporting the trend in better general health for LS1 was the greater likelihood of being in a healthy BMI category (18.6 – 24.9 Kg/m2) (46.9%), with LS4 having a greater likelihood of being obese (≥30 kg/m2) (34.3%) (χ^2=73.848, d.f.=9, p<.001). In addition, LS1 were most likely to report having no limitation in lifting groceries (χ^2=28.00, d.f.=6, p<.001), climbing one (χ^2=56.559, d.f.=6, p<.001) or several (χ^2=131.666, d.f.=6, p < .001) flights of stairs, walking one mile (χ^2=95.121, d.f.=6, p < .001) or kneeling (χ^2=65.771, d.f.=6, p<.001). These data are presented in more detail in Table 3.

Table 3: Self-reported restrictions in physical capacity by Pearson's chi-squared test (χ^2), Omitted responses given in brackets Groups: (1)

Group	1		2		3		4		Total		
	n	%	n	%	n	%	n	%	n	%	P*
Restricted in:											
Lifting groceries (Limited a lot/a little)											
Not at all	691	88	327	84.3	1205	82.3	682	78.5	2905	82.9	< .001
Climbing one flight of stairs (Limited a lot/a little)											
Not at all	739	94.3	351	91.4	1288	87.7	721	82.9	3099	88.4	< .001
Climbing several flights of stairs (Limited a lot/a little)											
Not at all	652	83.3	295	76.2	1015	69.2	529	60.7	2491	71	< .001
Walking one mile (Limited a lot/a little)											
Not at all	719	91.5	336	87	1184	80.8	642	74	2881	82.2	< .001
Bending or kneeling (Limited a lot/a little)											
Not at all	621	79.1	274	70.8	1021	69.5	531	61	2447	69.7	< .001

Groups: (1) Meeting the recommended guidelines or above for both leisure time activity and sleep; (2) Meeting the recommended guidelines or above for leisure time activity but with poor sleep; (3) Meeting the recommended guidelines or above for sleep but not leisure time activity; and (3) Not meeting the recommended guidelines for both leisure time activity and sleep,
n - number, % - percentage of total group,
*Pearson's Chi-squared

Table 4: Association between disease and adherence to physical activity and sleep recommendations

Group	2			3			4			
	OR	CI	p	OR	CI	p	OR	CI	p	p*
Anxiety	1.34	.95-1.90	0.097	1.12	.88-1.48	0.329	1.56	1.19-2.06	0.001	0.006
Cervical cancer	2.18	1.22-3.92	0.009	1.05	.63-1.70	0.867	1.22	.71-2.11	0.474	0.023
Congestive heart failure	2.07	.86-5.02	0.107	0.91	.41-1.99	0.803	0.54	.19-1.49	0.231	0.056
Depression	1.6	1.21-2.12	0.001	1.38	1.12-1.70	0.003	1.76	1.41-2.21	>.001	>.001
Elevated triglycerides	1.2	.74-1.94	0.464	1.52	1.08-2.15	0.016	1.83	1.28-2.63	0.001	0.007
Elevated cholesterol	1.57	1.12-2.22	0.009	1.52	1.18-1.97	0.001	1.92	1.46-2.52	>.001	>.001
High blood pressure	1.29	.90-1.84	0.163	1.2	.92-1.56	0.176	1.56	1.18-2.06	0.002	0.015
Osteoarthritis	1.86	1.17-2.96	0.009	1.69	1.18-2.43	0.005	2.29	1.57-3.34	>.001	>.001

Groups: (1) Meeting the recommended guidelines or above for both leisure time activity and sleep; (2) Meeting the recommended guidelines or above for leisure time activity but with poor sleep; (3) Meeting the recommended guidelines or above for sleep but not leisure time activity; and (3) Not meeting the recommended guidelines for both leisure time activity and sleep, Group 1 are the reference group and the association is presence of disease, OR – Odds Ratio, CI – 95% confidence interval, p – significance by binary logistic regression between group and the reference group, p* model significance by binary logistic regression

Disease

For disease, LS1 were most likely to report no history of anxiety (87.8%) (χ^2=12.385 d.f.=12, p=.006) and osteoarthritis (94.8%) (χ^2=19.196, d.f.=3, p<.001). LS2 was most likely to report a history of cervical cancer (6.2%) (χ^2=9.911, d.f.=3, p<.019) and congestive heart failure (2.6%) (χ^2=8.197, d.f.=3, p<.042). LS4 were most likely to report a history of depression (31.1%) (χ^2=26.019, d.f.=3, p<.001), elevated triglycerides (10.7%) (χ^2=12.178, d.f.=3, p<.007), cholesterol (20.3%)

(χ^2=22.313, d.f.=3, p<.001) and high blood pressure (17.3%) (χ^2=10.478, d.f.=3, p<.015). Logistic regression analyses for diseases (Table 4) demonstrated LS1 had a significantly reduced risk for osteoarthritis, elevated cholesterol and depression compared to all other groups (p≤.009).

Discussion

This study demonstrates significant benefit for nurses physically active and sleeping at or above the recommended level. Specifically, the findings conclusively show that those attaining the recommended physical activity and sleep profile are most likely to be productive, experience reduced barriers to workplace and external physical activities, have a reduced risk of disease and be more likely to report 'better' health. Moreover, we hypothesize these "healthier" nurses would have a greater capacity for caring. To this end, affirmed are the benefits to nurses that actively pursue personal wellbeing and to the efforts of employers who support employee healthy lifestyle promotion.

Across all populations physical inactivity and sedentary behaviour are established precursors to premature mortality; and poor sleeping patterns are linked to reduced wellbeing, increased morbidity and diminished productivity [11,13,14]. For nurses, the impact of daytime fatigue associated to poor sleep, reduces workplace productivity and lowers cognitive function [14,28]. When coupled with shift-work, consistent poor sleep has been shown to play a significant role in reducing work and post-work safety, and specifically the increased risk of post-shift road fatality [20]. In our study, 32% of the sample reported getting less than optimal sleep, which is consistent with norms that report greater than one third of adult populations have poor sleeping patterns [27].

As a countermeasure, there have been a number of reported strategies targeting improved sleep. Recently, Steffen et al. [29] demonstrated the value of an 8-week workplace healthy sleep program, where following a 1 hour session per week that delivered improved sleep technique education, participants reported reduced stress and fewer nights of "poor sleep", as well as an improved quality of life and energy levels. Other strategies specific to nurses that have been successful have included structured workplace napping and permanent night or day duty rosters [30]. Given the extended duration of nurse shifts and the impact of rotating rosters on life balance, workplace interventions hold potential for improved sleeping profiles [20,31]. These considerations should also be extended to physical activity. Workplace based interventions and/or educational seminars either; (a) targeting improved activity participation, or (b) lobbying holistic healthy lifestyle behaviours, have been consistently demonstrated successful [32-36]. For participants, workplace interventions are convenient to access and are reported to improve markers of disease and quality of life as well as reduce job stress and improve productivity [34,37]. For the employer, the investment of delivering workplace interventions is associated with reduced absenteeism and staff turnover [33].

The current study findings indicate that when physical activity participation is coupled with good sleep practice, nurses achieve a psychosomatic benefit. With the exception of congestive heart failure, LS1 reported an enhanced level of disease resistance to all other groups for osteoarthritis, elevated cholesterol and depression. Moreover, when compared to those not achieving sufficient sleep and physical activity, the LS1 health profile extended to a reduced risk of high blood

pressure, elevated triglycerides and anxiety. This disease disparity between those with the highest profile and those with the lowest, speaks to the value of a healthy lifestyle. With increased disease risk comes other personal and financial implications [38]. For osteoarthritis alone, individuals can incur medical cost 28% - 30% higher than their non-arthritic counterparts, with the cost increasing in the presence of a secondary diagnosis such as high blood pressure [39]. With an ageing population, and the increase in chronic illness and complex health care needs, the demand for nursing services will increase [40]. Therefore, the promotion of a healthy nurse workforce is paramount to meet the increased demands for services and reducing the potential for nurses prematurely being consumers of health care services themselves.

Work to date demonstrates that within the nursing profession, turnover is high and consistently associated with reduced patient care and nurse burnout [41]. Recent work by Wang et al. [42] reported emotional exhaustion and depersonalization as underlying factors in nurse burnout. Supported by previous research, Wang et al. urged workforce administrators to seek means of improving nurse self-efficacy and reduce environmental stressors [10,42]. This and previous work undertaken by our group, has consistently demonstrated an association between improved workplace vitality, emotional capacity and general health among nurses adhering to one or multiple lifestyle health behaviour [8,21]. Workforce administrators need to take note of this if they wish to reduce nurse staff turnover, extend staff workforce retention and the attendant quality of care.

The present study limitations include the following. Firstly, data are self-reported and the development of the sub-grouped units of analysis is informed by a two stage categorization process in a convenience sample. However, this form of delivery is common in epidemiological evaluation, with large internet population-based surveys and other web-based questionnaires having demonstrated acceptance and feasibility. In an electronic age, web-based surveys have greater accessibility and integrity, with improved cost-effective outcomes over traditional telephone contact and/or face-to-face collections [22]. For this work, categorization is substantiated by that BMI increased across groups (LS1-4) as would be expected with decreasing levels of physical activity participation [43]. In addition, the cohort figures for physical activity (<28%) and sleep (>70%) guideline adherence are consistent with national estimates [27,44]. While barriers to participation are an important consideration not discussed here, for workforce administrators looking to intervene in poor nurse health the underlying fact delivered by this work is that adherence and participation play an undisputable role in an individual's health and wellbeing. Finally, the current data was drawn from nurses working in the southern hemisphere and the findings reported here may not be generalizable to nurses working elsewhere. That said, similar results have been reported in a study of nurses working in the northern hemisphere [9].

Conclusion

This study demonstrates the benefits to nurses of meeting and exceeding the recommended guidelines for physical activity and sleep. These benefits are further contextualized against measures of disease, workplace productivity and general health and wellbeing, especially when compare to nurses who do not adhere to the recommendations. The majority of nurses were insufficiently engaged in physical activity, but were achieving the recommended level of sleep. However, it is the combination of attaining the two recommendations that affords the greatest benefit. The implications of not adhering to recommended levels of sleep and activity extends to individual wellbeing and would be assumed to reduce capacity for patient care. The findings from this study are an important reminder to employers seeking to bolster their nurse recruitment and retention efforts. For example, effective workplace activity based programs are likely to yield significant benefits to workers, patients and the organization's 'bottom line'.

Funding Statement

Funding support for the Nurse and Midwives e-Cohort study was received from the Australian Research Council (LP0562102), (SR0566924), Australian National Health and Medical Research Council (2005002108) and New Zealand Health Research Council (456163). Industry Partners providing additional funding include: Queensland Health, the South Australian Department of Health, Injury Prevention and Control Australia (Pty Ltd), Nursing Council of New Zealand and the Macquarie Bank Foundation. No specific funding was received to undertake the analysis described in this article.

Acknowledgement

The data on which this article is based was collected as part of the Nurse and Midwives e-Cohort study (http://e-cohort.net) at The University of Queensland. Industry partners providing in-kind support to the e-Cohort study include: Queensland Nursing Council, Nurses and Midwives Board of New South Wales, Nurses Board of Tasmania, Nurses Board of Western Australia, Nurses Board of the Australian Capital Territory and the Nursing Council of New Zealand, Corporate sponsors include Virgin Blue, Virgin Atlantic and Message Net.

References

1. Blake H, Malik S, Mo PK, Pisano C (2011) 'Do as say, but not as I do': are next generation nurses role models for health? Perspect Public Health 131: 231-239.

2. Malik S, Blake H, Batt M (2011) How healthy are our nurses? New and registered nurses compared. Br J Nurs 20: 489-496.

3. Zapka JM, Lemon SC, Magner RP, Hale J (2009) Lifestyle behaviours and weight among hospital-based nurses. J Nurs Manag 17: 853-860.

4. Alimoglu MK, Donmez L (2005) Daylight exposure and the other predictors of burnout among nurses in a University Hospital. Int J Nurs Stud 42: 549-555.

5. Poissonnet CM, Véron M (2000) Health effects of work schedules in healthcare professions. J Clin Nurs 9: 13-23.

6. Wong H, Wong MCS, Wong SYS, Lee A. (2010) The association between shift duty and abnormal eating behavior among nurses working in a major hospital: a cross-sectional study. Int J Nurs Stud. 47:1021-7.

7. Hawker CL (2012) Physical activity and mental well-being in student nurses. Nurse Educ Today 32: 325-331.

8. Henwood T, Tuckett A, Turner C (2012) What makes a healthier nurse, workplace or leisure physical activity? Informed by the Australian and New Zealand e-Cohort Study. J Clin Nurs 21: 1746-1754.

9. Sveinsdóttir H, Gunnarsdóttir HK (2008) Predictors of self-assessed physical and mental health of Icelandic nurses: results from a national survey. Int J Nurs Stud 45: 1479-1489.

10. Vahey DC, Aiken LH, Sloane DM, Clarke SP, Vargas D (2004) Nurse burnout and patient satisfaction. Med Care 42: II57-66.

11. World Health Organistaion. Global Recommendations On Physical Activity For Health. 2010.

12. Owen N, Healy GN, Matthews CE, Dunstan DW (2010) Too much sitting: the population health science of sedentary behavior. Exerc Sport Sci Rev 38: 105-113.

13. Hillman DR, Lack LC (2013) Public health implications of sleep loss: the community burden. Med J Aust 199: S7-10.

14. Petersen H, Kecklund G, D'Onofrio P, Nilsson J, Åkerstedt T (2013) Stress vulnerability and the effects of moderate daily stress on sleep polysomnography and subjective sleepiness. J Sleep Res 22: 50-57.

15. Chan MF (2009) Factors associated with perceived sleep quality of nurses working on rotating shifts. J Clin Nurs 18: 285-293.

16. Hsieh ML, Li YM, Chang ET, Lai HL, Wang WH, et al. (2011) Sleep disorder in Taiwanese nurses: a random sample survey. Nurs Health Sci 13: 468-474.

17. Mah CD, Mah KE, Kezirian EJ, Dement WC (2011) The effects of sleep extension on the athletic performance of collegiate basketball players. Sleep 34: 943-950.

18. Sagaspe P, Taillard J, Chaumet G, Moore N, Bioulac B, et al. (2007) Aging and nocturnal driving: better with coffee or a nap? A randomized study. Sleep 30: 1808-1813.

19. Signal TL, Gander PH, Anderson H, Brash S (2009) Scheduled napping as a countermeasure to sleepiness in air traffic controllers. J Sleep Res 18: 11-19.

20. Ftouni S, Sletten TL, Howard M, Anderson C, Lenné MG, et al. (2013) Objective and subjective measures of sleepiness, and their associations with on-road driving events in shift workers. J Sleep Res 22: 58-69.

21. Tuckett A, Henwood T. (2014) The impact of five lifestyle factors on nurses' and midwives' health: the Australian and New Zealand nurses' and midwives' e-cohort study. Int J Health Promot Educ 1-13.

22. Turner C, Bain C, Schluter PJ, Yorkston E, Bogossian F, et al. (2009) Cohort Profile: The Nurses and Midwives e-Cohort Study--a novel electronic longitudinal study. Int J Epidemiol 38: 53-60.

23. Huntington A, Gilmour J, Schluter P, Tuckett A, Bogossian F, et al. (2009) The Internet as a research site: establishment of a web-based longitudinal study of the nursing and midwifery workforce in three countries. J Adv Nurs 65: 1309-1317.

24. Schluter PJ, Turner C, Huntington AD, Bain CJ, McClure RJ (2011) Work/life balance and health: the Nurses and Midwives e-cohort Study. Int Nurs Rev 58: 28-36.

25. Ainsworth BE, Bassett DR Jr, Strath SJ, Swartz AM, O'Brien WL, et al. (2000) Comparison of three methods for measuring the time spent in physical activity. Med Sci Sports Exerc 32: S457-464.

26. Garber CE, Blissmer B, Deschenes MR, et al. (2011) American College of Sports Medicine position stand. Quantity and quality of exercise for developing and maintaining cardiorespiratory, musculoskeletal, and neuromotor fitness in apparently healthy adults: guidance for prescribing exercise. Med Sci Sports Exerc. 43:1334-59.

27. The Division of Sleep Medicine at Harvard Medical School. Get Sleep: Steps you can take to get good sleep and improve health, work, and life. Available from: http://healthysleep.med.harvard.edu/need-sleep/whats-in-it-for-you/mood; 24.1.2014.

28. de Lange AH, Kompier MA, Taris TW, Geurts SA, Beckers DG, et al. (2009) A hard day's night: a longitudinal study on the relationships among job demands and job control, sleep quality and fatigue. J Sleep Res 18: 374-383.

29. Steffen MW, Hazelton AC, Moore WR, Jenkins SM, Clark MM, et al. (2015) Improving sleep: outcomes from a worksite healthy sleep program. J Occup Environ Med 57: 1-5.

30. Alward RR, Monk TH (1990) A comparison of rotating-shift and permanent night nurses. Int J Nurs Stud 27: 297-302.

31. Smith-Coggins R, Howard SK, Mac DT, Wang C, Kwan S, et al. (2006) Improving alertness and performance in emergency department physicians and nurses: the use of planned naps. Ann Emerg Med 48: 596-604, 604.

32. Anderson LM, Quinn TA, Glanz K, Ramirez G, Kahwati LC, et al. (2009) The effectiveness of worksite nutrition and physical activity interventions

for controlling employee overweight and obesity: a systematic review. Am J Prev Med 37: 340-357.

33. Cancelliere C, Cassidy JD, Ammendolia C, Côté P (2011) Are workplace health promotion programs effective at improving presenteeism in workers? A systematic review and best evidence synthesis of the literature. BMC Public Health 11: 395.

34. Morgan PJ, Collins CE, Plotnikoff RC, Cook AT, Berthon B, et al. (2012) The impact of a workplace-based weight loss program on work-related outcomes in overweight male shift workers. J Occup Environ Med 54: 122-127.

35. Peterson M (2004) What men and women value at work: implications for workplace health. Gend Med 1: 106-124.

36. Whitehead D (2006) Workplace health promotion: the role and responsibility of health care managers. J Nurs Manag 14: 59-68.

37. Flannery K, Resnick B, McMullen TL (2012) The impact of the Worksite Heart Health Improvement Project on work ability: a pilot study. J Occup Environ Med 54: 1406-1412.

38. Katzmarzyk PT, Janssen I (2004) The economic costs associated with physical inactivity and obesity in Canada: an update. Can J Appl Physiol 29: 90-115.

39. Maetzel A, Li LC, Pencharz J, Tomlinson G, Bombardier C; Community Hypertension and Arthritis Project Study Team (2004) The economic burden associated with osteoarthritis, rheumatoid arthritis, and hypertension: a comparative study. Ann Rheum Dis 63: 395-401.

40. Goss. J (2008) Projection of Australain health care expenditure by disease, 2003 to 2033. In: Australian Institute of Health and Welfare. AIHW, Canberra.

41. Hsu HY, Chen SH, Yu HY, Lou JH (2010) Job stress, achievement motivation and occupational burnout among male nurses. J Adv Nurs 66: 1592-1601.

42. Wang S, Liu Y, Wang L (2015) Nurse burnout: personal and environmental factors as predictors. Int J Nurs Pract 21: 78-86.

43. Bonnefoy M, Cornu C, Normand S, et al. (2003) The effects of exercise and protein-energy supplements on body composition and muscle function in frail elderly individuals: a long-term controlled randomised study. British Journal of Nutrition. 89:731-9.

44. Physical Activity in Australia: A Snapshot, 2007-08 (2011) In: Australian Bureau of Statistics, ABS, Canberra.

7

Effectiveness of a Nursing Shift Information System on a Surgical Ward in Taiwan

Bi Lian Chen*

Department of Nursing, Taichung Veterans General Hospital, Taiwan

*Corresponding author: Bi Lian Chen, Department of Nursing, Taichung Veterans General Hospital, Taiwan, E-mail: blchen25@gmail.com

Abstract

Background: Nurse Shift is a routine but essential operation in hospital management. Classically, paper records have been used in nurse shift but these procedures are time consuming and inefficient. For efficiency and quality nursing care, as well as patients' wellbeing, a computerized nurse shifting information system is essential.

Objective: This study aimed to estimate the performance of a computerized nurse shifting information system (CNSIS) designed to simplify the nurse shifting procedures.

Methods: Seventeen female nursing staffs were recruited into this study. Two thousand and one hundred sixty six nursing shift data related to 142 inpatients from one ward during the period of November 20, 2007 to January 4, 2008, were also used in the analysis. ANOVA was used in analysing the time consumed before and after CNSIS implementation.

Results: On application of CNSIS, time needed for shift (TNS) during 2nd (p<000), 3rd (p<000) and 4th week (p<000) had decreased significantly. Besides, only one incomplete intake and output event was reported.

Conclusions: The CNSIS appears to increase the efficiency of nursing administration. Implementation of CNSIS is promising and worth to be practically used in nursing administration.

Keywords: Computerized nurse shifting information system (CNSIS); Nursing information system; Hand over; Nursing administration

Background

Work shift in nursing care is part of the health management process. As a routine, patients' health information is to be completely transferred from a nurse to another, so that the patients are being cared on a continuous basis [1-3]. This allows the nursing staffs who take over the duty to arrange duty priority between caring and the patients. Incorrect or incomplete transfer, misunderstood or missing of information, may cause unwanted complications in patients [4]. In the perspective of a hospital administrator, a proper nurse shift is an issue of work efficacy and labor-salary [5].

The use of computerized nurse shifting system has the advantages to provide correct, on time, complete and integrated information, which reduce length of stay of the patients and chances to make errors. Classically, patients' information are transferred by verbal, written and taped methods [1,5,6]. These methods require well established forms and rules. The Kardex written shift, a classic shift method, is time consuming and may not be literally recognizable. Sexton et al. found that only 84.6% of contents in written shift were related to the necessary information. In addition, 30% of the patients' information was incorrectly transferred. Tape shift is a time saving method, but lacking of face-to-face communication. As a result, the transferred information may not be correct and in time, and lack of feedback from both sides. For the considerations of cost and safety, it would be appropriate to integrate patients' past history and high risk events by computerized system to reduce errors between shifts [2,6].

Computer and wireless technologies have been explored as a possible solution to improve the shift report process and, subsequently, health care outcomes and patient safety [2,6]. Statistics of The Joint Commission on Accreditation of Health Care Organizations (JCAHO) on 2000 demonstrated that, more than 50% of shifting sentinel events had caused lethal events in patients, e.g., a note of patient's penicillin allergy on nursing record which had not been orally reported and thus caused penicillin lethal event [6]. The Joint Commission identified communication as with handoffs playing a "role in an estimated 80% of serious preventable adverse events" [2] Such events strengthen the need of a proper communication during nurse shifting. In addition, current Taiwan joint Commission on Hospital Accreditation and Quality improvement requires a clear information transfer in nurse shifts and a respect of patients' subjective feelings. To resolve the existing problems in classic nurse shift method, we developed a computerized nurse shifting information system (CNSIS) that suits our environments and analyzed the performance of the system.

Methods and Materials

This study was an intervention study, data collection were including before and after of CNSIS implementation. We adopted purposeful sampling (judgment sampling) design to recruit research subjects from a ward who cared for patients admitted for surgery or treatment for none surgery health problems. The nurses recruited in this study were all board qualified (defined board qualified stands for the nurse who take care patient and worked over three months). New employees (less than 3 months employment), head nurse and administrative assistant were excluded from the study to avoid bias in work experiences. Finally, 142 inpatients were recruited in this study and 2166 records of shift data were collected between 20 November 2007 and 4 January 2008. Time needed for shift (TNS) and completeness of shift (COS) was used for the evaluation of the performance of the CNSIS. The TNS and COS were measured at 3 periods (12 December 2007 to 18 December 2007, 19 December 2007 to 25 December 2007, and 26 December 2007 to 4 January 2008). COS included 15 items, namely, allergies, pertinent history, status during admission and past history, therapeutic prescription, none therapeutic treatment, examinations that need pre-arrangements, vital signs, nursing records (patients' complains, nurse's observation, nursing procedures and routine care, etc.), use of tube/drain, physical activity, disclosure of truth (disclosure of exact disease status to patient), request for do not resuscitation (DNR), dying, pharmacy dispensing for chemotherapy and treatment prohibition (to avoid harms in particular conditions, e.g., do not measure blood pressure when artery-vein shunt is implanted). Data collection tools that the interface calculated the time needed to accomplish reporting the 15 items, and the operator (the nurse) could not made further changes on confirmation of the report. The data were automatically stored and transferred into excel file. To compliment possible missing information when using CNSIS, we also designed a report for missing data to the next staff on duty, so that the information can be fulfilled. The report for missing was also included in our analysis.

Data analysis and management which simple statistics were used to describe the characters of variable included in this study, including COS. Analysis of variance (ANOVA) was used to evaluate effects of CNSIS implementation to TNS. Age, education, seniority, time of shift, and unit (the teams in which the nurses joined), were used as covariates. SPSS version 12.0 was used to conduct the statistics. This study was approved by the Institutional Review Board of the Taichung Veterans Hospital, Taiwan (IRB TCVGH No: 951204/C06272) and written Informed consents were obtained from the nursing staffs who joined to agree to participate.

Results

Demographics

Seventeen nurses were enrolled into this study. Their mean age was 31.5 ± 7.7. About 31% of the research subjects had worked in this hospital for 3 to 6 years, and 68.7% had a college education. Fifteen research subjects had completed the evaluations before and after CNSIS implementation, and 2 research subjects only completed the post examination. The number of patients recorded in this study was 142, and 2166 records were available for statistical analysis (Table 1).

Time	N	Mean ± SD	95% Confidence Interval		Min	Max
			Lower Bound	Upper Bound		
Baseline	30	1.94 ± 0.72	1.67	2.21	0.43	4.29
2nd week	24	0.98 ± 0.38	0.82	1.14	0.07	1.8
3rd week	32	1.13 ± 0.39	0.99	1.27	0.47	2.19
4th week	34	1.03 ± 0.41	0.89	1.18	0.22	1.9
Total	148	1.25 ± 0.75	1.13	1.38	0.05	6.43

Table 1: Demographic characteristics (n=2166).

Mean time used in nurse shift before CNSIS implementation was 1.93 ± 0.72 minutes. After CNSIS implementation, the means of time used in nurse shift were 1.13 ± 0.39, 1.03 ± 0.41, and 1.25 ± 0.75, respectively. Further stratification showed that all research subjects had saved time in day shift and evening shift, but not in night shift.

All nurses started to use the CNSIS in the first week. We compared the TNS at 2nd, 3rd and 4th week, with TNS at baseline. The statistical results of post-hoc comparisons are summarized in Table 2 and 3. TNS at 2nd (p<0.000), 3rd (p<0.000) and 4th week (p<0.000), were significantly less the baseline.

Shift	Time	Mean ± SE	95% Confidence Interval		Sig.
			Lower Bound	Upper Bound	
Day					
Baseline	2nd week	.21	0.92	1.77	0
	3rd week	1.06 .20	0.66	1.48	0
	4th week	1.21 .20	0.81	1.62	0
Evening					
Baseline	2nd week	.22	0.42	1.33	0
	3rd week	0.98 .19	0.58	1.38	0
	4th week	0.89 .19	0.49	1.29	0
Night					
Baseline	2nd week	0.71 .45	-0.2	1.62	0.12
	3rd week	0.55 .43	-0.32	1.43	0.21
	4th week	0.74 .40	-0.07	1.56	0.07

Table 2: Post-hoc comparisons (LSD) of time used in shift in second, third and fourth week Day, evening, nightwith the baseline.

Time	Mean Difference (I-J)	Std. Error	95% Confidence Interval	
			Lower Bound	Upper Bound
2nd week	0.95609	0.19	0.59	1.32*
3rd week	0.80817	0.17	0.47	1.15*

| 4th week | 0.90486 | 0.17 | 0.6 | 1.24* |

Table 3: Post-hoc comparisons (Tukey's LSD) of time used in shift in second, third and fourth week with the baseline, I: initial mean of time; J: sequential mean of time; *p<0.000.

Discussion

Our study found that the CNSIS saved time during shift. The only item among the 15 that had been missed by some nurses was the input/output (i.e., daily food intake and excretion). Interestingly, input/output is the final item to be done before shift. It was quite possible that the nurses forgot to conduct the task or forgot to report records of the task. An enhancement on the input/output item is recommended. The CNSIS has successfully pointed out possible missing duties that should be done, which may not be noticed when using classic methods. This also implies a further saving in overtime pay, which is essential in hospital management; this is a new outcome in our study. Strople and Ottani estimated that the cost saved by computerization of shift procedures have saved to worth US $610,570.20 annually in US [3]. Our unpublished data on subjective estimation of the nurses included in this study suggests that implementation of CNSIS has saved 20 to 30% of their time. In addition to the time and cost effects [2,6] digitalization of shift information provides a database for statistical analysis in routine quality monitoring and research. This includes a benefit in the presentation of the quality of chart records which is routinely carried out between carried and every 3 months in our hospital.

One major behavioral change in work among the nurses is the use of computer instead of papers. Some nurses were uncomfortable with CNSIS at the beginning because it was totally a different way of communication. However, they were familiar with the new system in few weeks into the installation. One of the positive comments to the CNSIS from the nursing staff was that the system provides an all-in-one page shift, which is easy to handle and clear in information. On the other hand, they were also worry of possible computer break-down, which may cause chaos for the whole ward. Such problem can be avoided by setting data and power back-up system, and these have been set-up in the CNSIS of our emergency unit. Further discussion with the nurses included in this study indicates a need to integrate a camera system for recording patients' wounds instead of manual hand drawing, to be used as references for changing dressing. This will further improve the efficiency of nurse shift and quality of the health records.

This study has a few limitations. First, only nursing staffs of one ward were recruited in this study and generalization was limited. However, further implementation of the CNSIS appeared smooth among the nursing staffs. Second, this study focused work items related to nurse shift, possible confounding effects, e.g., diagnosis and severity of disease, have not been examined in this study. Third, effects on patients have not been evaluated in this study. Forth, our study was time limited, for the long term effect need more study to warrant.

For advantage, we conclude that CNSIS is an efficiency system for nurse shift. Besides from saving time and cost, the system also provides a platform for quality control and research. Also recommendation, further improvement on the system warrants better performance of nursing quality. Further study on patient care quality is suggested.

Declaration of Conflicting Interests, the author declared no potential conflicts of interest with respect to the research, authorship.

Acknowledgement

This study was supported by research grant from the Taichung Veterans General Hospital, Taiwan (grant no.: TCVGH- 967413A). We thank head nurse Ms. HN Huang and all nurses who joined this study. Also, we wish to express our appreciations to Dr. El-Wui Loh at National Health Research Institutes, Taiwan, for his advice on manuscript editing.

References

1. Bomba DT, Prakash R (2005) A description of handover processes in an Australian public hospital. Aust Health Rev 29: 68-79.
2. González Sánchez JA, Cosgaya García O, Simón García MJ, Blesa Malpica AL (2004) Nursing records: conventional versus computerized. Critical care unit. Enferm Intensiva 15: 53-62.
3. Baldwin L, McGinnis C (1994) A computer-generated shift report. Nurs Manage 25: 61-64.
4. Moody LE, Slocumb E, Berg B, Jackson D (2004) Electronic health records documentation in nursing: nurses' perceptions, attitudes, and preferences. Comput Inform Nurs 22: 337-344.
5. Popovich D (2011) 30-Second Head-to-Toe tool in pediatric nursing: cultivating safety in handoff communication. Pediatr Nurs 37: 55-59.
6. Sexton A, Chan C, Elliott M, Stuart J, Jayasuriya R, et al. (2004) Nursing handovers: do we really need them? J Nurs Manag 12: 37-42.

8

Effect of Nurse-Physician Teamwork in the Emergency Department Nurse and Physician Perception of Job Satisfaction

David O Ajeigbe[1*], Donna McNeese-Smith[2], Linda R Phillips[3] and Linda Searle Leach[4]

[1]Alumni University of California School of Nursing, Nurse Manage Ambulatory Managed Care Service, Inland Empire Health Plan, Rancho Cucamonga, California, USA

[2]Professor Emerita University of California School of Nursing, Los Angeles, CA, USA

[3]Sectional Chair, Acute and Chronic Health Services, University of California School of Nursing, Los Angeles, CA, USA

[4]Assistant Professor, University of California School of Nursing, Los Angeles, CA, USA

*Corresponding author: Alumni University of California School of Nursing, Los Angeles, California, Nurse Manage Ambulatory Managed Care Service, Inland Empire Health Plan, Rancho Cucamonga, California, 5974 Arlington Avenue, Riverside, CA, USA, E-mail: Box894@aol.com

Abstract

Introduction: Research studies in the military and aviation demonstrated that teamwork is essential to safety. However, there were limited studies dealing with the practice of teamwork between nurses and physicians in the emergency departments (EDs).

Aim: The aim of this cross-sectional, quasi-interventional study was to compare nurses and physicians (staff) who worked in the interventional group emergency departments and those who worked in the control group emergency departments on the effect of teamwork on staff job satisfaction.

Methodology: Data were collected over a three-year span (2009-2011) for a seven-day period in each participating hospital emergency departments using Revised Nurse Work Index, a four-point (1 to 4) Likert-type scaled instrument. Primary investigator and trained research assistants distributed surveys to ED staff who agreed to participate in the study. Completed surveys were returned into a locked box. Result: Staff who worked in the interventional group emergency departments showed significantly higher levels of staff job satisfaction associated with improved practice of teamwork (p<0.0001) than their counterparts who worked in the control group emergency departments which had no practice of teamwork. Discussion: Staff who worked in the interventional group EDs worked together and participated as equal partners in patient care leading to improved interpersonal relationships and suppression of hierarchical status among the members of both professions, however, this condition was not present in the control group.

Conclusion: Active teamwork practice was associated with an increased perception of higher levels of staff's perception of job satisfaction in the staff who worked in the interventional group EDs compared with those who worked in the control group EDs.

Keywords: Nurse-physician teamwork; Communication; Job satisfaction; Physician job satisfaction; Nurse job satisfaction

Introduction

In recent years, healthcare organizations have faced shortages of health personnel, resulting in managers and hospital administrators working to create environments favorable to recruiting and retaining staff. Studies showed that satisfied staff were happier with their jobs, enjoyed their work, had less burnout, and had a greater tendency to stay on the job [1-3]. Therefore; teamwork has been considered by organizations as one of the means of providing an environment to foster satisfied staff. Other studies also showed relationships between the practice of teamwork and improvements in staff cohesion and camaraderie. Quality of communication, quality of interactions, improved work environment, social networking, trust among staff, working towards common goals, job satisfaction, job enjoyment, reduced burnout, and improved longevity were shown to result from effective practice of teamwork [4-6].

However, despite common goals between nurses and physicians for providing quality health care and relief to patients, there is the traditional economic and gender hierarchical relational gap between nurses and physicians whereby physicians, (mainly males) have maintained dominance and the nurses, (mainly females) have displayed deference [7]. Nurses have learned to package their contributions for patient care in such a way to be acceptable to physicians in order for their contributions not to be summarily dismissed by the physicians [8,9]. This was contrary to teamwork behavior in another study that showed that when team members were able to express their thoughts, expand and achieve their potential, they were more likely to associate with and rely on the team, resulting in trust, commitment to the team, and job longevity [10].

Emergency departments operate under chaotic conditions with lack of adequate information regarding incoming patients, and this is compounded by rapid movements of events. It is, therefore, necessary for ED staff to realize that close working relationships and reliance on each other allow a team to do collectively what one staff member cannot do alone and could lead to positive outcomes for the staff and patients. The stressful conditions that are predominant in emergency departments could augment differences between medicine and nursing in their educational backgrounds, skills, and values [11]. However, teamwork training could reduce the differences to the point that both sides could work amicably for the benefit of the patients. As a result, organizations should understand that in order for team training and subsequent teamwork practice to be successful, factors such as leadership support and the learning environment must be supportive, and organizations must be committed to participate in growth and invest resources in changes driven by data [12]. This research is essential since there have been few studies dealing with nurse-physician teamwork in the emergency department.

The purpose of this cross-sectional quasi-interventional study was to compare nurses and physicians who worked in the interventional group emergency departments and those who worked in the control group emergency departments on their job satisfaction. The interventional group staff had previously undergone formal teamwork training and they stated teamwork was operationalized in their emergency departments. New staff members in those emergency departments were trained on teamwork process during their orientations and current staff receives yearly refresher courses. The staff in the control group did not participate in any formal nurse-physician teamwork training and teamwork was not operationalized in their emergency departments.

Literature Review

Adams and Bond found that work-group cohesion among nurses was associated with 51% of the nurse job satisfaction and staff-patient ratio was associated with 41% of nurse job satisfaction [13]. Group cohesion improved nurses' interests in assisting coworkers to cope with stressful patient issues [13,14]. A unit-based team-building strategy correlated with better work-group cohesion (N=300) with an increase in mean scores from 5.5 pretest to 6.01 posttest (scale of 1-10), (p≤0.001). In a post unit-based team building evaluation, nurse-nurse interaction scores increased (p=0.05); nurse-physician interaction improved significantly (p=0.05); job enjoyment also improved (p=0.05); and turnover decreased significantly by 33%. Perception of professional practice also improved (p<0.05) [4].

Kovner et al., found that factors such as work-group cohesion, work and family conflicts, variety of work, supervisor support, autonomy, distributive justice, promotional opportunities, and organizational constraints predicted more than 40% of nurse job satisfaction. Work-group cohesion was also associated with nurse job satisfaction (p<0.01) [6].

Doan-Wiggins et al., studied physician job satisfaction, attrition, and job related stress and found that job satisfaction among most resident and primary care physicians was related to their professional practice conditions, such as: job associated prestige; professional respect; and working relationships [15]. Some primary care physicians and some resident physicians felt burnt out with their jobs and some planned to leave emergency medicine. Physicians who reported a lower mean score of job satisfaction (p=0.0001) and higher burnout (p=0.001) planned to stop practicing [15].

Another study of physicians' job satisfaction, turnover, and job dissatisfaction, (N=5,704) revealed similarities in the levels of job satisfaction amongst the generalists and specialists with younger physicians reporting lower job satisfaction than their older counterparts. Physicians who reported lack of satisfaction with some

aspects of their jobs had a greater tendency to want to quit within two to five years than those with median levels of job satisfaction. Generalists who were not satisfied with their community relationships (p<0.0001) or with non-physician staff relationships in their offices (p<0.01) were more likely to plan to quit practice than those who had higher scores on job satisfaction measures (p<0.01) [16].

Conceptual Framework

The theoretical framework used in this study was based on Donabedian's structure-process-outcome model of quality care. Donabedian's theory was initially developed to measure quality of patient care. It consists of three components which are structure, process, and outcomes. Donabedian demonstrated that good structures increase the possibility of good processes and good processes enhance good outcomes [17,18]. In this study, the organization represents the structure, teamwork represents the process, and nurse-physician perception of teamwork and job satisfaction represent outcomes. This study revealed that the more positive the organizational participation, the more effective was teamwork practice and the more positive was the resulting outcome. Based on the conceptual framework and previous research evidence, a modified conceptual model was developed (Figure 1).

Research Design

This was a comparative cross-sectional quasi-interventional study of effects of emergency room nurse-physician teamwork on the interventional group emergency departments' staff with the staff who worked in the control group emergency departments. The study was developed after the Emergency Team Coordination Course (ETCC) was implemented. The ETCC was introduced in emergency departments by Morey et al. from May 1998 to March 1999 to evaluate the impact of the training on the successful practice of teamwork [19].

Teamwork training was conducted by Morey in each participating ED by a team of trained nurses and physicians in each interventional ED prior to the study, as part of their on-going operational training on teamwork practice. Participating staff in the interventional EDs were taught strategies to maintain the structure and climate of the team, communicate effectively with the team while applying strategies to solve problems, improve team skills, carry out plans, and manage workload.

Sample and inclusion criteria

The interventional group was comprised of a convenience sample of nurses and physicians from all shifts of each of the four interventional hospital emergency departments.

Control group was comprised of a convenience sample of nurses and physicians from all shifts of each of the four control hospital emergency departments. Invitations to participate in the study and complete survey questionnaires were given to all nurses (RNs, N=433) and physicians (MDs, N=105) at participating emergency departments. Staff who had been employed in the emergency departments for a minimum of six months and staff who had worked in full time or part-time positions was qualified to participate in the study. Staff who did not meet the criteria was excluded. Participants were told the purpose of the study and were given opportunities to participate or to refuse. Only that staffs that completed and returned questionnaires were considered to have consented to participate in the study.

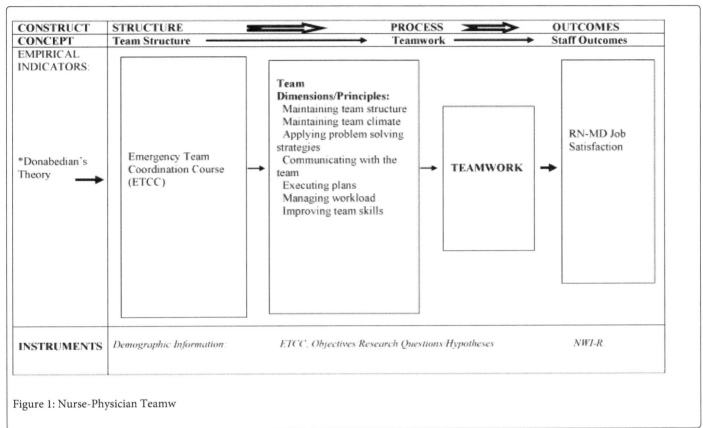

CONSTRUCT	STRUCTURE		PROCESS	OUTCOMES
CONCEPT	Team Structure		Teamwork	Staff Outcomes
EMPIRICAL INDICATORS:		Team Dimensions/Principles: Maintaining team structure Maintaining team climate Applying problem solving strategies Communicating with the team Executing plans Managing workload Improving team skills		RN-MD Job Satisfaction
*Donabedian's Theory	Emergency Team Coordination Course (ETCC)		TEAMWORK	
INSTRUMENTS	Demographic Information:	ETCC. Objectives Research Questions/Hypotheses		NWI-R

Figure 1: Nurse-Physician Teamw

*Adapted/Modified from Donabedian's Structure-Process-Outcome of Quality Care Model Donabedian, A (1988). The quality care: How can it be assessed: Journal of American Medical Association, 260: 1743-1748.

Instrument (Tool)

The instrument used to assess the effect of teamwork on staff job satisfaction was the Revised Nurse Work Index (NWI-R), a 4 point Likert-type scale with 1 being strongly disagree and 4 being strongly agree [21,22]. Psychometric information about NWI-R was described by Aiken and Patrician and reliability was estimated using Cronbach's alpha which equaled 0.96 for the entire NWI-R; the aggregated subscale alphas ranged from 0.84 to 0.91.

The original NWI has three subscales: autonomy consisting of five items, control over practice setting consisting of seven items, and nurse-physician relationship consisting of three items, two of which measure quality of nurse-physician relationships and quality of teamwork between nurses and physicians [20]. When revised a fourth subscale was added to depict organizational support for caregivers. The fourth subscale consists of ten items [21]. The subscale of interest of this study is the nurse-physician relationship (teamwork).

The original instrument demonstrated validity by its ability to differentiate nurses who worked within a professional practice environment from those who did not, and its capacity to predict differences in nurse burnout [22]. When revised to measure physician job satisfaction, every word "nurse" was changed to "physician" and

every word referring to "nursing" was changed to "medical." Content validity for the change was not performed; changing the words "nurse" to "physician" and "nursing" to "medical" was not expected to have changed content validity of the instrument for this study. Cronbach's alpha and reliability of the instrument were not determined for this study as those have been determined by the studies for which it has been previously used.

This instrument was selected for this research because of its ability to demonstrate significant differences between the interventional and the control groups. The findings of this research are from a different data set from the article published in the Journal of Nursing Administration which dealt with the impact of nurse-physician teamwork in the emergency department on perception of job environment, autonomy, and control over practice [23].

Research procedure

Morey suggested names of hospital emergency departments in California which had participated in the ETCC training as potential participants in the study. However, in order to get additional hospital emergency departments to participate as the controls, the primary researcher invited other emergency department managers and asked whether or not their emergency departments participated in formal teamwork training. Emergency departments in California which have undergone formal teamwork training at various periods between 1998 and 2011 and had operationalized its principles in their emergency departments were members of the interventional group (N=4) and those that have never participated in the formal teamwork training and did not operationalize its principles were members of the control group (N=4). The interventional group, as part of their annual competency, underwent annual review in-services to reinforce principles of teamwork. Both groups were invited to participate in the study and of all hospital emergency departments (about 21) in Northern and Southern California that were invited, eight agreed and were selected to participate (two interventional and two control hospitals from each area, Northern and Southern California). IRB approval was received from UCLA and from each of the eight participating hospitals.

Surveys were given by the primary researcher and trained research assistants to all participants who agreed to participate. Completed surveys were returned into a locked box that could be opened only by the primary researcher at the end of data collection. Data collection took seven days for 24 hours per day at each participating emergency department. Data collection occurred between 2009 and 2011 because of the length of time it took for IRB approval from each hospital. Staff demographic data collected were gender, age, educational level, shift worked, and work/employment status (Table 1).

Employment Status											
	Interventional Group	Percent	Missing Data	Percent	Total		Control Group	Percent	Missing Data	Percent	Total
MD	25	13%			191		40	13%			307
RN	166	87%					267	97%			

Gender											
	Interventional Group	Percent	Missing Data	Percent	Total		Control Group	Percent	Missing Data	Percent	Total
Male	58	30%	7	4%	191		84	27%	12	4%	307
Female	126	66%					211	69%			

Age of Participants (RN and MD)											
	Interventional Group	Missing Data	Mean	Std Dev	Total		Control Group	Missing Data	Mean	Std Dev	Total
	169	22	38	9.67	191	278	29	39	10.61	307	

Years in Current Unit											
	Interventional Group	Missing Data	Mean	Std Dev	Total		Control Group	Missing Data	Mean	Std Dev	Total
	177	14	6	6	191	287	20	7	6	307	

Shift Worked											
	Interventional Group	Day Shift	Evening Shift	Night Shift	Missing Data	Total	Control Group	Day Shift	Evening Shift	Night Shift	Missing Data	Total
	183	92	52	39	8	191	281	120	72	89	26	307

Table 1: Results - Participants' Demographics

One hundred and ninety one (191) staff of the interventional group emergency departments participated; 166 (86.9%) were nurses and 25 (13.1%) were physicians. Females comprised a majority of the participants with 6.3 average years working in the participating emergency department. The three shifts worked by the participating ED staff were night, evening and day shifts, but a majority worked day shift. The participants also had various educational levels. In the control group, 307 staff participated of which 267 were nurses and 40 were physicians. Two hundred and eleven (211) were female and 84 were male and they worked an average of 6.8 years in the participating emergency departments. A majority of them also worked day shift and had various educational levels. There were no significant differences demographically between the interventional and the control groups with regards to age, gender, (male/female), employment category (RN/MD), educational level, full-time/part-time, and day/evening/night shifts (Tables 1 and 2).

Data analysis

The Statistical Analysis Systems (SAS) program, release 9.2 (Cary, NC) was used for data analysis. The analysis used the two-sample, one-tailed t-test to identify significant differences between the interventional group and control groups (p=0.05).

Results

Nurse-Physician job satisfaction

Staff (nurses and physicians) job satisfaction data were collected using the NWI-R; on a Likert-type scale of 1 to 4; the interventional group had a mean score of 3.11, SD of 0.59 and the control group had a mean score of 2.88, SD of 0.53. There was a significant difference between the interventional group ED staff and the control group ED staff (p<0.0001), (Table 3). The effect size of the study was calculated and it was 0.21 indicating that staff in the interventional group was more satisfied than the staff in the control group by 21% of a standard deviation.

Participants' Educational Level										
	Diploma	Associate	BSN	Masters	DO	MD	Ph D	Other	Missing Data	Total
Interventional Group	7	62	81	11	0	15	1	3	11	191
Percent	4%	%	42%	6%	0%	8%	1%	2%	5%	100%
Control Group	9	107	121	16	1	35	0	1	17	307
Percent	3%	35%	39%	5%	0%	11%	0%	0%	6%	100%

Table 2: Results - Participants' Educational Level

Staff Job Satisfaction		
	Interventional Group	Control Group
Mean	3.11	2.88
95%	2.96	2.77
Std Dev	0.59	0.53
t Value	4.40	
P-Value	P < 0.0001	

Table 3: Results-Variables

Discussion

Referring back to Donabedian's structure-process-outcome model of quality care, it is apparent that the organizations (structure) of the interventional group emergency departments supported formal training and use of teamwork in their emergency departments. As a result of the support, staff in the interventional group emergency departments was able to learn, embrace, and practice active teamwork (process). Therefore, staff in the interventional group felt more surrounded by the presence of teamwork practice and were more satisfied with their job (outcomes) than the staff who worked in the control group emergency departments who did not get similar organizational support for formal teamwork training and were not practicing teamwork in their emergency departments. Training received by the interventional group EDs focused on problem solving strategies; communication; plan execution; workload management; team structure and climate maintenance; and skill improvement [24]. The result was also consistent with the findings of another study by Kalisch et al. which showed that participants' job satisfaction with their present position was rated higher when they felt a higher presence of teamwork in their present job [14].

Based on the findings of this study it could be deduced that the significant difference shown between the interventional group staff perception of job satisfaction was associated with teamwork. The practice of teamwork might have increased the frequency and quality of interactions between the nurses and physicians which helped each to understand the functions of the other so they were able to function side by side. Teamwork training received might have contributed to the strategies applied to improve effective communication between team members which might have improved team climate and thus increased the ability of the team members to solve problems, improve team skills, carry out plans, and manage workload collectively. The practice of teamwork appeared to increase the cohesiveness between the nurses and the physicians of the interventional EDs and thus removed hierarchical feelings of superiority between the nurses and the physicians.

Limitations

The study was conducted over a period of three years in multiple hospital emergency departments in Northern and Southern California, to assess the impact of nurse-physician teamwork on nurses and physicians. Regardless of the extent and diligence of data collection and analysis, certain limitations existed. First, the use of a cross-sectional quasi-interventional design provided a snapshot, which might not be reliable because participants' responses might be due to the emotional state and what was happening at the moment of responding to the surveys and could be different if the responses were taken longitudinally, over a period of time. Second, the study could not identify cause and effect relationships because the study was non-experimental. Third, there might be some departmental cultural issues that could not be accounted for that might have contributed to teamwork. Fourth, the degree and timeliness of the training and the number of staff who participated in the formal teamwork training that were still or not still working in the interventional group emergency departments could have confounded the findings. Fifth, not performing content validity and reliability of the instrument with the minor changes made to two words might have possibly had some effect on the content validity and reliability of the instrument. Sixth, recall bias could lead to misclassification of the findings and thus make generalization of the result unreliable. However, it is significant that in spite of the time since the educational intervention, those Emergency

Departments that had undergone teamwork training had significantly higher job satisfaction among nurses and physicians than in the Emergency Departments that had not undergone the training.

Conclusion/ Significance to Healthcare

This study demonstrated that the practice of effective nurse-physician teamwork in the emergency department was improved by the administrative support in providing staff with training on teamwork. It also showed that nurse-physician teamwork training and practice in the emergency department were associated with feelings among nurses and physicians of improved job satisfaction.

The results pointed to the need to invest resources in nurse-physician teamwork training and in operationalizing teamwork between nurses and physicians in the emergency department. Nurses and physicians could join their skills together in providing good quality care to the patients while maintaining a positive environment for both disciplines to thrive through teamwork practice.

Genuine teamwork between nurses and physicians in any healthcare setting could contribute to creating a work environment with reduced hierarchies between them, especially in the emergency department. Teamwork could also serve as an equalizer of hierarchies between nurses and physicians. When such an environment exists, the nurses and physicians could excel and coordinate their skills and efforts to deliver better quality care to the patients, resulting in increased teamwork and job satisfaction for both professions.

Future Study

Future studies should consider the effects of nurse-physician teamwork in the ED on the commission of errors in the emergency department. An effort to include the commission of errors in this study was aborted due to difficulties encountered in getting any hospital EDs to consent to having data collected on this variable.

Other studies should also focus on the effect of nurse-physician teamwork in the ED on patients' outcomes such as ED revisit within 24-48 hours of discharge from the ED, satisfaction with ED care, and willingness of patients to recommend the ED to their family members, friends, and acquaintances.

References

1. Khuwaja AK, Qureshi R, Andrades M, Fatmi Z, Khuwaja NK (2004) Comparison of job satisfaction and stress among male and female doctors in teaching hospitals of Karachi. J Ayub Med Coll Abbottabad 16: 23-27.

2. Manojlovich M (2005) Linking the practice environment to nurses' job satisfaction through nurse-physician communication. J Nurs Scholarsh 37: 367-373.

3. Simoens S, Scott A, Sibbald B (2002) Job satisfaction, work-related stress and intentions to quit of Scottish GPS. Scott Med J 47: 80-86.

4. DiMeglio K, Padula C, Piatek C, Korber S, Barrett A, et al. (2005) Group cohesion and nurse satisfaction: examination of a team-building approach. J Nurs Adm 35: 110-120.

5. Kalisch BJ, Lee KH (2010) The impact of teamwork on missed nursing care. Nurs Outlook 58: 233-241.

6. Kovner C, Brewer C, Wu YW, Cheng Y, Suzuki M (2006) Factors associated with work satisfaction of registered nurses. J Nurs Scholarsh 38: 71-79.

7. El Sayed KA, Sleem WF (2011) Nurse-physician collaboration: A Comparative study of the attitudes of nurses and physicians at Mansoura University Hospital. Life Science Journal 8: 104-46.

8. Vazirani S, Hays RD, Shapiro MF, Cowan M (2005) Effect of a multidisciplinary intervention on communication and collaboration among physicians and nurses. Am J Crit Care 14: 71-77.

9. Propp KM, Apker J, Zabava Ford WS, Wallace N, Serbenski M, et al. (2010) Meeting the complex needs of the health care team: identification of nurse-team communication practices perceived to enhance patient outcomes. Qual Health Res 20: 15-28.

10. Sheng CW, Tian YF, Chen MC. (2010) Relationships among teamwork behaviour, Trust, perceived team support, and team commitment. Social Behaviour and Personality 38: 1297-306.

11. Salas E, Almeida SA, Salisbury M, King H, Lazzara EH, et al. (2009) What are the critical success factors for team training in health care? Jt Comm J Qual Patient Saf 35: 398-405.

12. Stein-Parbury J, Liaschenko J (2007) Understanding collaboration between nurses and physicians as knowledge at work. Am J Crit Care 16: 470-477.

13. Adams A, Bond S (2000) Hospital nurses' job satisfaction, individual and organizational characteristics. J Adv Nurs 32: 536-543.

14. Kalisch BJ, Lee H, Rochman M (2010) Nursing staff teamwork and job satisfaction. J Nurs Manag 18: 938-947.

15. Doan-Wiggins L, Zun L, Cooper MA, Meyers DL, Chen EH (1995) Practice satisfaction, occupational stress, and attrition of emergency physicians. Wellness Task Force, Illinois College of Emergency Physicians. Acad Emerg Med 2: 556-563.

16. Pathman DE, Konrad TR, Williams ES, Scheckler WE, Linzer M, et al. (2002) Physician job satisfaction, dissatisfaction, and turnover. J Fam Pract 51: 593.

17. Donabedian A (1966) Evaluating the quality of medical care. Milbank Mem Fund Q 44: Suppl:166-206.

18. Donabedian A (1988) The quality of care. How can it be assessed? JAMA 260: 1743-1748.

19. Morey JC, Simon R, Jay GD, Wears RL, Salisbury M, et al. (2002) Error reduction and performance improvement in the emergency department through formal teamwork training: evaluation results of the MedTeams project. Health Serv Res 37: 1553-1581.

20. Kramer M, Hafner LP (1989) Shared values: impact on staff nurse job satisfaction and perceived productivity. Nurs Res 38: 172-177.

21. Aiken LH, Smith HL, Lake ET (1994) Lower Medicare mortality among a set of hospitals known for good nursing care. Med Care 32: 771-787.

22. Aiken LH, Patrician PA (2000) Measuring organizational traits of hospitals: the Revised Nursing Work Index. Nurs Res 49: 146-153.

23. Ajeigbe DO, McNeese-Smith D, Leach LS, Phillips LR (2013) Nurse-physician teamwork in the emergency department: impact on perceptions of job environment, autonomy, and control over practice. J Nurs Adm 43: 142-148.

24. Brannick MT, Prince A, Prince C, Salas E (1995) The measurement of team process. Hum Factors 37: 641-651.

9

Emergency Department Nurses' Perceptions toward Factors Influencing the Occurrence of Medication Administration Errors

Naglaa Abd El- Aziz El Seesy* and Faten El Sebaey

Alexandria University , Department of Nursing Administration, Faculty of Nursing , Alexandria , Egypt

*Corresponding author: Naglaa Abd El- Aziz El Seesy, Alexandria University , Department of Nursing Administration, Faculty of Nursing , Alexandria ,Egypt, E-mail: nona20102002@ yahoo.com

Abstract

Background: Significant efforts have been directed to understand medication errors causes in recent years because it contributes directly to patient morbidity and mortality. This study was conducted to determine the factors influencing the occurrence of medication administration errors, as perceived by nurses in emergency department (ED).

Aim: The current study aimed to assess emergency department nurses' perceptions toward factors influencing the occurrence of medication administration errors.

Design: The study followed a cross-sectional descriptive design.

Setting: The present study was carried out at ED in teaching Main University Hospital in Alexandria governorate, Egypt.

Subjects: 84 nursing staff worked in the previous mentioned setting.

Tool: The data gathering tool was Medication Administration Errors (MAEs) Reporting Questionnaire which was developed by Wakefield in 1998 [1]. It contains 16 items regarding reasons why medication errors occur.

Results: This study suggested four categories for reasons of why MAEs occur in emergency department and the leading cause of medication errors was due to nurses- physicians' communication.

Conclusion: Medication errors are common in emergency department. A wide range of factors perceived as contributing factors of the occurrence of medication administration errors were identified such as nurses- physicians communication, medication packaging, pharmacy processes and nurse staffing. This information could be used to improve the medication system in emergency department in Egypt.

Recommendations: This study recommended for provision of safe work environment that encourage good physicians-nurses team work relationship, dissemination of safety guidelines in all hospital department specially nursing and pharmacy, on-going education and training on safe medication administration and supervision of newly hired nursing staff during medication administration process and provision of adequate staffing and fair scheduling for nursing staff working in a highly urgent care departments.

Keywords: Medication administration errors; Emergency department; Nurses; Perception

Introduction

MAE is one of the factors causing death and harm to patients and the most common important challenges threatening healthcare system in all countries worldwide [2]. The definition typically cited in literature that is authored by nurses defines MAE as mistakes associated with drugs and intravenous solutions that are made during the prescription, transcription, dispensing, and administration phases of drug preparation and distribution [1,3]. Medication administration errors (MAEs) in the ED are common, with errors occurring most often in the prescribing and administration phase [4].

American Society of Health System Pharmacists (ASHP), (2003) recognizes that medication errors can be minimized by assessing the medication use process, identifying inadequacies within systems, and developing interventions to correct the recognized deficiencies.

A possible contributing factor to MAEs in the ED is the unique medication distribution system used. For example, on-pharmacy profiled automated dispensing cabinet (ADC), unit stock, or refrigerator, as the prescriber's order may not be reviewed by a pharmacist before the drugs are given (Flynn et al. 2010). However, high patient acuity, crowding, and frequent interruptions are pervasive in the ED's clinical environment. Interruptions in the ED are conservatively estimated to be as frequent as every minute for attending physicians and every 14 minutes for resident physicians.

Although the results are mixed, several studies suggest that links exist between medication error and systemic organizational factors. These include nurse staffing adequacy, hours worked per week, overtime, staffing mix (professional versus unregulated), and other factors reflecting how the work system is designed [5-7]. Evidence of links between stress in the clinical workplace and medication error is also emerging. For example, a recent study of nurses in Alberta and Ontario found that patient safety outcomes including medication error and other adverse events were associated with emotional exhaustion ('burnout') in nurses, which in turn was related to staffing inadequacy, poor nurse-physician relations, and other "work life" factors [8]. Clearly, adverse drug events that occur in the ED are a significant public health problem and need to be reduced, but this must be accomplished without making the ED less efficient [9].

Previous studies have examined important factors in refusal or act as barriers to report medication errors [10-13] or the analysis and improvement medication error reporting practices by emergency department physicians, nurses, and pharmacists [14]. However, few studies have focused only on the assessment of the occurrence and reasons of nursing medication errors, these studies recommended further studies to determine and investigate the causes of medication errors [15-18].

Understanding factors that contribute to medication error is the first step toward preventing it to ensure safety and quality of patient care. Therefore we have conducted this study to explore the most important factors influencing the occurrence of MAEs in ED from nurses' perspective which can lead to improve medication administration process, diminish the risks of adverse events that impact patient morbidity and mortality, improve patient safety, and lower cost of patient care.

Materials and Methods

Research Design

This study followed a cross-sectional descriptive design.

Setting

This study was carried out in emergency department at teaching Main University Hospital in Alexandria governorate, Egypt which contains 42-bed during the period from June 2013 to the end of august 2013.

Subjects

All nursing staff (n=84) who were working in the previously mentioned setting and willing to participate in such study were included. All of them were responsible for providing nursing care for urgent cases.

Tool

Medication Administration Error Survey: It was developed by Wakefield in 1998 [1] included 16 items regarding reasons why medication errors occur. Respondents were asked to how much they believe they affect the occurrence of medication errors in the emergency department using a six points Likert type scale with fix values ranging from 6= strongly agree to 1= strongly disagree. In addition data were collected on nurses' sociodemographic data including sex, marital status, age, education level, years of experience, working unit, and the most frequent shift they work.

Procedures

The Ethics Committee of Faculty of Nursing, Alexandria University has approved the study protocol. They have determined that this survey does not fall under the committee's jurisdiction. The Medication Administration Error Survey was translated into Arabic language and accordingly, minor changes were made for a few unclear words. Also it was tested for content validity by five experts in the same field of the study of nursing at Alexandria Faculty of Nursing. The subscales' reliability values of these factors measured by Cronbach's coefficient Alpha, in which the internal consistency reliability ranged from 0.75 to 0.92, while the statistical significance level was set at p < 0.05.

Before embarking to data collection, an informed consent was obtained from each participant to share in the study. All participants were assured that their participation is voluntary. Also their privacy and confidentiality were maintained. A pilot study was carried out on 10 nurses who were working in other unit rather than the studied units and the necessary modifications were made. The questionnaire was hand delivered to each study participant in the morning and afternoon shifts and it was completed through self-report method. About 30 minutes were consumed to complete the questionnaire. Data collection took about three months from June 2013 till the end of august 2013.

Statistical Analysis

After data were collected it was revised, coded and fed to statistical software SPSS IBM version 20. The given graph was constructed using Microsoft excel software. All statistical analysis was done using two tailed tests and alpha error of 0.05. Discrete items concerning nurses responses for each domain were summed together to have the domain total score. Descriptive statistics in the form of frequencies and percent were used to describe the categorical data variables while mean and standard deviation was used to describe domains scores. To test for association between sample characteristics and their scores at different domains, independent samples t-test and One Way ANOVA were used. To identify the relative importance of each domain at committing error, factor analysis was used to express factor loading which is the correlation between each domain and the overall hidden factor.

Results

Table 1 illustrated the demographic characteristics of nursing staff at emergency department in Main University Hospital. The table reveals that the female nurses were the dominant, 85.7% of nursing staff were female, and more than half of them were in the age group from 20 to less than 30 years old, as well as 65.5% of them were married. It was observed that majority of nursing staff (79.8%) were permanent residents at Alexandria governorate, 72.6% of them had diploma secondary school degree, and 73.8% of them had less than 10 years of experience in their work unit. Moreover, it can be noticed that 54.8% of nursing staff always work variable shifts.

Socio demographic data	No	%
Age		
• 20-	48	57.1

• 30-	17	20.2
• 40+	19	22.6
Marital Status		
• Single	29	34.5
• Married	55	65.5
Sex		
• Male	12	14.3
• Female	72	85.7
Residence		
• Daily Travel	7	8.3
• Permanent Residence	67	79.8
• Temporary Residence	10	11.9
Education		
• Diploma Secondary School	61	72.6
• Nursing Institute	12	14.3
• B SN	11	13.1
Experience in Nursing (in years)		
• <10	38	45.2
• 10-19	24	28.6
• 20+	22	26.2
Experience in The Hospital (in years)		
• <10	42	50
• 10-19	21	25
• 20+	21	25
Experience in the Unit (in years)		
• <10	62	73.8
• 10-19	13	15.5
• 20+	9	10.7
Shift		
• Morning	33	39.3
• Evening	2	2.4
• Night	3	3.6
• Variable	46	54.8

Table 1: Distribution of nursing staff demographic characteristics at Main University Hospital Emergency Department

Figure 1 represents the perception of participants for why medication administration errors occur. Accordingly the ranking of the factors loading values of MAEs, participants reported that the physician-nurses' communication reasons (0.84) was perceived as the most important factor for reasons of MAEs occurrence. These included illegible physicians' medication orders, unclear physicians' medication, frequently change physicians' orders, poor communication between nurses and physicians. The second factor was medication packaging (0.79) such as look-alike/sound-alike medication names can result in medication errors. Misreading medication names that look similar is a common mistake. These look-alike medication names can lead to errors associated with verbal prescriptions. The third factor was pharmacy processes reason (0.76) for example, pharmacy delivers incorrect doses, and pharmacy does not prepare and label the medication correctly, as well as pharmacists unavailable 24 hours a day. The last factor was nurse staffing (0.72) was perceived as the least reason of MAEs occurrence.

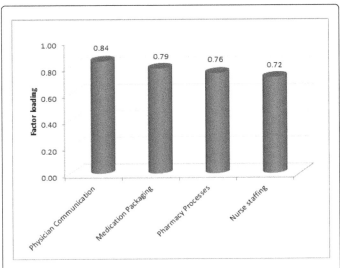

Figure 1: Relative ranks for causes of committing drug medication error according to nurses' perception

Table 2 describes the relationship of socio-demographic data with the four reasons of why medication administration errors occur. This study revealed no statistically significant relation between participants' sex, residence, and educational level and their experience in units with reasons of why MAEs occur. Concerning age, there were significant relation with only medication packaging reasons of MAEs at P<0.05. Regarding marital status, there was statistically significant relationship between participants and physician – nurse communication reason P<0.05 where the highest mean percent for single nurses agree that these reasons causing MAEs as well as statistically significant correlation for medication package reason of why MAEs occur P<0.05.In relation to nurses' experience, there were inverse statistically significant correlation between nurses experience for medication packing reasons of why MAEs occur at P<0.05. Furthermore, this study showed statistically significant correlation between participants' most frequent shift with medication packaging reasons of why MAEs occur P<0.05.

Socio Demographic characteristics	Physician communication		P	Medication packaging		P	Pharmacy processes		P	Nurse staffing		P
	Mean	SD	Mean	SD	Mean	SD	Mean	SD				
Age												
20-	53.5	23.9		68.6	30		71.9	31.7		44.3	23.2	
30-	52	21.7	0.581	52.5	33.3	0.006*	69.9	31.7	0.197	51.2	21.4	0.147
40+	46.3	31.3		41.7	33.6		86	28.4		56.6	27.3	
Marital Status												
Single	59.2	24.5	0.043*	71.3	26.3	0.015*	73.2	30.1	0.753	47	23.6	0.685
Married	47.5	24.8		52.9	34.8		75.5	32		49.2	24.5	
Sex												
Male	40	21.5	0.086	50	24.9	0.301	74.5	26.6	0.987	56.3	23.3	0.229
Female	53.5	25.4		60.8	34.2		74.7	32.1		47.2	24.1	
Residence												
Daily Travel	46.2	24.6		58.3	27.2		81	16.3		45.8	28.3	
Permanent Residence	50.1	25.1	0.185	56.5	33.9	0.151	73.8	32.7	0.84	49.6	24.8	0.658
Temporary Residence	65	23.9		78.3	27.6		76.1	30.2		42.5	15.7	
Education												
Diploma Secondary School	52.2	26.7		58.3	33.7		75.3	32.7		51.5	25	
Nursing Institute	50.8	26.1	0.899	71.5	33.2	0.303	84.7	20.4	0.16	41.7	22.6	0.164
BSN	48.5	14.9		50.8	28.7		60.1	29		39	16.7	
Experience in Nursing												
<10	51.8	24.1		65.6	29.7		70.5	31.4		44.7	23.8	
19-Oct	55.1	23.5	0.576	66.7	33.6	0.006*	71.8	33.5	0.188	47.7	22.6	0.236
20+	47.3	29.1		40.2	32.2		85.1	26.9		55.7	25.6	
Experience in The Hospital												
<10	51.3	23.7		62.7	30		68.5	32.4		44.3	23.7	
19-Oct	56.3	23.4	0.5	70.2	34.2	0.010*	75.7	30.6	0.11	49.4	21.8	0.205
20+	47.1	29.9		41.3	32.5		86	27.3		55.8	26.2	
Experience in the Unit												
<10	51.7	25.5		60.5	32.1		71	33.1		48.1	24.4	
19-Oct	55.6	22.4	0.594	63.5	35.9	0.356	77.8	26.1	0.077	39.7	18.3	0.065
20+	44.4	27.9		44.4	36.1		95.7	9.5		63.9	24.3	
Shift												
Morning	48.8	27.5	0.327	46	31.7	0.016*	81.6	28.5	0.118	53.9	26.3	0.368
Evening	41.7	35.4		50	23.6		58.3	58.9		37.5	29.5	

| Night | 75.6 | 33.7 | | 83.3 | 22 | | 100 | 0 | | 51.4 | 12 | |
| Variable | 52.4 | 22.5 | | 67.6 | 32.2 | | 68.7 | 31.9 | | 44.8 | 22.6 | |

Table 2: Distribution of the studied nurses according to their socio demographic characteristics in relation to medication administration errors causes domains

Discussion

In this study, results of the factor analysis ranked four categories of factors influencing the occurrence of MAEs in emergency department. In descending order of magnitude, these categories included physician communication, followed by medication package, then pharmacy processing and finally nurse staffing. Finding of the current study illustrated that participants perceived physician communication reason as the highest ranked factor influencing the occurrence of MAEs. This finding was relevant and consistent with Dumo in 2012 [19] who reported that poor nurse/physician relationships may cause MAEs due to physicians don't spend enough time discussing care options with nurses. Many nurses still feel that physicians don't understand, respect, or care to listen to nursing perspectives on patient care that lead to misunderstanding and conflict between nurses and physicians. While, Al-Youssif in 2013 [11] illustrated that participants perceived physician-nurse relationship reason as the fourth category of MAEs. Moreover, poor communication accounts for more than 60% of the root causes of sentinel events reported to the Joint Commission (JC) Anderson and Townsend in 2010 [20].

Participants also ranked medication package as the second factor influencing the occurrence of MAEs .This result could be in the same line with Mrayyan in 2007 [21] who suggested that the medications' labels and packages may be confusingly the healthcare personnel due to do not place important information prominently and small font size of displaying text, which may lead to poor readability. In addition, Peth in 2003 [22] in USA reported that the explosion of new drugs appearing in the marketplace has made it virtually impossible for physicians, nurses, and pharmacists to keep abreast of all of the latest data concerning the indications, contraindications, drug interactions, and adverse effects associated with each new drug. Moreover, all medications have side effects, and rare but potentially fatal side effects are unlikely to show up in preliminary clinical trials. In fact, once a medication has been removed from its packaging, it's hard to identify and can be easily confused with another one [11].

The present study factor analysis for MAEs causes ranked pharmacy processing as the third factor influencing the occurrence of MAEs in ED .Ideally, the pharmacist should collaborate with the prescriber in developing, implementing, and monitoring a therapeutic plan to produce defined therapeutic outcomes for the patient.

Surprising that nurse staffing was the least ranked factor influencing the occurrence of MAEs although inadequate staffing mentioned by Egyptian nurses due to high nurse/patient ratio in ED. This finding is consistent with Wakefield in 2000 [23], who showed that workload and type of care delivery system, and other factors such as number of consecutive hours worked, rotating shifts, staffing mix and numbers, nurse-to-patient ratios, assignment of floating nurses to unfamiliar units . In addition heavier workloads also are associated with medication errors. The nursing shortage has increased workloads by increasing the number of patients for which a nurse is responsible. Also Anderson and Townsend in 2010 [20] reported that, nurses

perform many tasks that take them away from the patient's bedside, such as indirect activities, answering the telephone. Absence of nurses from the bedside is directly linked to compromised patient care. In addition, Al-Shara in 2011[24] found that the highest level of medication errors were 48.4%, 31.7% and 11.1% related to nurses, physicians and pharmacists, respectively. Furthermore, the leading causes of medication errors were due to heavy workload (41.4%) and new staff (20.6%).

Based on the nurse perception, the results of the current study showed that regarding demographic characteristics, there was no relation between participants' age, marital status and their experience in units with nurse staffing and pharmacy processing factors that influencing the occurrence of MAEs. This means that all nurses are almost ranking these factors influencing the occurrence of MAEs regardless of their age, marital status or years of experience. Also, the finding of this study showed a significant difference between nurses' marital status and physician communication as factor influencing occurrence of MAEs, since single nurses had higher ranking for this factor than married ones. This could be due to physicians either male or female underestimating nursing as profession which result in poor relationship between younger nurses and physicians however, as new graduated nurses become older and experience nurses receive more respect from them.

An interesting finding in this section of the study, in relation to nurses' experience in nursing and hospital, there were statistically significant relationship between nurses experience and medication packing reasons of why MAEs occur, in which nurses who have more working experience highly perceived that medication packaging is factor causing the occurrence of MAEs compared to nurses who have worked less years of experience. This result may note that experience is important factor affect the occurrence of MAEs. This result is consistent with the study of Flor et al in 2012, Zein Eldin and Abd Elaal in 2013 [25,26].This result is in contrast with Al-Youssif et al. in 2013 [11] who reported that there was no relation between participants' experience with reasons of why MAEs occur or not reporting.

This study showed statistically significant correlation between participants' most frequent shift with medication packaging reasons of why MAEs occur where nurses who are working night shift has highest mean for perception that medication packaging is the most factor causing MAEs. Anderson and Townsend in 2010 [20] mentioned that fatigue and sleep deprivation are linked to decreases in vigilance, memory, information processing, reaction time, and decision making. A person who works a 12-hour shift and has a long commute may need to stay awake for up to 18 consecutive hours. Moreover, Tully in 2009 and Hartel et al in 2011 [27,28] stated that fatigue and sleep deprivation also may diminish a nurse's ability to recognize subtle patient changes. As a result, the nurse may not notice an adverse reaction to a drug quickly enough to avoid a devastating outcome. When medication errors occur, multifactorial causes in a badly shaped system affect their occurrence, as well as manual prescriptions, lack of bar codes, stress, fatigue, lack of attention and lack of ability.

Conclusion

In conclusion, this study determined the factors influencing the occurrence of medication administration errors, as perceived by nurses in emergency department. The data of this study suggested the ranking of four reasons of why MAEs occur; nurse - physician communication reasons, medication packaging, pharmacy reasons and finally nurse staffing. Additionally, medication errors are common in emergency department. Actually, reducing these errors requires the commitment of everyone with a stake in keeping patients safe. The physician who wrote the prescribed medications, pharmacist who dispensed it and the nurse who received the medications and administered to the patient, all play an important role in preventing MAEs.

Recommendations

The current study suggested the need to improve factors influencing MAEs by nurses through; Designing safe work environment that encourage good physician-nurses' communication conducive for patient care delivery and reduce the occurrence of MAEs, healthcare organizations should ensure that all medications are provided in clearly labelled unit-dose packages for institutional use. Top management should provide adequate staffing and fair scheduling for all urgent care to provide fair workload between nursing staff that reduce the occurrence of MAEs. Developing and disseminating the patient safety guidelines in all hospital setting especially in nursing and pharmacy departments. The researchers recommended for provision of on-going education & training on practice of safe medication administration for all nurses especially in urgent care units.

In summary, the findings from this study highlight the need to further examination on how hospital management is addressing the problem of MAEs occurrence in ED and the role of the nurse managers in preventing medication errors through participation in quality management processes. Alternate methods may need to be created for a supportive unit culture that encourages multidisciplinary team from nurse, physician, and pharmacist to prevent medication errors and improve patient safety in the ER hospital setting.

References

1. Wakefield BJ, Wakefield DS, Uden-Holman T, Blegen MA (1998) Nurses' perceptions of why medication administration errors occur. Medsurg Nurs 7: 39-44.
2. Sanghera IS, Franklin BD, Dhillon S (2007) The attitudes and beliefs of healthcare professionals on the causes and reporting of medication errors in a UK Intensive care unit. Anaesthesia 62: 53-61.
3. Peris-Lopez P, Orfila A, Mitrokotsa A, van der Lubbe JC (2011) A comprehensive RFID solution to enhance inpatient medication safety. Int J Med Inform 80: 13-24.
4. Flynn EA, Barker K, Barker B (2010) Medication-administration errors in an emergency department. Am J Health Syst Pharm 67: 347-348.
5. Rogers AE, Hwang WT, Scott LD, Aiken LH, Dinges DF (2004) The working hours of hospital staff nurses and patient safety. Health Aff (Millwood) 23: 202-212.
6. McGillis Hall L, Doran D, Pink GH (2004) Nurse staffing models, nursing hours, and patient safety outcomes. J Nurs Adm 34: 41-45.
7. Whitman GR, Kim Y, Davidson LJ, Wolf GA, Wang SL (2002) The impact of staffing on patient outcomes across specialty units. J Nurs Adm 32: 633-639.
8. Spence Laschinger HK, Leiter MP (2006) The impact of nursing work environments on patient safety outcomes: the mediating role of burnout/engagement. J Nurs Adm 36: 259-267.
9. Fairbanks RJ, Hays DP, Webster DF, Spillane LL (2004) Clinical pharmacy services in an emergency department. Am J Health Syst Pharm 61: 934-937.
10. Mostafaei D, Barati Marnani A2, Mosavi Esfahani H3, Estebsari F4, Shahzaidi S5, et al. (2014) Medication errors of nurses and factors in refusal to report medication errors among nurses in a teaching medical center of iran in 2012. Iran Red Crescent Med J 16: e16600.
11. Al-Youssif S, Mohamed L, Mohamed N (2013) Nurses' Experiences toward Perception of Medication Administration Errors Reporting. Journal of Nursing and Health Science 1: 56-70
12. Abou Hashish E, El-Bialy G (2013) Nurses' Perceptions of Safety Climate and Barriers to Report Medication Errors. Life Science Journal 10: 2160-2168.
13. Baker M, Attala H (2012) Medications errors, causes, and reporting behaviors as perceived by nurses. Journal of pharmaceutical and biomedical sciences 19: 1-7.
14. Lisa D (2009) Medication error reporting by physicians, nurses, and pharmacists in a Level 1 Trauma Center Emergency Department.
15. Kamel S (2008) Studying medication administration errors in Ain – Shams University Hospital. MSCs. Thesis. Faculty of Medicine Ain Shams University, Egypt.
16. Abo El-Maged N, Gaber E, El-Maghraby M (2002) Relationship between work setting and the occurrence of medication errors among nurses of Assiut University Hospital, Egypt. Assuit Med.J 26: 55- 66.
17. Mousa S (2000) Assessment of nursing medication errors factors causing them in the critical care unit At El Manial University Hospital, Egypt.
18. Abdou H, Saber K (2011). A baseline assessment of patient safety culture among nurses at Student University Hospital. World Journal of Medical Sciences 6: 17-26
19. Dumo MA (2012) Factors Affecting Medication Errors among Staff Nurses: Basis in the Formulation of Medication Information Guide. IAMURE International J of Health Education 1: 1-62.
20. Anderson P, Townsend T (2010) Medication errors: Don't let them happen to you Mistakes can occur in any setting, at any step of the drug administration continuum. Here's how to prevent them. American Nurse Today 5: 23-28.
21. Mrayyan MT, Shishani K, Al-Faouri I (2007) Rate, causes and reporting of medication errors in Jordan: nurses' perspectives. J Nurs Manag 15: 659-670.
22. Peth HA (2003) Medication errors in the emergency department: a systems approach to minimizing risk. Emerg Med Clin North Am 21: 141-158.
23. Wakefield J B, Uden-Holman T, and Wakefield S D (2000) Development and Validation of the Medication Administration Error Reporting Survey, Journal of Advances in Patient Safety 4: 475-89.
24. Al-Shara M (2011) Factors contributing to medication errors in Jordan: a nursing perspective. Iran J Nurs Midwifery Res 16: 158-161.
25. N. Flor (2012) Ateneo de Manila University. Retrieved February 2012, from Ateneo de Manila University
26. Zein ElDin YK , Abd ElAal HN (2013) The Relationship between Perceived Safety Climate, Nurses' Work Environment and Barriers to Medication Administration Errors Reporting. Life Science Journal, 10: 950-62.
27. Tully MP, Ashcroft DM, Dornan T, Lewis PJ, Taylor D, et al. (2009) The causes of and factors associated with prescribing errors in hospital inpatients: a systematic review. Drug Saf 32: 819-836.
28. Hartel MJ, Staub LP, Röder C, Eggli S (2011) High incidence of medication documentation errors in a Swiss university hospital due to the handwritten prescription process. BMC Health Serv Res 11: 199.

10

Environmental Biodecontamination: When a Procedure Performed by the Nursing Staff has an Economic Impact in ICU Rooms

Ragusa R[1-3*], **Lombardo A**[1,2,4], **Bruno A**[4], **Sciacca A**[2,6] and **Lupo L**[1,7]

[1]Heath Technology Assessment Committee, University Hospital, Italy

[2]Committee against nosocomial infection, University Hospital "G. Rodolico" Catania, Italy

[3]Direzione Medica di Presidio, University Hospital "G. Rodolico" Catania, Italy

[4]Nursing for the Control of Hospital Infections, University Hospital "G. Rodolico" Catania, Italy

[5]Science of Health Professions Technical Diagnostic, University of Catania, Italy

[6]Department of Biomedical and Biotechnological Sciences, University of Catania, Italy

[7]Department of Medical and Surgical Sciences and advanced technologies, University of Catania, Italy

*Corresponding author: Rosalia Ragusa, Via Rosso di San Secondo, 3 - Catania 95128 Italy, E-mail: ragusar@unict.it

Abstract

Objective: The transmission of hospital-acquired infections most commonly occurs by means of healthcare workers coming into contact with contaminated surfaces or patients during routine care and the lack of or poor implementation of hygiene procedures. We present this study to assess the efficacy of a new environmental infection control system, managed by a nurse in charge of infection control, in terms of safety, clinical outcome and hospital/healthcare costs.

Methods: The following is an observational retrospective study performed at University Hospital of Catania; containing data on HAI infections from years 2013 and 2014, before and after a new disinfection procedure was introduced. The procedure used a no-touch technology for the indoor environment, using micronebulized hydrogen peroxide and silver cations. Cases of infections concerned adult inpatients with hospitalization time being greater than three days. The efficacy of the procedure was evaluated by comparing the decrease in number of infections, related deaths, and changes in antimicrobial load, whereas economic impact of the new procedure was assessed by a cost-effectiveness analysis. User satisfaction and environmental safety issue were also addressed.

Results: A total of 489 patients were hospitalized in the ICU between January 1, 2013 and December 31, 2014. The introduction of the procedure coincided with a significant decrease overall in infection-related deaths, as well as hospital days (16.95 ± 20.46 (mean $\pm$ SD) to 11.55 ± 10.03 (mean $\pm$ SD: p value <0.05). Bacterial load in samples from CVC and from broncho-alveolar lavage decreased, as well.

The incremental cost-effective ratio resulted in € 807.80 to be added for each infection-related death avoided.

Conclusion: We demonstrated that HyperDRYMist technology with hydrogen peroxide and silver cations is effective, safe and cost-effective without evidence of safety risk. Biodecontamination performed by motivated and experienced nurses could be useful in reducing microbial load and nosocomial infections. The system can contribute to improving the ICU patient's final outcome.

Keywords: Nosocomial infection; Biodecontamination; Infections control nurse; Cost-effectiveness analysis; Hydrogen peroxide; Indoor environment; Economic impact; ICER

Introduction

Nosocomial infections are among the most frequent causes of morbidity and mortality in the hospital environment accounting for a 5-10% increased risk of infection, and a ten-fold further increase in critical care departments, such as in the ICU, where invasive, diagnostic and therapeutic procedures are more frequent, and where patients receiving immunosuppressive therapies are more vulnerable.

The transmission of hospital-acquired infections (HAI) most commonly occurs by means of healthcare workers coming into contact with contaminated surfaces or patients during routine care and the lack of/or poor implementation of hygiene procedures [1-3].

Moreover, the long-term persistence and selection of resistant infections (Meticillin-resistant *Staphylococcus aureus*, *Clostridium difficile*, *Acinetobacter baumanii*, Vancomycin-Resistant Enterococci, *Pseudomonas aeruginosa*, *Klebsiella pneumoniae*, *Mycobacterium tuberculosis*) is further fostered by the extensive administration of unnecessary antibiotic therapy and the consequent selection of resistant strains, making their eradication throughout hospital wards more difficult [4-6].

Approximately 30% of care-associated infections are preventable by adopting specific care practices such as hand hygiene, prudent antibiotic prescription, isolation of infected patients and appropriate use of gloves and other equipment [7].

Conventional cleaning is generally achieved by use of ammonium (or other surfactant-based) detergents applied by housekeeping staff to high-touch surfaces, such as bathrooms and floors and surfaces surrounding patients, but has proven to be inadequate (difficult-to-reach multiplanar surfaces, incorrect dilution of detergent, cleaning rounds, variability of materials used to manufacture components/surfaces of furniture and devices) and in some cases, even inducing vegetative forms of virus that can survive for many months in the environment.

The issue of environmental disinfection has been addressed by a large number of studies which have evidenced that best results are achieved on several levels starting from educating cleaning staff and, implementing consistent cleaning protocols, to adopting more effective environmental disinfection control systems such as aerosolized hydrogen peroxide (aHP) systems, H_2O_2 vapor systems, ultraviolet C radiation (UVC) systems, and NTD system based on pulsed-xenon UV (PX-UV) radiation [8,9].

In the attempt to reduce avoidable costs and the improve the quality of healthcare services provided in our hospital, we decided to evaluate the effectiveness of an indoor nebulisation system using hydrogen peroxide and silver cations as an alternative to conventional decontamination procedures [10-13]. The infections control nurse has been trained in the use of the device.

Hence, the aim of the present study was to compare clinical and economic impact of this system in the intensive care unit before (2013 data) and after (2014 data) introducing the new procedure for environmental decontamination.

Methods

The presented work was a prospective observational study performed at the ICU of the University Hospital "G. Rodolico", considering data from January–December, 2014 and the previous year January-December, 2013 (control). The environmental disinfection procedure under evaluation was adopted and implemented throughout 2014 and was performed for all rooms that had been occupied by patients showing clinical manifestations of infection (after at least 3 days from admission, in accordance with definition of nosocomial infections), as soon as the room became vacant.

The ICU was composed of 3 rooms with 2 beds each. Whenever an infection was suspected, patient was isolated, while the patient occupying the other bed was transferred to another room.

Hygiene status of ICU was periodically monitored by sampling in areas throughout the ward (hallways, patient rooms and service room). Efficacy of disinfection procedure was evaluated by difference in microbial load (measured as CFU/cm^2), before and after decontamination.

The nursing staff of the department collected samples for most high-touch surfaces (specifically: bedrails, bell switches, servant tables, blood pressure cuffs, intravenous pumps, urinary collection bags) and sent them to the Microbiological Laboratory for analysis.

Efficacy of clinical outcome was evaluated by difference in frequency and type of infections occurring in 2014 in comparison to 2013 when the procedure was still not in use.

Data was collected from medical records for patients admitted to the ICU between 2013 and 2014 and included age, days in hospital, positive microbial cultures, outcome/death, treatment and therapies. In 2013 a total of 244 patients were hospitalized in the ICU (88 patients>3 day stay; 48 infection-related deaths). In 2014 a total of 245 patients (98 patients>3 day stay; 42 infection-related deaths) were hospitalized. Samples for patients with a suspected infection came from blood, bronchoalveolar lavage (BAL) and central venous catheter (CVC), as representatives of supposedly sterile sources and which are most often associated with adverse outcome; specimens from urine and stool were not considered. All cultures with positive outcome were clinically defined as sepsis.

For our pharmaco-economical evaluation, we assessed the consumption of drugs (Defined Daily Dose, DDD) for HAI treatment over the two-year period and the cost of the drugs used for second level infections. Drugs considered for the evaluation were those used in treatments: teicoplanin, tigecycline, daptomycin, colistin, anidulafungin, voriconazole, vancomycin, fluconazole.

Environmental disinfection procedure

After the doctor's report of a case of infectious disease or "alert organism" isolation, nursing staff of the ICU rooms, required the infection control nurse to perform the decontamination.

Environmental decontamination was performed using the 99MA system manufactured by 99 Technologies (Lugano, Switzerland). This system employs the new HyperDRYMist® technology, which nebulises a mix of hydrogen peroxide in the concentration of 5-8% and silver cations at a concentration of 60 mg/L. The highly-reactive hydroxyl free radical of hydrogen peroxide acts on the microorganism's membrane lipids, DNA and other important cellular components, while the silver cations inhibit microbial protein synthesis.

Before decontamination, room doors and vents were sealed and the air ventilation was turned off. The disinfectant solution was prepared according to the manufacturer's instructions, in order to achieve the required concentration of 7 ppm. The device was positioned in a corner facing the room. Time of treatment was established based on the room volume (application time is directly proportional to volume, thus the bigger the volume to decontaminate, the longer the time for treatment). At the end of the process, the room was reopened and ventilation or air-conditioning system reactivated.

Finally, we assessed user-satisfaction by administering a structured questionnaire to the nursing and cleaning staff, enquiring on the presence of any perceived irritation to eyes, skin or respiratory tract.

Statistical analysis

The normality distribution of the variables was tested by the Kolmogorov-Smirnov test. Proportions and means were obtained using the X^2 and Mann–Whitney tests, respectively. All variables are expressed as mean and standard deviation.

Cost-effectiveness measures and outcomes

Clinical outcomes (number of infections and deaths) were compared for the two years in order to perform an economic evaluation of the decontamination procedure. The X^2 test was used and data was summarized using averages and standard deviation.

Cost-effectiveness analysis for the economic impact was performed, and Incremental Cost Effectiveness Ratio (ICER) was calculated. This indicator is calculated using the following formula: ICER=(C1-C2)/(E1-E2) where C indicates the cost and E indicates the effectiveness of the treatment [14,15].

To assess the costs, we calculated the differential between the costs borne in the two years for the following parameters: C1 (2013): cost drugs; C2 (2014): cost drugs+cost device+cost material+hourly cost of staff; E1: number deaths in 2013; E2: number deaths in 2014.

Results

Microbiological environmental data

We measured the efficacy of the procedure in the reduction of the bacterial and fungal load in the environment. The most heavily contaminated areas in the ICU rooms were servant tables, urine collection bags, buzzers and bed linens (Table 1). After treatment with 99T, contaminated residues had been completely eliminated.

Surfaces Analyzed Using Environmental Swabs	TBC 37°C (cfu/cm^2)		TBC 22°C (cfu/cm^2)		M (cfu/cm^2)	
	PRE (a)	POST(b)	PRE (a)	POST(b)	PRE (a)	POST(b)
Bedrails	3	0.1	2,6	0	1.8	0
Bedlinen	2.2	0.2	3,2	0.3	0.7	0
Table servant	7.4	0.4	6,6	0	6.8	0
Blood pressure cuffs	3.4	0	2	0.1	1.4	0.1
Intravenous pumps	1.6	0	0.8	0.1	1	0
Nurse call buttons	4.5	0	3.7	0.1	4.2	0
Bag of urine collection	8	0.3	8.5	0.1	4	0

Table 1: Bacterial and mycetic load measured throughout the intensive care before and after use of the 99MA System, Legend a) before use of 99MA System, b) after use of 99MA System, TBC, Total Bacterial Count; M, total mycetum count, For each sampling, different temperatures allowed to evidence bacterial load originating from environmental infections and those from human host.

Clinical outcome

The patient population admitted to the ICU between 2013 and 2014 was quite homogeneous in reference to demographic and clinical characteristics (Table 2).

Clinical Characteristics	Year	Year
	2013	2014
No. of total admitted patients	244	245
No. of patient >3 days stay	88	98
No. of total deaths	68	60
No. of deaths patients >3 days	48	42
Days of hospitalization	1796	1431
Average hospital stays	7.4 ± 14.2	5.8 ± 7.9
Average patient age	64 ± 17	65 ± 18
Male	147	147
Female	97	98

Table 2: Clinical patient characteristics of total ICU patient population.

As compared to 2013, in 2014 there was a significant decrease in number of deaths caused by infections compared to deaths for other causes—decreasing from 59% to 38% (χ^2=4,02; P= 0,045) (Figure 1). In 2013, out of 34 patients with positive cultures, 8 were found with multiple infections (7 deaths, 1 survival) whereas in 2014, only 5 were multiple infections.

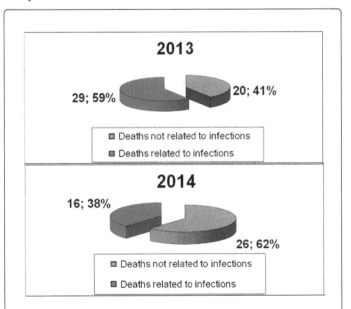

Figure 1: Decrease in number of deaths related or not to infections between adult inpatients with hospitalization >3 days in different years.

The causative agents most frequently isolated were *A. baumannii*, followed by *S. epidermidis*, *Candida* spp., *P. aeruginosa*, *E. coli*, *S. maltophiliae*, *K. pneumoniae*.

As compared to 2013, the Mann-Whitney test showed a significant reduction in 2014 in hospitalization days (Figure 2), which decreased from 16.95 ± 20.46 (mean ± SD) to 11.55 ± 10.03 (mean ± SD: p value<0.05).

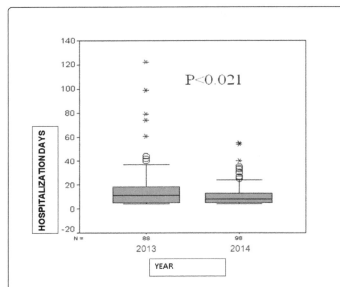

Figure 2: Mann Whitney test showed a significant reduction in hospitalization days between 2013 and 2014.

The number of disinfection interventions performed with HyperDRYMist in 2014 was 44 (approximately one after each death).

Assessment cost-effectiveness

To calculate ICER the following costs were identified: (i) Cost of drugs dedicated to the treatment of infections of the 2nd and 3rd level claimed in patients hospitalized for at least three days. Cost of antibiotics treatment from the first day to the third was excluded. (ii) Device cost (depreciation charge=25% yearly); (iii) Cost of consumables; (iv) Hourly cost of personnel responsible for biodecontamination.

ICER was calculated as follows: ICER=(C1-C2)/(E1-E2) where C1-C2 is the differential cost and E1-E2 is the efficacy differential.

C1 cost in 2013 was €54,620; C2 cost in 2014 was €49,773 (€47,223 for drugs, €1,500 for device, €600 for consumables, €540 for the personnel dedicated to the bio-decontamination). Differential Cost (C1-C2) was €4,847.

As an effectiveness indicator, we considered the number of patients who died after three days of hospitalization. In 2013 the number of deaths was 48 (E1) and in 2014 the number of deaths amounted to 42 (E2). Efficiency differential, E1-E2, is equal to:

Efficacy Differential (E1-E2)=48 deaths-42 deaths=6 deaths

The ratio between the cost differential and the efficacy differential returns ICER, the incremental costs for saving on deaths in infected ICU patients, is €807.83 per death-related infection.

Figure 3 illustrates that ICER value is positioned in the first quadrant, thus confirming the study to be cost-effective, as it has higher costs but is more effective.

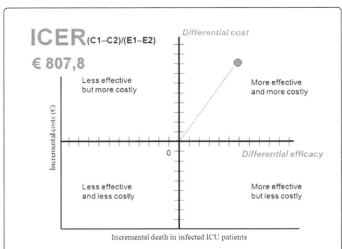

Figure 3: Incremental cost for saving death in infected ICU patients. The figure illustrated that ICER value is positioned in the first quadrant, thus confirming to be cost-effective, as it has higher costs but is more effective.

Discussion

A high frequency of nosocomial infections is an indicator of poor quality of health services provided and a source of avoidable costs.

Since 2011 in our Hospital there has been a hand-hygiene protocol, as suggested by WHO recommendations, focusing on high risk transmission practice.

Sometimes the isolation procedure cannot be performed, the disinfection of hands is not properly done, or the proper use of gloves is not properly performed, even in the presence of severe infectious disease [16]. Despite many interventions, hand disinfection rate remains very bad, as described by observation or more recently by videotaping [17].

Our study aimed to evaluate the efficacy of a new system to reduce HAIs, in particular infections brought by most common resistant and threatening infections that can further compromise the conditions of already critically ill patients.

Accurate cleaning and decontamination of hospital environments is essential to reduce contamination, but does not completely remove the bacteria from all surfaces [18].

This may depend on many factors, including the efficacy of the decontamination protocols in use, the poor observance by the operators, the inefficacy of the treatments on the surfaces complex shapes, the improper use and choice of agents in relation to the materials and environments undergoing decontaminated.

Environment plays a central role in the transmission of pathogens acquired in the hospital. Some bacteria can survive for several months in a hospital setting —particularly in those areas most in proximity of patients (bedrails, bed linen, table's servant, blood pressure cuffs, intravenous pumps, nurse call buttons, bags of urine collection) — adapting and becoming resistant to antimicrobial actions [1,2,19-21].

Hence it is important to choose an easy-to-implement and effective method, that is less operator dependent and that acts on bacterial walls in a relatively short time, without leaving pollutants or residues in the air.

A number of studies in literature have reported the use of hydrogen peroxide in several disinfection systems and its effectiveness in significantly reducing environmental microbial load [22-24].

Indeed, our data confirms a decrease in the number of infections since the introduction of this new technology. In general, 2014 did not show infections of *S. epidermidis*, *Candida* spp., or *P. aeruginosa*, although it appears that infection by *A. baumannii* remained steady over 2013 and 2014. However, these infections did not appear to be linked to each other and their frequency of occurrence could be due to an increased epidemiological trend of this agent in 2014.

A health technology assessment for see a global evaluation of effectiveness, safety, costs [25] and organizational impact was done; our results showed a significant decrease in infections and confirmed safety and user satisfaction of the procedure. Satisfaction with the ease of use of the equipment and environmental safety has been highlighted by the questionnaire to operators and nursing staff, after the intervention of disinfection.

A strong support by this system can certainly be given in hospital clustering of cases, when infection occurs in multiple bedrooms or eventually at discharge of patients infected or colonized with resistant germs or multiple microorganisms. ICER Value confirms that the new approach is cost effective as it has higher costs but is more effective: environmental biodecontamination has reduced costs in the global management of the ICU rooms.

In conclusion we can say that this practice, coordinated by the nursing staff, can be useful for reducing microbial load and nosocomial infections and it is also an opportunity to increase communication between medical and nursing staff.

The infection control nurse, that acquired the knowledge base to use the biodecontamination device, became aware of its role and could increase the active practice of decontamination in the proper manner.

This procedure could improve global quality of care and the final outcomes.

We intend to adopt this system in other critical care units.

Acknowledgement

The authors are grateful to Pencil and Papers Italy and Mallory Wolfe for language editing of the paper.

References

1. Otter JA, Yezli S, French GL (2011) The role played by contaminated surface in the transmission of nosocomial pathogens. Infect Control Hosp Epidemiol 32: 687-699.
2. Weber DJ, Rutala WA, Miller MB, Huslage K, Sickbert-Bennett E (2010) Role of hospital surfaces in the transmission of emerging health care-associated pathogens: norovirus, *Clostridium difficile* and Acinetobacter species. Am J Infect Control 38: S25-33.
3. Hayden MK, Blom DW, Lyle EA, Moore CG, Weinstein RA (2008) Risk of hand or glove contamination after contact with patient colonized with vancomycin-resistant Enterococcus or the colonized patient's environment. Infect Control Hosp Epidemiol 29:149-54.
4. Abreu AC, Tavares RR, Borges A, Mergulhão F, Simões M (2013) Current and emergent strategies for disinfection of hospital environments. J Antimicrob Chemother 68: 2718-2732.
5. Zarb P, Coignard B, Griskeviciene J, Muller A, Vankerckhoven V, et al. (2012) The European Centre for Disease Prevention and Control (ECDC) pilot point prevalence survey of healthcare-associated infections and antimicrobial use. Euro Surveill 17.
6. Dancer SJ (2008) Importance of the environment in meticillin-resistant *Staphylococcus aureus* acquisition: The case for hospital cleaning. Lancet Infect Dis 8:101–113.
7. Richards MJ, Edwards JR, Culver DH, Gaynes RP (2000) Nosocomial infections in combined medical-surgical intensive care units in the United States. Infect Control Hosp Epidemiol 21: 510-515.
8. Havill NL (2013) Best practices in disinfection of noncritical surfaces in the health care setting: Creating a bundle for success. Am J Infect Control 41: S26-30.
9. Weber DJ, Anderson D, Rutala WA (2013) The role of the surface environment in healthcare-associated infections. Curr Opin Infect Dis 26: 338-344.
10. French GL, Otter JA, Shannon KP, Adams NM, Watling D, et al. (2004) Tackling contamination of the hospital environment by methicillin-resistant *Staphylococcus aureus* (MRSA): A comparison between conventional terminal clearing and hydrogen peroxide vapour decontamination. J Hosp Infect 57: 31-37.
11. Hardy KJ, Gossain S, Henderson N, Drugan C, Oppenheim BA, et al. (2007) Rapid recontamination with MRSA of the environment of an intensive care unit after decontamination with hydrogen peroxide vapour. J Hosp Infect 66: 360-368.
12. Otter JA, Yezli S, Perl TM, Barbut F, French GL (2013) The role of 'no-touch' automated room disinfection systems in infection prevention and control. J Hosp Infect 83: 1-13.
13. Davies A, Pottage T, Bennett A, Walker J (2011) Gaseous and air decontamination technologies for *Clostridium difficile* in the health care environment. J Hosp Infect 77: 199-203.
14. Drummond M, Torrance G, Mason J (1993) Cost-effectiveness league tables: More harm than good? Social Science and Medicine 37: 33-40.
15. Eichler H, Kong S, Gerth W, Mavros P, Jönsson B (2004) Use of cost-effectiveness analysis in health care resource allocation decision-making: How are cost-effectiveness thresholds expected to emerge? Value in Health 7: 518–528.
16. Marranzano M, Ragusa R, Platania M, Faro G, Coniglio M (2013) Knowledge, attitudes and practices towards patients with HIV/AIDS in staff nurses in one university hospital in Sicily. Epidemiol Biostat Public Health 10: e 8731-1 -6.
17. Boudjema S, Reynier P, Dufour JC, Florea O, Patouraux P, et al.(2016) Hand hygiene analyzed by video recording. J Nurs Care 5:2
18. Cahill OJ, Claro T, O'Connor N, Cafolla AA, Stevens NT, et al.(2014) Cold air plasma to decontaminate inanimate surfaces of the hospital environment. Applied and Environmental Microbiology 80: 2004–2010.
19. Huang SS, Datta R, Platt R (2006) Risk of acquiring antibiotic-resistant bacteria from prior room occupants. Arch Intern Med 166: 1945-1951.
20. Kramer A, Schwebke I, Kampf G (2006) How long do nosocomial pathogens persist on inanimate surfaces? A systematic review. BMC Infect Dis 6: 130.
21. Boyce JM. (2007) Environmental contamination makes an important contribution to hospital infection. Journal of Hospital Infection 65: 50-54.
22. Blazejewski C, Wallet F, Rouzé A, Le Guern R, Ponthieux S, et al. (2015) Efficiency of hydrogen peroxide in improving disinfection of ICU rooms. Crit Care 19: 30.
23. Fu TY, Gent P, Kumar V (2012) Efficacy, efficiency and safety aspects of hydrogen peroxide vapour and aerosolized hydrogen peroxide room disinfection systems. J Hosp Infect 80:199–205.

24. Passeretti CL, Otter JA, Reich NG (2013) An evaluation of environmental decontamination with hydrogen peroxide vapor for reducing the risk of patient acquisition of multidrug-resistant organisms. Clinical Infectious Disease 56: 27-35.

25. Ragusa R, Lupo L, Lombardo A, Sciacca A, Venuto V, et al. (2013) Biodecontaminazione ambientale in ambienti protetti: Valutazione dei costi. Hospital based HTA session pag.43 6th National Congress of SIHTA Bari 7-9 Novembre 2013.

11

Experiences of Critical Care Nurses of Death and Dying in an Intensive Care Unit: A Phenomenological Study

Vasanthrie Naidoo[1*] and Sibiya MN[2]

[1]School of Nursing, Department of Medical and Surgical Nursing, Life College of Learning-KZN, South Africa

[2]School of Nursing, Faculty of Health Sciences, Durban University of Technology, South Africa

*Corresponding author: Vasanthrie Naidoo, School of Nursing, Department of Medical and Surgical Nursing, Life College of Learning-KZN, South Africa, E-mail: vasie.naidoo2@lifehealthcare.co.za

Abstract

Background: Working in the intensive care unit can be traumatic for nursing personnel. Critical care nurses are faced with repeated exposure to death and dying as they are involved in caring for patients who are actively dying, have a terminal illness or face impending death. These nurses relate in different ways to the phenomena of death and dying within their nursing profession and their scope of practice. Critical care nurses often have a difficult time coping with the stress that comes with caring for those who are dying or relating to loved ones of those that are dying.

Aim of the study: The aim of the study was to explore the critical care nurse's experiences of death and dying.

Methods: A qualitative, descriptive phenomenological research approach was used to guide the study. Approval to conduct the study was obtained from Durban University of Technology Faculty Research Committee, the eThekwini District Health Research Unit, and the Nursing Service Manager of the participating hospital. The study population comprised of nurses working in the Critical care unit of the participating hospital.

Results: Findings of this study revealed that issues such as communication, multicultural diversity, education and coping mechanisms relating to caring for the critically ill and dying patient are essential in nursing education and practice.

Conclusions : Critical care nurses need to have support networks in place, not only to assist in providing care, but also for their own emotional support and well-being.

Keywords: Critical care nurse; Death; Dying

Introduction and Background Information

According to Prompahakul, Nilmanat, and Kongsuwan it was noted that the most important aspect of nursing is caring and this is even more so in an intensive care unit (ICU) [1]. In a study done by Farrell, it was noted that critical care units of today are totally dedicated to saving lives by offering specialized disease and surgical management to many patients [2]. Not only must the critical care nurse be able to deliver high quality medical care skilfully, using all appropriate technologies, she must also be able to apply psychosocial and other holistic approaches when planning and delivering care [3]. According to Urden, Stacy and Lough critical care nurses fulfil speciality roles that require their clinical teaching, leadership, research and consultative abilities. According to Alspach [4], the scope of practice for acute and critical care nursing is defined by the dynamic interaction with the acutely and critically ill patient. Hay and Oken further argue that the psychological burdens placed on critical care nurses are extraordinary often the situation these nurses face on a regular basis can be likened to that of a soldier serving with a combat group [5]. Critical care nurses are continuously championing the needs of the critically ill patient, the family or significant others [6]. A study that was conducted by Dracup and Bryan-Brown, revealed that

while much attention was focused on the critical care nurse's role to assist others in the end-of-life or dying process, little attention was paid to the critical care nurse's psychological, cultural, and spiritual well-being when dealing with death and dying or end-of-life issues [7].

Problem statement

Even though a nurse can celebrate the positive effects that nursing care has on a patient, there may still be no closure when death, dying and despair are witnessed. Therefore, understanding critical care nurses' experiences of death and dying can help the health care delivery system prepare and educate these nurses on issues relating to the needs of the dying or terminally ill patient and also teach them how to effectively deal with such issues.

Aim of study

The aim of this study was to explore the critical care nurse's experiences with death and dying.

Research question

There was only one central research question that was posed to all the participants which guided the study, "What are the critical care nurses' experiences of death and dying in an ICU?" Further probing questions were based on the responses from the central research question.

Significance of study

Understanding critical care nurses' experiences of death and dying will help the health care delivery system prepare and educate nurses working in a critical care environment to the needs of the dying or terminally ill patient, as well as, assisting her in promoting quality end-of-life care in an ICU and how to deal effectively with the stress that these situations can cause.

Research Methodology

Research design

A qualitative study using a descriptive phenomenological approach was used to guide the study. This type of approach was useful in describing the subjective experiences of the participants and in examining the beliefs and cultures that impact on the death and dying experiences of the subjects. A phenomenological paradigm is concerned with understanding human behaviour from the participant's own frame of reference [8].

Study setting

This study was conducted in the intensive care unit of a provincial hospital in the eThekwini District in the province of KwaZulu-Natal.

Sampling process

A purposive sampling of all consenting professional nurses employed in the ICU of the participating hospital was done.

Data collection

A qualitative data gathering method was employed. In-depth interviews were conducted with the use of an interview guide containing a demographic section as well as a central question to focus the discussion. The initial question that was asked was "What are the critical care nurses' experiences of death and dying in an ICU?" Probing questions were then used to elicit more information.

Data analysis

Giorgi's four steps for data analysis were used to identify themes regarding experiences of death and dying. The goal was to keep the richness of the experience that each participant had with the patients that they cared for whilst exploring the descriptive meanings of such experiences, through identification of essential themes [9].

Trustworthiness

According to Polit and Beck, researchers want their findings to reflect the truth. Research that is inaccurate or holds a biased viewpoint cannot be of any benefit to nursing practice [10]. To enhance trustworthiness, the following four principles outlined by Guba's strategies of credibility, transferability, dependability and confirmability were applied [11].

Ethical consideration

Before commencement of the study, ethical clearance was obtained from the Durban University of Technology Faculty Research Committee (FHSEC039/10). Written consent was obtained from Nursing Service Manager of the participating hospital and eThekwini District Health Research Unit (HRKM189/10). All the participants made an informed, voluntary decision to participate in the study. The nature of the study, the right to refuse to participate, the risks as well as the benefits was fully described to them.

Research Findings

Participant's demographic profile

The sample in the study comprised of four participants. Of the four participants, only 1(25%) was within the 20-25 years age group and 3(75%) fell into 38 years and above age group. With regards to the duration of the experience in ICU, 2(50%) had 4-7 years' experience and the remaining 2(50%) had above eight years' experience in ICU.

Critical care nurses' thoughts about caring for a dying patient

It was apparent from the participants' responses that the thoughts on death of an elderly or aged patient often crossed a critical care nurse's mind. The concept of death being inevitable or real seemed to provide some measure of comfort to the nurse caring for the patient. When youngsters or children died, it becomes very sad and unmanageable at times for all staff in an ICU. The fact that it was a young person involved tends to make the whole situation highly emotional.

The age of the nurse caring for such a patient seemed to have a bearing on the way the nurse copes with the event. Younger nurses were found to be task orientated, and lacked the empathy, respect and psychosocial aspect of patient care. Older nurses were considered to be the most suitable candidates to deal with death and dying issues in the unit as they have more 'humane attributes and qualities stemming from her life's experiences as well as having sound technical and theoretical skills'.

Critical care nurses' feelings about caring for a dying patient

The pain of watching a loved one die or caring for a loved one throughout the dying process can evoke feelings of despair, anger and even denial. Apart from playing the important role of being a patient advocate, the findings of this study revealed that the critical care nurse felt ethically responsible to do his or her best. Feelings of preparedness allowed the nurse to foresee or predict, using their nursing knowledge, the prognosis of a critically ill patient in their care. This helped them prepare themselves and others for what to expect.

Critical care nurses' communication with dying patients

The findings of this study also revealed that the nurse who provided verbal and non-verbal communication with her patients, allowed her to become more in tune with the needs of the patient and their desires as they neared death. According to Lee, Anderson and Hill [12], sometimes culture plays a vital part in end-of-life decision-making. Responses from participants demonstrated that a critical care nurse needed to be aware of cultural attitudes, behaviours and traits of patients to enhance the caring component in critical care nursing.

Past experiences with death and dying and the impact it had on the critical care nurse

Michell also felt that repetitive exposure to resuscitative measures, end-of-life care needs, prolonging life by pharmacological and mechanical means results in psychological disorders such as post-traumatic stress disorder [13]. All the participants that were interviewed felt that a critical care nurse's personal experiences with death and dying impacted on the way she communicated or related to her patients and their loved ones. Participants further stated that the knowledge and skills gained from their personal experiences of caring for a dying family member or any other person that they were associated with impacted on the way they communicated verbally and non-verbally with their patients and the family of their patients.

Support systems that enable the critical care nurse to cope with the trauma of death and dying

The findings of this study also showed that the ICU nurse experiences death in a critical care environment as a series of inter-relationships between patients, nurses, doctors and other members of the multidisciplinary team. This enabled them not only to support the dying patient or the patients' family, but also to support each other in the face of grief. According to Kirchhoff and Beckstrand [14], the collaboration between ICU caregivers and member of the multidisciplinary team can result in timelier decisions regarding life-sustaining treatments. The Table 1 below provides a summary of themes and sub-themes identified in the study.

Main Themes Identified	Sub-themes Identified
Thoughts of a critical care nurse	Age of patient and its role in death acceptance
	Age of nurse and its role in determining maturity and understanding.
Feelings of a critical care nurse	Feelings of grief when coping with the dying or dead patient.
	Feelings of knowing when to prepare for inevitable death of a patient
Communication of a critical care nurse	Communication with dying patient
	Communication with loved ones of dying patient
	Communication of cultural awareness
	Non-verbal communication
Experiences of a critical care nurse with death and dying	The personal impact of death and dying on the critical care nurse
	Exposure of critical care nurse to death and dying and the role it plays in coping.
Support Systems to cope with death and dying in a critical care unit	lack of workplace structures
	use of spirituality as support and guidance
	lack of nurse education on death and dying issues

Table 1: Summary of themes and sub-themes identified in the study.

Discussion on the Experiences of Critical Care Nurses of Death and Dying in an Intensive Care Unit

Acute grief following the death of a loved one or a patient in ICU is often intensely painful but diminishes over time as the loss becomes integrated into ongoing life and the general nursing routine [15]. Despite advances in the healthcare sector, the critical care nurse is not being sufficiently equipped with skills to deal with death and dying in their professional practice, especially if the nurse had little or no exposure dealing with death and dying issues. The knowledge and skills deficit of recently qualified ICU nurses dealing with death and dying issues was another feeling shared by all those interviewed.

There were also strong viewpoints regarding the active participation of the patient's attending doctor in the end-of -life care of their patients, as well as in keeping the patient and relatives fully informed of the patient's progress. Participants felt that the skills that had been acquired by them were learned through their personal and life's experiences. It was also felt that other resources such as social workers, counsellors and designated grieving areas were needs that were still outstanding in the hospital ICU set-up.

Conclusion

Death takes an emotional toll on all persons caring for the dying and therefore, critical care nurses need to have support networks in place, not only to assist in providing care, but also for their own emotional wellbeing. Irrespective of religion, culture or race, spirituality plays a huge role when caring for the dying and provides a resource for coping with death and dying for participants in this study. A nurse's age and level of maturity, as well as past experiences with dying and death plays a key role in providing care at end-of-life.

Recommendations

Nursing education

Nursing as an academic discipline can, and should be concerned with the generation of new research about nursing practice, but this will remain meaningless if not integrated into learning and teaching especially in the clinical practice and setting. End-of-life or death education should be emphasised in undergraduate nursing curriculum and continue to be integrated to post-graduate or post basic nurse training. This should include skills specifically related to end-of-life care or dying in an ICU.

Institutional management and practice

Nursing as a profession needs to create a support network made up of the multidisciplinary team. Health care settings that have an ICU should have a separate grieving area that can facilitate the comfort needs of the family or loved ones of the deceased. Professional assistance and advice should be readily available to all ICU staff requiring debriefing from traumatic ICU events.

Policy development and implementation

All nursing staff allocated to work in an ICU environment should undergo an ICU orientation programme on the death and dying policies and protocols in an ICU. These policies should comply with the ethical and legal guidelines laid down by the laws of the country such as information on termination of life support, brain stem death testing and information of organ donation [16-18].

Further Research

Further research is recommended to ascertain whether the present South African Diploma in Medical and Surgical Nursing-Critical Care nursing curriculum adequately addresses the issues of death and dying in an ICU. Research into the expectations of the grieving family and the dying patient from the ICU nurse will serve as useful sources for future research reference.

Strengths and Limitations

This study focused on a fundamental phenomenon (death and dying) in critical care nursing. Using a phenomenological research methodology, the researcher was unable to anticipate how the study was going to evolve. Much of the research design appeared to come about during the data collection and analysis process. Using this approach, helped the researcher examine the human experience based on the descriptions provided by the persons involved and what meanings these descriptions held for them for them alone.

References

1. Prompahakul BSN, Nilmanat K, Kongsuwan W (2011) Factors relating to nurses' caring behaviours for dying patients. Nurse Media Journal of Nursing 1: 15-27.

2. Farrell M (1989) Dying and bereavement. The role of the critical care nurse. Intensive Care Nurs 5: 39-45.

3. Thelan LA, Davie JK, Urden LD (1994) Critical care nursing: Diagnosis and management. (2ndedn). St Louis: Mosby.

4. Alspach JG (2006) Core curriculum for critical care nursing. 6th ed. Philadelphia: W.B Saunders Company.

5. Hay D, Oken D (1972) The psychological stresses of intensive care unit nursing. Psychosom Med 34: 109-118.

6. Hov R, Hedelin B, Athlin E (2005) Being an intensive care nurse related to questions of withholding or withdrawing curative treatment. J Clin Nurs 16: 203-211.

7. Hudak MC, Morton GP, Fontaine KD, Gallo MB (2008) Critical care nursing: A holistic approach. (8thedn). Philadelphia: Lippincott Williams & Wilkins.

8. Dracup K, Bryan-Brown CW (2005) Dying in the intensive care unit. Am J Crit Care 14: 456-458.

9. George JB (2011) Nursing Theories: The Base for Professional Nursing Practice. (6thedn). New Jersey: Pearson Education.

10. Polit DF, Hungler BP (2004) Nursing research: Principles and methods. (6thedn). Philadelphia: Lippincott Williams and Wilkins.

11. Polit DF, Beck CT (2008) Nursing research: Generating and assessing evidence for nursing practice. (8thedn). Philadelphia: Lippincott Williams and Wilkins.

12. Lincoln YS, Guba EG (1985) Naturalistic inquiry. Newbury Park: Sage Publications.

13. Lee CA, Anderson MA, Hill PD (2006) Cultural sensitivity education for nurses: a pilot study. J Contin Educ Nurs 37: 137-141.

14. Michell L (2010) Crash and burn. Southern African Journal of Critical Care 26: 34.

15. Kirchhoff KT, Beckstrand RL (2000) Critical care nurses' perceptions of obstacles and helpful behaviors in providing end-of-life care to dying patients. American Journal of Critical Care 9: 1-10.

16. Carlson KK (2009) Advanced critical care nursing. Canada: Saunders.

17. Liebert M (2011) Follow-up study of complicated grief amongst parents eighteen months after a child's death in the paediatric intensive care unit. Journal of Palliative Medicine 14: 207-214.

18. Urden LD, StacyKM, Lough ME (2010) Critical care nursing: Diagnosis and management. (6thedn). St Louis: Mosby.

12

Factors in the Critical Thinking Disposition and Skills of Intensive Care Nurses

Nurdan Gezer[1*], Belgin Yildirim[2] and Esma Özaydın[3]

[1]Medical Surgical Nursing Department, Nursing Faculty, Adnan Menderes University, Aydın, Turkey

[2]Health Nursing Department, Nursing Faculty, Adnan Menderes University, Aydın, Turkey

[3]Adnan Menderes University Hospital Intensive Care Unit, Aydın, Turkey

*Corresponding author: Nurdan Gezer, Adnan Menderes Üniversitesi, Hemşirelik Fakültesi Gençlik Cd. No: 709100 Aydın, Turkey,
E-mail: ngezer@adu.edu.tr

Abstract

Aim: The aim of this study is to define and evaluate factors related to the California Critical Thinking Disposition Inventory (CCTDI) of intensive care unit nurses working at Adnan Menderes University.

Methodology: The population of the study consisted of 60 nurses studying and at working at university hospitals. The sample size consisted of 40 nurses who volunteered to participate in the study. The data were collected from January to March 2012. The Socio-demographic Features Data Form and the CCTDI were used as data collection tools. This inventory was developed based on the results of the Delphi Report in which critical thinking and disposition toward critical thinking were conceptualized by a group of critical thinking experts. The original CCTDI includes 75 items loaded on seven constructs. These are inquisitiveness, open-mindedness, systematicity, analyticity, truth-seeking, critical thinking self-confidence, and maturity. The SPSS 15.0 package software was used in the evaluation of data, which employed numbers, percentage estimations, arithmetic means, the Kruskal-Wallis Test, the t test and Pearson's correlation analysis.

Results: When total score means are examined, it is seen that the mean score obtained by the nurses was 190,90 ± 20,23. The CCTDI score means of the nurses taken into the scope of the study reveal that the mean score on the "truth-seeking" subscale was 21,50 ± 5,62; the mean score on the "Open-mindedness" subscale was 36.95 ± 7.32; the mean score on the "systematicity" subscale was 19,32 ± 3,56; the mean score on the "Self-confidence" subscale was 27,75 ± 6,02; the mean score on the "Inquisitiveness" subscale was 34,47 ± 6,00.

It was determined that there was no statistically significant difference between the CCDTI scale mean scores and the nurses' ages, years of study, income levels, and education levels ($p > 0.05$).

Conclusion: This study found the nurses' critical thinking dispositions to be at a low level. To ensure the development of a critical thinking disposition in nursing, educational opportunities must be provided inside and outside the institution.

Keywords: Critical thinking; Intensive care; Nursing

Introduction

The concept of critical thinking has been discussed and defined by philosophers, psychologists and educators, all of whom have differing but related definitions. Socrates, Plato and Aristotle provided the important foundations for the concept of critical thinking, the idea of questioning assumptions, analyzing rationally and using empirical experience [1].

There is no universally accepted definition of critical thinking. However, the Delphi report published by the American Philosophical Association gives us a description of critical thinking in terms of cognitive skills and affective dispositions that is generic with no domain-specific implications. This has resulted in a definition of critical thinking as, "the process of purposeful, self-regulatory judgment; an interactive, reflective, reasoning process" [2].

Kataoka-Yahiro and Saylor argue that in nursing, "the critical thinking process is reflective and reasonable thinking about nursing problems without a single solution is focused on deciding what to believe and do. According to Yıldırım, critical thinking is "the process of searching, obtaining, evaluating, analyzing, synthesizing and conceptualizing information as a guide for developing one's thinking with self-awareness, and the ability to use this information by adding creativity and taking risks " [3,4].

Critical thinking needs to be a central and vital component of nursing practice. Its significance for nursing is that improved critical thinking skills can also improve educational theory and psycho-motor nursing skills. Critical thinking disposition and skills can have a positive effect on patient care and outcomes. Critical thinking should thus be a basic component of nurses' work, especially in intensive care units [5,4].

In intensive care units, patients with severe physical conditions are monitored, their life functions are supported, care staff use special treatment methods, and the most complex biomedical devices are employed. Therefore, these units require a considerable amount of attention [6,7]. For this reason, the intensive care unit is an environment in which quick and sound decisions should be taken in cases where the life of a patient is in danger. While intensive care nurses provide care to often unstable patients who suffer from complex medical or surgical conditions, they also administer an increasingly complicated environment and deal with situations while juggling multiple priorities [6,8]. Team members, and especially nurses, working in such an environment must take responsibility in making quick and rational decisions [9].

As members of a profession that makes them the first to determine changes in patients' status, nurses working in intensive care units are required to make rapid decisions when faced with emergency situations or immediate, complex and unexpected problems. In addition to their overall knowledge of nursing, intensive care nurses who make rapid decisions must use the power of critical thinking based on knowledge peculiar to science as an essential and critical element for maintaining patients' lives [3,9].

Along with clinical skills, within the stressful intensive care environment, critical thinking skills help nurses to believe in themselves, provide secure nursing care and ensure competence. Because critical thinking is an important component of decision-making and clinical case management, it is important to help nurses improve their critical thinking skills at every level [8].

Therefore, in intensive care environments, where complex patient care is provided, critical thinking plays an important role owing to the fact that nurses perform a crucial function in inpatient care [8,10].

Objective

The purpose of this descriptive study was to determine the factors affecting the critical thinking disposition and skills of nurses working in the intensive care units of Adnan Menderes University Hospital, Aydin, Turkey.

Methodology

The study's population and sample

The universe of the study comprised a total of 55 nurses working in the intensive care units of Adnan Menderes University Hospital in Aydın, Turkey. Study data were collected from January to March 2012 between the hours of 8:00-16:00. Seven nurses did not agree to participate in the study. One of the nurses was on sick leave; 2 had just had babies. Three of the nurses were on annual leave. One of the nurses died; another one was assigned to another department. The study sample consisted of 40 nurses who agreed to participate. The flowchart of the study is provided in Figure 1. Before initiating this study, the written and verbal informed consent of the participating nurses as well as institutional permission were obtained.

As data collection tools, the study used a Socio-demographic Characteristics Data Form developed by the researchers after reviewing the relevant literature, and the California Critical Thinking Disposition Inventory (CCTDI). The Socio-demographic Characteristics Data Form consisted of ten questions. The data form included questions about nurses' age, sex, marital status, educational status, spouse's educational status and jobs, activities attended, and status of having attended in-service training or congresses. The CCTDI

was developed within the scope of the Delphi project carried out by the American Philosophical Association.

This 75-item scale has 7 sub-scales that were theoretically determined and have been psychometrically tested: inquisitiveness, open-mindedness, systematicity, analyticity, truth-seeking, critical thinking self-confidence and maturity. The inquisitiveness construct includes 10 items that measures one's intellectual curiosity and one's desire for learning without regard for profit. The open-mindedness construct contains 12 items that measure tolerance of divergent views and sensitivity to the possibility of one's own bias. The systematicity construct has 11 items and measures the extent to which a person is organized, orderly, focused and diligent in inquiry. The analyticity construct has 11 items that address reasoning and the use of evidence to resolve problems.

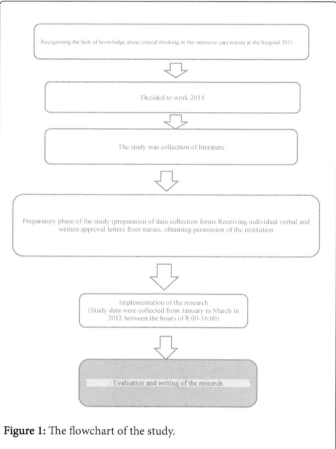

Figure 1: The flowchart of the study.

The truth-seeking construct includes 12 items and measures eagerness to seek the best knowledge in a given context, the courage to ask questions, and honesty and objectivity in inquiry. The critical thinking self-confidence construct has 10 items that measure trust in the soundness of one's reasoning processes. Finally, the maturity construct has 10 items that measure cognitive maturity and judiciousness in decision-making [11]. Kökdemir adapted this inventory, addressing cultural concerns in the Turkish version. Eight persons, including six psychologists, a simultaneous translator and the researcher himself translated the items Turkish and it was administered to 913 students in the faculty of economic and administrative sciences. Item-total score correlations were estimated and 19 items with correlations under 20 were eliminated from the scale. Factor analysis of the shortened scale found that five items had factor loadings lower than 32 and the items under the open-mindedness and maturity constructs were loaded on one construct. Finally 51 items with six constructs were kept in the scale. The reliability of the entire scale was 88. The reliability coefficients of the subscales ranged from 61 to 78.

In this study, this scale was administered to the nurses with 51 items in six constructs. The reliability of the entire scale was 76. The reliability coefficients of the subscales ranged from 61 to 75. The CCDTI scale and subscale Cronbach alpha values are shown in Table 1. Data were analyzed using SPSS 15.0 software (IBM Analytics) and were evaluated in terms of numbers, percentages, Reliability Statistics, ANOVA, Pearson's correlation, and Regression analysis.

Researchers	Years	Scale Total (α)	Truth-seeking (α)	Open-mindedness (α)	Analyticity (α)	Systematicity (α)	Self-confidence (α)	Inquisitiveness (α)
Facione, Facione and Giancarlo (n=267)	1998	0.92	0.71	0.73	0.72	0.74	0.78	0.80
Kökdemir (n=193)	2000	0.88	0.61	0.75	0.75	0.63	0.77	0.78
Topçu and Beşer (n=231)	2005	0.84	0.59	0.60	0.63	0.63	0.82	0.76
Dirimeşe (n=56)	2006	0.87	0.66	0.68	0.68	0.39	0.85	0.77
Yıldırım and Özsoy (n=78)	2010	0.90	0.70	0.73	0.68	0.68	0.78	0.76
This Study (n=40)	2012	0.81	0.70	0.64	0.73	0.63	0.85	0.76

Table 1: CCDTI scale and subscale Cronbach alpha values researchers.

Results

In this study, the mean age of nurses was 28.97 ± 5.56. Of the intensive care nurses, 45%, 30% and 25% had worked for 0-5, 6-10 and ≥ 11 years, respectively. Of the nurses, 5% graduated from a vocational school of health and 95% had bachelor's degrees. Of the participating nurses, 10% worked as a chief nurse and the rest worked as intensive care nurses. Of the nurses, 82.5% stated that they had intermediate socioeconomic status and 37.5% said they had attended different levels of training, respectively. This study determined that the nurses' mean score on the CCTDI was relatively low (190.90 ± 20.23) (Table 2). This study revealed that the nurses' scores on the truth-seeking, open-mindedness, analyticity, systematicity, self-confidence and inquisitiveness subscales were 21.50 ± 5.62, 36.95 ± 7.32, 50.90 ± 6.94, 19.32 ± 3.56, 27.75 ± 6.02, and 34.47 ± 6.00, respectively (Table 2).

	Frequency	Percent
Age Mean	28.97 ± 5.56	
Marital Status		
Married	20	50%
Single	20	50%
Education Status		
High School	3	7.5%
University	37	92.5%
Study Year		
0-5 years	18	45%
6-10 years	12	30%
11 and years above	10	25%

Socio-Economic Level		
Low	5	12.5%
Medium	33	82.50%
High	2	5%
Critical Thinking Different Levels of Trainings		
Yes	15	37.50%
No	25	62.50%
Total	40	100%

Table 2: Socio-demographic characteristics data, * column percentage.

The study did not find a statistically significant difference between the nurses' CCTDI mean scores when adjusted for age, working years, economic status or educational background (p>0.05).

Discussion

Critical thinking is fundamental to nursing practice. National nursing organizations, nurses and intensive care nurses in the workplace identify critical thinking disposition and skills as essential to competent nursing.

Nurses in intensive care units have always needed to be safe, competent and skilful practitioners who are able to make valid judgments concerning their patients' care. This is becoming increasingly difficult due to the ever-increasing complexity and sensitivity of most health care settings. Therefore, critical thinking needs to be a central and vital component of nurses' work in intensive care units.

The mean age of the participating intensive care nurses was 28.97 ± 5.56 years. Of these, 45%, 30% and 25% had worked for 0-5, 6-10 or ≥ 11 years, respectively. However, it was encouraging that 95% of the nurses had bachelor's degrees. Of the nurses, 10% worked as chief nurses and the rest worked as intensive care nurses. Of the nurses, 82.5% stated that they were of middle socioeconomic status, and 37.5% had attended different levels of training in critical thinking. The socio-demographic characteristics data are given in Table 2.

This study determined that the nurses' mean score on the CCTDI was relatively low (190.90 ± 20.23) (Table 3). In Turkey, other studies conducted with nurses, namely Kıranşal et al. [12], Eşer et al. [13], Arslan et al. [14], Yıldırım et al. [15] similarly found that nurses scored low in critical thinking dispositions and skills (198.57 ± 15.61, 191.01 ± 30.14, 200.08 ± 21.95 and 189.00 ± 18.21, for the four studies). Yıldırım et al. [15], Dirimeşe and Dicle [16], Yıldırım-Özeruz [17] similarly found that nurses scored low on critical thinking dispositions and skills [18-20] (Table 4). Ip et al. [21], Shin et al. [22], Topçu and Beşer [23] found medium-level scores in critical thinking dispositions and skills (Table 4).

	N	Minimum	Maximum	Mean	Std. Deviation
Scale Total	40	148,00	243,00	19,09,000	20,23,047
Truth-seeking	40	9,00	35,00	2,15,000	5,62,959
Open-mindedness	40	22,00	54,00	3,69,500	7,32,033
Analyticity	40	36,00	65,00	5,09,000	6,94,225
Systematicity	40	14,00	29,00	1,93,250	3,56,182
Self-confidence	40	14,00	40,00	2,77,500	6,02,878
Inquisitiveness	40	21,00	47,00	3,44,750	6,00,422

Table 3: CCDTI scale points.

Researchers using CCDTI	Country	Scale Total	Truth-seeking	Open-mindedness	Analyticity	Systematicity	self-confidence	Inquisitiveness
Ip et al. [21] (n=122)	China	264.70 ± 24.01	31.88 ± 24.01	31.88 ± 4.44	36.84 ± 4.92	38.30 ± 6.48	42.12 ± 6.60	38.30 ± 6.48
Shin et al. [22] (n=305)	China	263.20 ± 18.24	30.12 ± 4.06	36.91 ± 3.35	40.42 ± 4.09	35.70 ± 4.19	40.98 ± 5.12	44.64 ± 5.19
Topçu and Beşer [23] (n=231)	Turkey	267.30 ± 24.9	42.00 ± 6.95	46.25 ± 4.6	50.1 ± 4.1	46.8 ± 6.5	43.4 ± 6.1	48.65 ± 5.8
Dirimeşe and Dicle [16] (n=56)	Turkey	277.00 ± 19.7	44.0 ± 7.0	47.9 ± 5.9	48.8 ± 5.3	46.7 ± 4.8	41.4 ± 4.2	48.0 ± 5.5
Şenturan and Alpar [24] (n=1124)	Turkey	216.33 ± 24.82	26.11 ± 5.2	51.30 ± 8.5	46.52 ± 6.52	25.56 ± 4.47	27.49 ± 5.36	39.31 ± 6.81
Yıldırım [25] (n=78)	Turkey	207.26 ± 13.79	25.83 ± 3.81	43.45 ± 5.13	52.01 ± 5.62	20.31 ± 2.07	27.45 ± 4.48	33.61 ± 4.35
Yıldırım et al. [15]	Turkey	188.72 ± 20.71	21.43 ± 5.06	40.70 ± 6.38	50.77 ± 8.08	19.21 ± 3.21	27.84 ± 5.07	32.85 ± 5,85
This Study (2012) (n=40)	Turkey	190.90 ± 20.23	21.50 ± 5.62	36.95 ± 7.32	50.90 ± 6.94	19.32 ± 3.56	27.75 ± 6.02	34.47 ± 6.00

Table 4: Distribution of findings of studies that used CCDTI.

These findings are in line with those of the present study. Furthermore, Dirimeşe and Dicle [16] conducted a study that determined that nurses scored at an intermediate level in terms of critical thinking disposition (261.1 ± 23.4) In Turkey, nursing services are provided by nurses with different levels of education [18]. For this reason, strengthening nursing care services is much more important issue. According to numerous study findings, it is clear that nurses who are required to use critical thinking skills based on science are in need of strengthening these abilities.

Critical thinking is a cognitive activity that is a composite of knowledge, disposition, skills and attitudes. Intensive care nurses use critical thinking disposition and skills to deliver safe, competent nursing care. As part of problem-solving and decision-making processes, intensive care nurses collect and assess data to address intensive care patient problems.

This study revealed that nurses scored 21.50 ± 5.62, 36.95 ± 7.32, 50.90 ± 6.94, 19.32 ± 3.56, 27.75 ± 6.02, 34.47 ± 6.00 n the truth-seeking, open-mindedness, analyticity, systematicity, self-confidence and inquisitiveness subscales respectively (Table 3).

Critical thinking subscale scores obtained from studies by Eşer et al. [13], Şenturan and Alpar [24], Yıldırım et al. [15] show similarities with the present study findings.

As the results of both this and other studies show, nurses' critical thinking disposition scores are not satisfactory, indicating that nurses should be trained in this set of skills. It is necessary not only for nurses, but also for nursing students, to receive education about critical thinking from the moment they start their nursing education [4,23].

Critical thinking is required in intensive care nursing because of its increased responsibilities. In addition, clinical problem solving and decision-making are among the most crucial tasks intensive care nurses perform. Critical thinking and decision-making and problem-solving skills have been described as closely related [23,24].

Nowadays, intensive care nurses face a rapidly changing healthcare landscape, shifting student and patient demographics, an explosion of technology and the globalization of healthcare. Given the multiple financial constraints of managed care, the delivery of appropriate care remains one of the most complex issues in nursing today [15,25].

In the literature, it has been reported that critical thinking can be affected by individual and environmental factors [1,25]. In this study, a statistically significant difference among nurses' CCTDI mean scores by age, working years, economic status and educational backgrounds was not found ($p>0.05$). This study did obtain similar results to those of studies conducted by Eşer et al. [13], Yıldırım et al. [15].

Conclusion and Recommendations

This study found that the participating nurses' critical thinking disposition scores were at low levels. These results suggest that educational opportunities should be provided both inside and outside institutions, that nurses should be encouraged to participate, and that improving their abilities will afford nurses greater opportunities to apply their critical thinking disposition and skills.

Intensive care nurses, nurses, nurse educators and scholars should engage in research about how students learn to apply critical thinking in clinical and intensive care practices. Currently, nurse educators and scholars know very little about how the use of critical thinking in clinical settings is learned.

Further studies are needed in order to more fully explore the meaning of critical thinking in nursing. Future nursing research should focus on the following areas of interest.

1. Exploring the impact of culture on critical thinking.
2. Nurses should be provided training in critical thinking and the impact of this explored.
3. The relationship between happiness and critical thinking.
4. The relationship between depression and critical thinking.
5. Studies involving many nurse scholars should be conducted in order to determine the advisability of developing a consensus definition of critical thinking for nursing. Future studies should focus on identifying the core components of critical thinking in order to develop flexible, usable structures that explain critical thinking, but do not limit nurses to narrow interpretations of the concept.

Finally, future studies should explore the impact of transcultural nursing experiences on critical thinking dispositions and skills. They might also examine which aspects of transcultural experiences have the greatest impact on critical thinking, and which facets of critical thinking are most affected by transcultural experiences.

Study Limitations

The study's limitation was that it was conducted in only one institution and in intensive care units.

References

1. Norris S (1985) Synthesis of research on critical thinking. Educational Leadership.
2. Facione PA (1990) Critical thinking: A statement of expert consensus for purposes of educational assessment and instructions. Research Findings and Recommendations, The California Academic Press, Millbrae, CA.
3. Katoaka-Yahiro M, Saylor CA (1994) A critical thinking model for nursing judgement. J Nurs Educ 33: 351-356.
4. Özkahraman S, Yıldırım B (2011) An overview of critical thinking in nursing and education. Am Int J Contemp Res 1: 190-196.
5. Yıldırım-ozeruz B (2010) Applied approach to critical thinking in nursing, Özsoy S.A. (eds.,) Tuna Matbaacılık, Aydın, 41-53.
6. Akansel N (2004) Investigation of the noise effects on patients in intensive care. Ege Üniversitesi Sağlık Bilimleri Enstitüsü Yayınlanmamış Doktora Tezi, İzmir.
7. Khorshid L, Demir Y (2006) Communication problems with patients during mechanical ventilation treatment in intensive care unit. İzmir Tepecik Education Hospital Magazine 16: 47-54.
8. Swinny B (2010) Assessing and developing criticalthinking skills in the intensive care unit. Crit Care Nurs Quart 33: 12-19.
9. Kaya H (1998) Critical reasoning power in University students. Istanbul University Health Sciences Institute, Unpublished Doctorate Thesis, Istanbul.
10. Hicks FD, Merritt SL, Elstein AS (2003) Critical thinking and clinical decision making in critical care nursing: A pilot study. Heart and Lung 32: 169-80.
11. Kökdemir D (2003) Decision making and problem solving in uncertainty, Ankara University Social Sciences University. Unpublished Doctorate Thesis, Ankara.
12. Kıranşal N, Adana F, Erdağı S (2006) Investigation of the effective factors of critical thinking tendency in nurses 42: 1-5.
13. Eşer İ, Khorshid L, Demir Y (2007) Investigation of critical thinking tendency and factors affecting intensive care nurses. C U J Nurs School 11: 13-22.
14. Arslan GG, Demir Y, Eşer İ, (2007) Investigation of factors affecting the trend of critical thinking in nurses 4th International and 11th National Nursing Congress Congress Book, Ankara.
15. Yıldırım B, Özkahraman Ş, Ersoy S (2012) Investigation of critical thinking disposition in nurses working in public hospitals. Int J Bus Hum Tecn 2: 61-67.
16. Dirimeşe E, Dicle A (2006) An investigation of critical thinking trends of nurses and student nurses. Dokuz Eylül University Institute of Health Sciences Surgical Diseases Nursing Unpublished Master Thesis, İzmir.
17. Yıldırım-Özeruz B (2011) Critical thinking in health professionals. Nobel Tıp Kitabevleri, İstanbul.
18. Allen PA (1992) Critical thinking behaviors in baccalaurate degree, associate degree and diploma prepared graduate nurses. Duquesne University, Unpublished Master Thesis.
19. Burnard P (1995) Learning human skills. Oxford: Butterworth-Heinermann, Ltd.
20. Akınoğlu O (2003) Critical thinking as a training value. Values Education Magazine 1: 7-26.
21. Ip WY, Lee D, Lee I, Chau, JPC, Wootton YSY, et al. (2000) Disposition towards critical thinking: A study of Chinese undergraduate nursing students. J Adv Nurs 32: 84-90.
22. Shin K, Jung DY, Shin S, Kim MS (2006) Critical thinking dispositions and skills of senior nursing students in associate, baccalaureate and RN-to_BSN programs. J Nurs Educ 45: 233-237.
23. Topçu S, Beşer A (2005) Analysis of critical thinking trends of students of Dokuz Eylül University School of Nursing. II Active Education Congress DEÜ Publications, Izmir, pp: 394-409.
24. Şenturan L, Alpar ŞE (2008) Critical thinking in nursing students. Cumhuriyet University Nursing School Magazine 12: 22-30.
25. Yıldırım B (2010) The effect of skill-based critical thinking teaching on the development of critical thinking in student nurses. Ege University Institute of Health Sciences Public Health Nursing USA, Thesis Advisor Prof. Dr. Süheyla Altuğ Özsoy, Published PhD Thesis.

13

How Nurses in Hospital in Vietnam Learn to Improve their Own Nursing Competency: An Ethnographic Study

Do Thi Ha and **Khanitta Nuntaboot**

Faculty of Nursing, Khon Kaen University, Vietnam

Corresponding author: Do Thi Ha, Student of Doctor of Philosophy in Nursing, Faculty of Nursing, Khon Kaen University, Thailand and Lecturer of Faculty of Nursing and Medical Technology, Pham Ngoc Thach University, Vietnam, E-mail: dohapnt@gmail.com

Abstract

Background: Competency affects several aspects of the quality of nursing care and has a significant contribution to the patient outcomes. There exists little up to date information concerning nursing profession as well as how nurses employing in clinical settings in Vietnam learn to improve their own competencies.

Objectives: To investigate the ways Vietnamese nurses practicing in clinical settings have learned to improve their own competencies.

Methods: A qualitative study, ethnographic method, comprised of the participant-observation, in-depth interview, and focus group discussion with multidisciplinary groups of nurses employing in Cho Ray Hospital, Vietnam, managers/administrators, nurse teachers, other health care personnel which derived from purposeful sampling technique. Content analysis was used to analyze the data.

Findings: The two ways of learning in order to develop competencies among nurses were identified by the participants through the data collection in this study, including formal and informal learning. Nurses have received their formal training in nursing education programs in nursing schools after graduation to upgrade their nursing professional level was identified as formal learning. However, in the situation of nursing education in Vietnam, there has been rare of formal nursing education programs in bachelor level and higher, informal learning included continuing nursing education, learning from working experience, learning from daily reflective process, and coaching and mentoring was a vital learning strategy for nurses to apply in order to enhance their competencies.

Conclusion: The findings from this study provide valuable information and understanding of the ways Vietnamese nurses working in hospital context have learned to improve individual competencies. It would assist to establish an effectively and appropriately strategy in an effort of enhancing nursing competency among nurses in Vietnam.

Keywords: Competency development; In-depth interview; Nurses; Vietnam

Introduction

Across a broad field of care, health issues, health care needs as well as the current health care system and nursing workforce issues stipulate that nurses be capable of performing optimally and assuming mounting responsibilities. Throughout the course of providing care to patients, nurses must be proficient in adjusting, applying critical thinking and problem-solving skills and corresponding efficiently with multidisciplinary team members. For nurses to be able to meet the complex blend of nursing practice, clinical nurses need to further acquire various knowledge and skills, beyond the focus of basic knowledge and technical foundation skills that they have been educated and trained on during their nursing education courses, in order to become competent individuals [1].

According to literature review, previous studies have identified that nurses practicing in clinical settings apply numerous of strategies in order to improve their individual competencies [2,3]. Nurses use both formal and informal learning strategies to enhance their capacities [3].

Merriam and colleagues mentioned that formal learning takes place in educational institutions, leading to degrees or credits [4]. This is relative to nurses receiving their formal training in nursing education programs. Marsick and Watkins suggested that formal learning is typically institutionally sponsored, classroom-based, and highly structured [4].

On the other hand, informal learning refers to the "experiences of everyday living from which we learn something" [3]. Marsick and Watkins proposed that informal learning may occur in institutions, but is not typically classroom-based or highly structured, and control of the learning rests primarily in the hands of the learner. It is typically experiential and non-institutionally based, rather a planned learning opportunity [4]. In a qualitative research, Sharoff interviewed 10 nurses employing in hospital to explore how experienced certified holistic nurses learned to become competent holistic nurse practitioners. The findings showed that the nurses used informal learning strategies including learning from experience, from self-reflection, mentoring, or learning from colleagues and others to help them achieve expectation competency [1].

In Vietnam, nurses encompass the largest group of healthcare personnel employed in the health sector [5]. Undoubtedly, they exhibit a vital role in providing health care services to clients. Unfortunately, a large number of Vietnamese nurses possess just a secondary level in nursing education accounting for around 70%, so they work in hospitals and clinical setting as workers and focus on medical techniques [5,6]. In addition, the traditional nursing in Vietnam is very technical and task-oriented; extremely focused on completion of a goal. The health care tasks of both physicians and nurses in clinical settings are focused entirely on the disease process [7]. Meanwhile, holistic nursing, applying in the national level, affords nurses the opportunities go to beyond this focus by reconnecting to self and others on a deeper level [8]. These require nurses in Vietnam need to develop their individual competencies in order to meet the requirements.

Over the years, in order to stay with the changing pattern of diseases and increasing of health care needs in Vietnam, the Vietnamese health care sector has strengthened and applied model equipment, and high technologies in terms of diagnosis, treatment and caring for patients. Indeed, the health care service has achieved certain successfulness; nonetheless, it has been faced with many challenges [5]. These require health care professionals including nurses in Vietnam to be well prepared and competent so as to serve the health care needs and demands of population.

At present, there are three main educational preparations for nurses in Vietnam, including secondary nursing education (two years), college nursing education (three years), and baccalaureate nursing education (four years), in which baccalaureate degree still remains limited. Recently introduced were post-graduation educations in nursing such as specialty level I and master degrees; however, still rarely [5]. There exists little up to date information concerning nursing competencies in Vietnam as well as how nurses acquire the needed knowledge, skills and attitudes in order to foster their proficiencies.

The purpose of this study is to provide an understanding of strategies that nurses practicing in clinical settings in Vietnam have applied in order to develop their individual competencies. Understanding how nurses develop their competencies in particular cultural and social contexts in Vietnam would indeed benefit development and innovating strategies to improve nurse competencies in Vietnam; thereby having a positive effect in enhancing quality of nursing care.

Research Methodology

Design: A qualitative research with the ethnographic approach was selected in this study by allowing the voice and experience of Vietnamese nurses practicing in clinical settings to be heard, thusly providing opportunity to actually truly discover how nurses develop their own competencies. Qualitative research methods have become increasingly important as models of inquiry among various disciplines such as sociology, psychology, education and nursing [7]. The purpose of this approach is not to test or verify researcher hypotheses on a given topic; rather, it is to obtain a deep understanding of participants' perception and experience and the meaning they take from that experience. Qualitative research is used for the understanding of what lies behind the phenomena as well as providing intricate details of the phenomena that are difficult to convey quantitatively [8]. The purpose of this study was to obtain a succinct understanding of the ways that Vietnamese nurses practicing in clinical settings have learned to improve their own competencies. By applying the qualitative approach, the researcher believed that rich and accurate information with regards the research topic would arise.

Setting and sample: Derived from purposive sampling, there were twenty-four participants who participated in this study. Of these participants, there were sixteen nurses as the key informants who were working in the clinical units in the Hospital with at least two years of experience in nursing profession. Other participants included nurse managers, administrators, teachers, and medical doctors. The study was conducted at Cho Ray Hospital, one of the two biggest national general hospitals in Vietnam under the Ministry of Health of Vietnam which is located in District 5 of Ho Chi Minh City.

Ethical considerations: Ethical approval was both obtained from the Khon Kaen University Ethics Committee in Human Research and the Research Division of Cho Ray Hospital. An information sheet, invitation letter, and consent form were sent to all participants directly with a clearly explanation about purpose, methods, procedures, potential risks and benefits of the study. Participation was voluntary and written informed consent was obtained or verbally consents. Participants were free to withdraw from the study at any time.

Data collection: Data had been collected during seven months starting in 2015. After obtaining permission for collecting data, the researcher entered the sites for establishing a rapport and developing a trusting relationship with nurses and other healthcare personnel in the setting. The data were gathered through participant-observations, in-depth interviews and focus group discussions. The researcher accompanied the nurse participants during their working shifts in the hospital as well as some other relevant activities outside the field to observe and learn how they acquire knowledge and skills in order to enhance their proficiencies.

There were twenty-two individual in-depth interviews and three focus group discussions were produced. Each interview participants in this study gave one to two times of interview, lasting from 30 to 45 min for this session. The interviews took place at a venue convenient to the participants in an effort of increasing the convenience and comfort to the participants as well as the successfulness of the interview. Each focus group discussion was composed of four to six members. Many of these participants had been involved in the in-depth interview situation before. The researcher acted as moderator to direct the participants regarding the topic to be discussed and to ensure that all voices of the participants to be heard. All the interviews were digitally recorded, with the participants' permission, and supplemented with detailed take notes. The research participants were asked to describe the ways nurses develop their competencies.

Data analysis: Content analysis was applied to analyze the data. The analysis and synthesis process were immediately conducted at the completion of each participant-observation, individual interview and focus group discussion session. For The data gathered from in-depth interview and focus group discussion, the tape recorders were heard and transcribed carefully. All of the transcriptions were then read several times and the key words or terms throughout the transcription were highlighted and noted. The coding then was made. The final emerging themes and categories were established.

Findings

The research participants indicated using formal and/or informal learning strategies to help nurses to improve competencies. The strategies of development competencies among nurses are presented in Figure 1.

Formal learning

The nurse participants described that they have used a variety of learning situations to foster their learning process. Many of them have chosen upgrading nursing level by attending higher nursing education programs in nursing schools, identified as formal learning. The programs included secondary level; associate degree; bachelor degree both full time and part-time education; specialty level I in nursing, master and doctoral degree (planning in the future).

"I attended the bachelor of nursing to improve my competence. Before, when studied in secondary level, I had just been learned about nursing technical skills. I could not understand the mechanisms. However, when I studied bachelor degree I understood more about this. When we understand the mechanisms we will know the way to care for clients better". (ID 03)

Meanwhile, the nurse participant (ID 09) expressed that besides gaining nursing knowledge from his formal learning program, his critical thinking, emotional control, or his compassion manner have been also improved and changed towards positively:

"I have learned from this course (bachelor of nursing) a lot. Before attending this course, I sometimes have trouble in controlling my emotion. However, by this course, I have changed my mind and my emotion control toward positively. I understand the patients more and especially improve my communication skills".

In the same line, a female nurse expressed how positively shift in her life through her formal learning course (ID 12):

"I felt so happy during my course (bachelor nursing course)...There I had many new friends, much better than when I just worked in my institution. Before joining this class, I rarely smile...You see, now, I smile very often. It's so nice. My competency has been also improved significantly..."

"We encouraged and sent them (the primary or secondary nurses) to nursing school to upgrade their nursing levels to be higher...that was an important way to help them to develop their capacities...Just secondary level or less...could not care for patients effectively". (Mentioned the nurse manager ID 22)

"I wish I have opportunity to upgrade my nursing level from secondary to bachelor and higher. Now, I am in secondary level... insufficient knowledge and skills to care of patients...". (Stated the secondary nurse ID 14)

Although there has been limited of nursing education programs in bachelor level and higher in the situation of nursing education in Vietnam currently which results nurses lacking of opportunities to upgrade their nursing certificates as well as competencies, most participants in this study concerned that formal learning was an essential strategy to help nurses achieving their expectation competencies.

Informal learning

The majority of learning opportunities that the research participants identified were informal learning. In the situation of nursing education in Vietnam, which have been rare of formal nursing education programs in bachelor level and higher; informal learning was an essential learning strategy for nurses to use in order to enhance their competencies. There were several types of informal learning strategy identified by the research participants included continuing nursing education; learning with and through others (colleagues, role models, mentors, patients); learning from experience and self-reflection process; learning from mentoring or coaching; and self-study.

Continuing nursing educations, as learned from this study, included both in-service education, including both hospital and department levels, and out-service education, such as attending short training courses in nursing schools, workshops or conferences.

"I attended short courses that trained for nurses held by the hospital. In my department has also established continuing education classes trained for nurses of my department. We could propose the topics that we thought needed. Such as, the topic: reading ECG. We have been trained how to read an ECG. When perform an ECG for patient, we could recognize the informal signals in order to inform the doctors promptly...that is the ways we develop our competencies". (ID 04)

Developing competencies by attending some particular patient education projects was also shared by the participants:

"We (nurses) have attended the front-line supporting projects...We have been trained through Face-to-face program. We are provided tablet computers which had been already installed needed programs by the doctors and we have been trained to address these. We then applied acquired knowledge and skills to provide education to our patients directly and answer for all concerns from patients. This program improved our knowledge and skills very much...We are very confident when educate to patients and their relatives. Be confident front of patients and colleagues...enhance our clinical knowledge and skills..." (ID 07)

Not only in-service training, out-service is also one of the important strategies that have been applied in order to enhance competencies among nurses practicing in the hospital.

"...We send them (nurses) to attend specific training programs, attend workshops and conferences that relevant to their field to improve their competencies of knowledge and skills..." (Stated the administrator medical doctor ID 13)

The research participants also identified and explained how the process of learning with and through significant others, including role models, colleagues, mentors, patients as well as significant others, assisted their improving competencies. Interestingly, not all participants experienced the same way of learning with and have been learned by others as a strategy of enhancing nurses' capacities.

"I have learned from my colleagues...In many cases, I could not recognize these issues; however, others (medical doctors, nurses) they could recognize. I learned from their experiences. It's very significant for my competency development". (ID 09)

"I have learned from the nurse seniors...the knowledge and skills that I have gained from nursing school were not enough. Because each working environment is particular ...not the same...I mean different diseases and issues. For example, I have learned from the seniors in my department who are experts in taking care of patients after skeletal surgery...how to recognize complications and solve difficult solutions" (ID 24)

Working in team was identified by all nurse participants as one of the most effectively strategies to enhance their competencies.

"...worked with others in a health care team would enhance my capacity quickly. If you just depend on your experiences without collaborating with other colleagues your competency would be improved slowly and you might not recognized your faults, you could not learn from other experiences. I have learned from my working in team with other a lot; such as how to organized the activities scientifically, how to communicate with others effectively, how to work in a group with others. I also observed experienced doctor's performances to learn from him because he was an expert. I discussed with team members to find the appropriate way to care for patients... It's the most important strategy to improve our nursing competency". (ID 08)

Besides learning with and through colleagues in the same working facility, nurses also learned with and through colleagues from other hospitals or institutions:

"I often went to other hospitals to exchange experiences with my friends (the nurses working in others medical organizations). We went to coffee shops to enjoy and discuss together regarding our concerns, including sharing updated nursing information and experiences. I am very interested in this type of activities. We could share and learn from each other".

Role model and mentoring were identified as significant figures in the journey of nurses of seeking knowledge, skills, and positive attitude as a good nurse.

"...You see, before working with them (the nurse seniors) I thought that I were a good nurse because I took care of patients with all my heart and so carefully. However, when I had opportunities working together with them I found that I was not good enough as my feeling. They took care of patients much better than me, more careful than what I did. They loved patients very much. I admired them very much and I love them. They gradually became my mirrors, became shining examples to me to follow...as role models. You see, they have brought knowledge, skills, caring as well as loving to me. I have learned... learned a lot of significant things through these role models". (ID 02)

Attentively, numerous nurse participants described that the patients were the best ones who brought them knowledge, skills and significant experiences in their journey of enhancing competencies. The capacities of nurses would not be improved without learning from patients and family relatives. Furthermore, learning through experience and self-reflection were also significant strategies to improve competencies that the research participants experienced. They have learned from daily nursing activities, from particular situation, during taking care of patients and contacting with patients and others. The participants expressed that starting with the basic knowledge that they have been equipped in nursing schools, combined with experiences that they have learned every day at the field of nursing practice, needed knowledge and skills would be formed.

"I have learned from all my patients that I have cared for. I have learned from their issues, from the diseases or illnesses that they got. I have learned from the patients' complaints or even they argued me, because from their complaints I would reflect myself and investigated the causes that made them to be unsatisfied...the patients and the relatives were the most significant teachers who improved my competencies". (ID 04)

In order to improve competency, self-reflection was an important manner that the research participants described.

"I have improved my competency by listening to others' comments and self-reflecting on this in order to do it better". (ID 19)

"...I have learned from my working...self-reflection and learned from these. Even I learned from my mistakes. I reflected myself on that faults and learned from those...and I would do better". (ID 09)

"...If you (nurses) just wait for help or supporting from others such as medical doctors or experienced nurses, it would not foster your capacity. You needs also self-reflect on your daily activities..." (ID 21)

Self-learning was another strategy that all participant concerned and applied in order to develop their individual competencies. Most of the participants indicated that, in the situation of overload working among nurses in Vietnam, they could not wait from outside supporting. Indeed, they should self-prepare in an effort of raising their competencies.

"We are so busy during our working shift...In some cases, I have questions however, I could not answer at that time, no one could help me to answer my concerns at the busy time. I then investigated myself by searching information from internet or reading books..." (ID 10)

The experiences shared from participants in the individual interview sessions were also supported by the data of focus group discussion and participant-observation sessions.

"In the context of lacking of bachelor and higher levels of nursing education in Vietnam, attending the short training course is essential to foster nurses' competencies". (FDG participant ID 17)

"...Burnt out...overload working...Not enough time to self-reflect on our work at working place, Just try to finish our tasks. So self-study, such as at home or every time we have opportunities, is a significant way of improving our knowledge and skills" (FDG participant ID 11)

During the fieldwork, the researcher had opportunities to company the nurse participants attending workshops and some particular short course training programs. Indicating that, informal learning was an important strategy of competency development among nurses practicing in clinical setting in Vietnam (Figure 1).

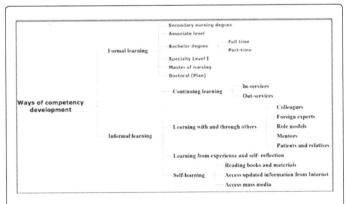

Figure 1: The ways of competency development among nurses.

With a slot of rich information derived from participant-observations, in-depth interviews, and focus group discussions, the journey of competency development among nurses included both formal and informal learning strategies. Although there has been limited of bachelor as well as post graduate nursing education programs in Vietnam, all participants in this study viewed that formal learning was the trend and significant strategy that helped nurses to acquire advanced knowledge and skills. Furthermore, informal learning, including continuing nursing education, learning from working experience, learning from daily reflective process, and coaching and mentoring, was an important and indispensable way that the nurses applied during their journey of competency development.

Discussion

The methods of improving nurses' proficiencies, as identified by the participants, included both formal and/or informal learning strategies to help them improve their individuals' competencies. Attending higher nursing education programs in nursing schools was identified as formal learning that nurses used to satisfy both qualification and competency requirements. In the situation of nursing education in Vietnam, which have been rare of formal nursing education programs in bachelor level and higher; informal learning was an essential learning strategy for nurses to use in order to enhance their competencies. The participants described that they have used a variety of learning situations to foster their capabilities that were identified as informal learning strategy included continuing nursing education, with both types of in-service as well as out-service; learning with and through others such as colleagues, role models, mentors, patients; learning from daily working experiences and self-reflection process; learning from mentoring or coaching, and self-study. Informal learning is an essential learning strategy for nurses to use in order to gain knowledge, skills and attitudes that will foster their capabilities.

Knowledge generated from this study was supported by the findings of previous studies. Nurses practicing in clinical settings used both formal and informal learning strategies to enhance their capabilities [2]. In the study of Sharoff, the findings revealed that as the adult learners, nurse practitioners employing in clinical environments focused on using informal learning strategy to help them reach optimal competency [1]. The informal learning strategy included various methods that facilitated the nurse practitioners to achieve expectation competencies. They acquired advanced nursing knowledge and skills through learning from their daily working experiences, learning from self-reflection on their practices as a nurse or clinical situations. The nurses also improved their proficiencies through mentoring, or learning from working together with colleagues and other significant healthcare personnel [1].

In the recent decades, Vietnam has opened the geopolitical boundaries to reinforce the relations with many countries. Socioeconomic in Vietnam recently has been dramatically improved. The health care needs have been increased quickly. The Ministry of Health of Vietnam has begun to concern and encourage as well as require nurses to advance their qualifications and capacities in order to response to the increasing of the health care needs [6]. These have been one of the reasons encouraged nurses to improve their individual competencies by applying formal learning strategy to meet the requirements.

Informal learning is enhanced when individuals are proactive, creative, and engage in critical reflection [4]. These characteristics were identified in this study as needed requirements to become competent nurses. Learning is a personal active process that entails an integration of knowledge and doing [9,10]. Nurses engaged in this personal activity by utilizing various strategies and then incorporating that knowledge into an action in order to learn to become competent individuals. Wan also indicated that learning from experience involves

changing both what we do and how we see thing [11]. The competent nurses need to be able to learn effective behaviors and gain meaningful interpretations of the experience because performance is the integration of knowing and doing [10], a learning where the nurse is actively engaged and involved. Furthermore, throughout self-reflection, nurses reflect upon the experience to develop an interpretation and understanding of the experience and then generate new skills, knowledge and attitudes that are brought into each new challenge and situation [11]. According to Boud et al. (2013), what we learn from experience does not simply add new information, but transforms our way of experiencing [12].

Throughout process of interpersonal interaction with other was identified as one of the significant strategies the nurses has applied to enhance their capacities. This interpersonal relationship could take the form of learning with and through others, including colleagues, role models, mentors as well as patients and family care takers. Role models and mentoring were important to the nurses in their journey of self-competency completing. In an atmosphere of care and support, the role of mentor is to challenge student to examine their conceptions of self and the world and to formulate new, more develop perspectives [3]. In order for nurses to become competent health personnel, needs for a connection with other significant individuals were concerned. Mentoring requires that both mentor and learner is critically reflective. Mentors who are able to critically reflect on their own experiences and learn from them are best able to model critical reflection in their mentoring interactions. Nurses intuitively seek out relationship with others, especially experienced health care personnel such as physicians or senior nurses [13].

In order for nurses practicing in clinical settings to improve their competencies, a variety of learning strategies they have applied. In addition to continuing learning both in-service and out-services and learn from and through from others, learning from daily working experiences and self-reflection process as well as self-study have been used. Strategies of establishing a variety of nursing education and training programs for nurses to develop their nursing competencies are implicated. Furthermore, facilitating nurses on their journey of enhancing nursing capacities is needed.

Limitation and Recommendation

The main limitation of this study is that the study was undertaken in the context of only one national general public hospital. The contexts, working environments or nurses' characteristics as well as the strategies of competency development among nurses practicing in other clinical settings in Vietnam such as specialty hospitals, provincial or district hospitals, private facilities, and etc. might have some differences from the studied hospital. It is recommended that further study should be included nurses in other working environments and across settings of the country. The knowledge generated helps further the understanding of significant ways that nurses practicing in clinical settings in specific socio-political and cultural contexts in Vietnam to develop their individual competencies. The appropriate strategies regarding the development of competencies among nurses practicing in clinical settings should be considered.

Acknowledgement

This paper was part of the research program conducted by Do Thi Ha in the fulfilment of a PhD degree in Nursing at Khon Kaen University, Thailand under the supervisor of Associate Professor Dr.

Khanitta Nuntaboot. The researcher thanks all the participants who participated in the study and all persons who facilitated made this research possible.

References

1. Sharoff LA (2006) Qualitative study of how experienced certified holistic nurses learn to become competent practitioners. J Holist Nurs 24: 116-124.

2. Sirotnik M (2006) Continuing competence in nursing: A study of issues and perceptions. A dissertation submitted of University of Toronto.

3. Merriam SB, Caffarella RS, Baumgartner LM (2012) Learning in adulthood: A comprehensive guide. John Wiley and Sons.

4. Marsick V, Watkins K (2015) Informal and incidental learning in the workplace. Routledge. Routledge: Reissue edition.

5. Ministry of Health [MOH] (2015) Kế hoạch phát triển nhân lực trong hệ thống khám bệnh, chữa bệnh giai đoạn 2015–2020.

6. Jones PS, O'Toole MT, Hoa N, Chau TT, Muc PD (2000) Empowerment of nursing as a socially significant profession in Vietnam. Journal of Nursing Scholarship 32: 317-321.

7. Leininger MM (1985) Qualitative research methods in nursing. Saunders.

8. Strauss AL, Corbin JM (1990) Basics of qualitative research: Grounded theory procedures and techniques, Sage Publications.

9. MOH (2016). Báo cáo chung tổng quan ngành y tế (jahr) năm 2015.

10. Hutchings P, Wutzdorff A (1988) Experiential learning across the curriculum: Assumptions and principles. New Directions for Teaching and Learning 35: 5-19.

11. Wan KE (2015) Learning to learn from experience, SUNY Press.

12. Boud D, Keogh R, Walker D (2013) Reflection: Turning experience into learning, Routledge.

13. Zachary LJ (2011) The mentor's guide: Facilitating effective learning relationships, John Wiley and Sons.

14

Implantation of Adult Stem Cells in Patients with Heart Disease: Clinical Practice Implications for Nurses

Tereza Cristina Guimaraes Felippe[1] and Deyse Conceicao Santoro[2*]

[1]Coordinator of the Heart Failure and Cardiac Transplantation of the National Institute of Cardiology / Rio de Janeiro, Brazil

[2]Department of Medical Surgical EEAN / UFRJ, Brazil

*Corresponding author : Deyse Conceicao Santoro, PhD in Nursing Cardiovascular from USP, Associate Professor, Department of Medical Surgical EEAN / UFRJ, Brazil; E-mail: deysesantoro@yahoo.com.br

Abstract

This is a systematic review that aims to identify scientific publications in databases that cover the bone marrow-derived adult stem cells implantation in heart disease patient with changes in ejection fraction. For the study were used the databases LILACS, MEDLINE, Cochrane, Embase, CINAHL, PubMed and Ovid. In the five eligible trials with 279 patients, bone marrow – derived adult stem cells implantation indicates that there is statistical significance, although the number of studies are not conclusive for expressive statements to allow inferences about the effectiveness of the outcome. Based on the results we point out that the nurse should be focused on promoting adherence to treatment through conventional education measures.

Keywords: Nurse; Cardiology; Stem Cells; Systematic review

Background

Heart diseases are considered one of the major risk factors for deaths in the population, both in developed and in those in underdevelopment. Most patients with heart disease, when they survive this health problem, evolve to a heart failure frame (HF), which reduces considerably the quality of life of these patients [1].

Despite recent advances in health, in Brazil, the main cause of heart failure is acute or chronic ischemic heart disease associated with hypertension, therefore, in many cases, patients do not respond to conventional treatments, and justified the growing search for new researches associated with the HF treatment [2]. Cell therapy is an innovative idea, with a huge perspective to contribute to the acute and chronic heart diseases treatment, to improve the heart muscle performance. From several studies of various specialties, cardiology studies have developed from stem cells, which are a promising research area in the cardiac muscle regeneration [3].

To address the care of nurses to patients with cardiovascular disease who are undergoing experimental treatment with adult stem cells, it is necessary to have knowledge of research currently in progress with bone marrow-derived adult stem cells implantation in these patients.

Given that premise, the study question: "What is shown by the scientific publications about bone marrow derived - adult stem cells implantation in heart disease patients with changes in ejection fraction (EF)?

Objectives

The paper aims to identify through evidence found in scientific publications the use of bone marrow derived - adult stem cells in a heart disease patient with changes in EF

Methods

This is a systematic review.

Work Plan

Sample

Were randomized controlled trials that address the patient with cardiomyopathy underwent CT-MO implantation published until March - December 2009.

Identification and selection of articles

Inclusion criteria

- Participant: adult cardiomyopathy patients with ejection fraction below 50%.
- Intervention: Therapy with bone marrow derived – intracoronary or intramyocardial adult stem cells implantation.
- Outcomes: ejection fraction.

Exclusion criteria

- The use of stem cells which were cultured prior to implantation and use of cell stimulating factors.
- Follow-up less than 06 months.
- Use of stem cells combined with coronary artery bypass grafting.
- methodological quality according to the Jadad scale less than 3 points.

Search strategy and identification of studies

Search strategy for studies: We used the Lilacs, SciELO, Pub Med / Medline, Embase, Cochrane Register of Controlled Trials (Evidence Portal), and OVID CINAHL databases from 2000 to 2009.

Terms used: standardized by the Medical Subject Heading (MESH) and Descriptors in Health Sciences (MeSH). The descriptor Stem cells were combined using the Boolean operator AND with the following terms: heart failure, acute myocardial infarction, controlled clinical trial, and bone marrow. Terms in Portuguese and English language were applied. For each database the following filters were used: title, subject, and type of publication (Figure 1)

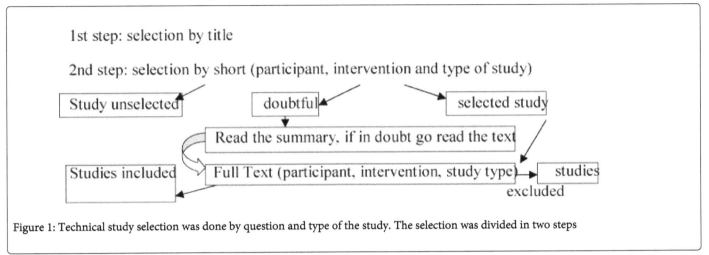

Figure 1: Technical study selection was done by question and type of the study. The selection was divided in two steps

Each study was assessed independently by two reviewers and the inclusion decision was by consensus based on the inclusion criteria and methodological quality of the Jadad scale. To systematize the analysis of the studies quality, a form for data collection with the following vestments was created: general information (title, year of publication, country of origin, language of publication, source of publication), eligibility data (criteria inclusion), methodological data (type of study, sample number, quantity of injected cells, numbers of centers, follow-up assessment, type of test used to assess ejection fraction and value of the Jadad scale) and outcome (value of the fraction ejection before and after stem cells administration in experimental and control groups).

Analysis

Data analysis was obtained by meta-analysis. The meta-analysis aims to combine the results of each study overall effect of the intervention, enabling the analysis of sources of heterogeneity. Data extracted from the studies were analyzed using STATA (version 11.0). Categorical variables were described as counts and the number and proportion as mean and standard deviation when normally distributed, and median and interquartile range in other cases. Effect measures used were the difference and the standardized difference between the experimental group and the control, modification of ejection fraction compared to baseline values. For the analysis of the standardized difference the g Hedges estimator and its standard error were calculated by the formula described by Hedges and Olkin. For each outcome random-effects meta-analysis by the method of DerSimonian and Laird was performed, weighted by the variance inverse, the result of which was exposed visually through graphic forest. The degree of heterogeneity between studies was assessed by Cochran Q test and I-squared.

Results

In total 2081 studies identified, 05 studies were selected by reviewers. The total number of studies were excluded in 2076, 106 of these are recurrent and 1962 are out of the inclusion criteria (such as animal studies, studies in phase I and II non-randomized). Besides these, we had 08 abstracts in other languages (06 Chinese and 02 German), which were not possible to retrieve the full articles when asked to Bireme and COMUT (the library UFRJ), because these journals are not registered.

Presentation of studies

Methodological quality

The JADAD scale was used for analysis of the studies and those who received score 4 points were selected.

Characterization of the population

The main clinical characteristics were similar between experimental and control group underwent percutaneous coronary intervention with improvement of blood flow in the coronary arteries and the participants were randomized three days after the intervention. Both groups had risk factors (RF) for coronary heart disease and average age between the two groups was 58 years.

Description of studies

The studies have diverse origins, despite having in common the same etiology-acute myocardial infarction.

Among the identified imaging studies that stratify the value of ejection fraction, echocardiography (Simpson's method) was used in two studies. The SPECT (Single Photon Emission Tomography / Computed Tomography single photon emission) was another imaging test used in two studies to evaluate the FE, and cardiac Magnetic Resonance (MR) was used in one study. Only the Dill study [4] was up longer than six months, making it as relevant to the management of treatment measures in an attempt to prevent remodeling cardiac. The Lund study [5] was that presented a higher number of participants in a single center. Mononuclear cells were used for implantation in four studies, as mononucleated cells characterized by being the primary portion among bone marrow cells and progenitor cells are the most common type of adult stem cells (Table 1).

Study	Year	Origin	Etiology	Exam	Center	Follow	Sample	Type of cells	Number (n16)
Lunde	2006	Norway	AMI	ECHO	only	6	100	mononucleate	68
Meluzin	2007	Czech Republic	AMI	SPECT	only	6	40	mononucleate	100
Dill	2009	Germany	AMI	MRI	multi	12	54	progenitor	100
Yao	2008	China	AMI	ECHO	only	6	47	mononucleate	120
Piepoli	2009	Italy	AMI	SPECT	only	6	38	mononucleate	418

Table 1: Description of studies

Description of Ejection Fraction Values

Studies with the primary outcome assessment of global left ventricular function from the EF evaluation and in both control and experimental groups were not statistically significant when compared to other outcomes, but their results highlight that there is statistical significance when the experimental group is evaluated separately, although there is no change from the infarcted area. Studies have demonstrated safety of the implantation stem cells procedure, without any adverse events. The studies presented as limiting the small number of patients in the study. Both groups showed an improvement in ejection fraction (Table 2).

Lunde	46.9	49	45.7	48.8
Meluzin	40	43	40	47
Dill	47.8	49.4	47.7	51.5
Yao	45.4	47.6	46.3	49.8
Piepoli	36.6	39.7	37.5	45

Table 2: Ejection fraction (EF) in the pre and post implantation of adult stem cells

Meta-analysis

Forest graphics values of ejection fraction (Figures 2 and 3).

Study	EF (pre) control	EF (post) control	EF (pre) exp	EF (post) exp

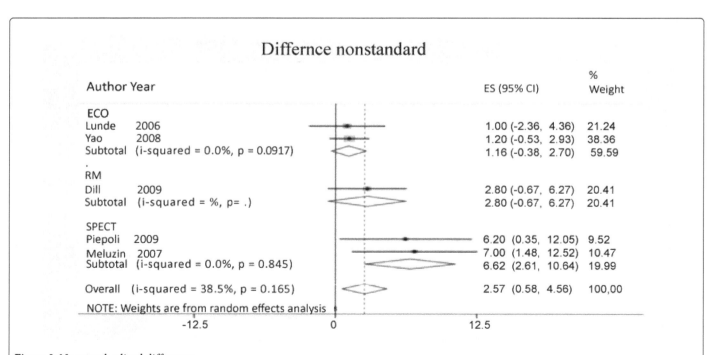

Figure 2: Nonstandardized difference

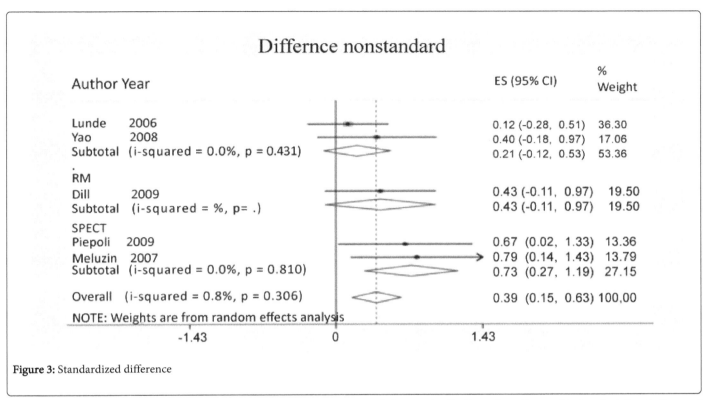

Figure 3: Standardized difference

Discussion

Whereas the horizontal lines of the studies represented in the graph of meta-analysis, with the exception of the line referring to studies Meluzin [6] and Piepoli [7], cross the vertical line, we can say that there is no statistical difference between the groups (experimental and control) When a study despite not cross the vertical line ends with arrow it means that the confidence interval extends beyond the graphs scale.

Therefore, the confidence interval increases as the sample size is small. In this sense, we can infer that the Meluzin study [6], while expressing its results in a significant improvement in ejection fraction in the experimental group can not claim that this improvement is effective for the intervention compared to other studies.

We can also observe that the central point of the horizontal lines of the studies is to the right of the graphic, which can be interpreted as not having the effect of the intervention size. Even in this analysis, we highlight the central point size, which indicates the relative weight of each study in the final result, which is based on the number of participants and the number of events. Whereas the central point of the horizontal lines is similar in terms of weight expressed in reduced form, we can interpret that the selected studies did not show relative weight on the end result.

In combination studies represented by the diamond at the bottom of the charts, the centerpiece has to be similar to these, and its extended form means an increase in the confidence interval, showing that even with the combination, studies of the sample remains small to affirm the effectiveness of the intervention on the outcome. When analyzing the results of related studies from the exams used to assess ejection fraction after implantation of stem cells it was observed the

need for standardization of results considering that the studies used different methodology examinations to assess the outcome (Figure 3).

When reading the subgroups from each examination carried out, it was found that among Lunde and Yao studies, there was no significant difference, being confirmed by the metadata. Dill study did not allow a comparative analysis as the only study to use MRI as the examination to evaluate the outcome [4,5,8].

Meluzin and Piepoli studies showed significant relation to the outcome both in subgroup analysis and the meta-analysis [6,7].

Comparing the results of meta-analyzes related to non-standardized and standardized difference, we observe a statistical significance, although the number of studies are not conclusive for expressive statements, not allowing inferences about the effectiveness in outcome related to EF. Thus, when analyzing more critically the graphs we found that Meluzin and Piepoli studies are responsible for the tendency of the diamond displacement to the right, giving margins for the interpretation of the implantation effectiveness [6,7].

Therefore, the results of this systematic review allow us to infer that although cell therapy show improvement in ejection fraction in each selected study, it is maintained at the same level or below 50% even in the Meluzin study with the highest percentage of improvement in the pre and post-implantation, which does not remove the characteristic picture of heart failure after myocardial infarction [6].

We consider in this meta-analysis that despite the small improvement in ejection fraction, suggesting less severe symptoms presented by the HF patient after AMI by the increase in ejection fraction, it does not imply changes in your lifestyle. However, the Hristov meta-analysis results showed a positive effect in FE before implanting adult stem cells in acute MI, but without statistical significance between the groups, noting that the studies presented number of stem cells and different segments despite present similarities related to the type of studies and clinical characteristics of the study population [9].

Heart failure (HF) is a marked functional limitation syndrome, it imposes worsening the life quality of patients. Although they are the most important causes of hospital readmission in this cardiac group, decompensation resulting from poor adherence to pharmacological and non-pharmacological are the predominant episodes [10]. Within this unfavorable scenario, one of the objectives of the HF management is to achieve and maintain clinical stability of patients at the expense of a very complex treatment regimen.

We believe the most important is to emphasize the consistency of the experimental studies, which demonstrated an improvement in ventricular function after implantation. However, only the most advanced and multicenter studies with many patients can determine the exact place of this type of therapy in clinical treatment and improve the life condition of heart failure patients [11-14].

Conclusion

This study allowed us to verify that it is not possible inference related to the stem cells effectiveness in cardiology, that leads to the need for better outcome assessment from the research development combined with other types of stem cells.

In addition to the studies that met the inclusion criteria for this meta-analysis, several other clinical trials of CT-MO implantation combined with surgery and use of cellular stimulation factors were fundamental to scientific trajectory, allowing evidence of change in EF, justifying the persistence in the pursuit of new studies that express results in order to target this intervention as a treatment in cardiology. Therefore, the studies show as consensus that the quantity and implanted stem cells lineage can affect the outcome of the ending.

The evolution of research involving stem cells in cardiology has played an important way to therapeutic innovation, generating demand for new knowledge for health professionals especially nurses that besides having the commitment to follow the progress technology they play an important role in monitoring changes in lifestyle necessary to everyday life of the patient and their subsequent life quality.

References

1. Woods S.L. (2004) Nursing Cardiology.4. ed. Sao Paulo: Manole.

2. Guideline 2-III congestive heart failure Review of the guidelines of the Brazilian Society of Cardiology for the diagnosis and treatment of chronic heart failure. Brazilian Archives of Cardiology, São Paulo, 2009.

3. MILK, R.S.; Dohmann, H. F (2004) Use of stem cells applied to cardiology. Journal of the Society of Cardiology of the State of São Paulo.

4. DILL Thorsten, Schächinger V, Rolf A, Möllmann S, Thiele H et al. (2009) Intracoronary administration of bone marrow derived progenitor cells improved left ventricular function in pacientes at risk for adverses remodeling after acute myocardial infarction-REPAIR-AMI. American Heart Journal, Saint Louis, March. Am Heart J 157: 541-547

5. Lunde K, Solheim S, Aakhus S, Arnesen H, Abdelnoor M, et al. (2006) Intracoronary injection of mononuclear bone marrow cells in acute myocardial infarction. N Engl J Med 355: 1199-1209.

6. Meluzín J, Janousek S, Mayer J, Groch L, Hornácek I, et al. (2008) Three-, 6-, and 12-month results of autologous transplantation of mononuclear bone marrow cells in patients with acute myocardial infarction. Int J Cardiol 128: 185-192.

7. 7-Piepoli M. F, Vallisa D, Arbasi M, Cavanna L, Cerri L et al. (2010) Bone marrow cell transplantation Improves cardiac, autonomic, and functional indexes in acute anterior myocardial infarction patients (Cardiac Study). Eur J Heart Fail 12: 172-180

8. Yao K, Huang R, Qian J, Cui J, Ge L, et al. (2008) Administration of intracoronary bone marrow mononuclear cells on chronic myocardial infarction improves diastolic function. Heart 94: 1147-1153.

9. Hristov M, Heussen N, Schober A, Weber C (2006) Intracoronary infusion of autologous bone marrow cells and left ventricular function after acute myocardial infarction: a meta-analysis. J Cell Mol Med 10: 727-733.

10. Rabelo ER, Aliti GB, Domingues FB, Ruschel KB, de Oliveira Brun A (2007) What to teach to patients with heart failure and why: the role of nurses in heart failure clinics. Rev Lat Am Enfermagem 15: 165-170.

11. Ferreira MC, Gallani MC (2005) [Heart failure: old syndrome, new concepts and nurse's role]. Rev Bras Enferm 58: 70-73.

12. Strömberg A (2002) Educating nurses and patients to manage heart failure. Eur J Cardiovasc Nurs 1: 33-40.

13. Jovicic A, Holroyd-Leduc JM, Straus SE (2006) Effects of self-management intervention on health outcomes of patients with heart failure: a systematic review of randomized controlled trials. BMC Cardiovasc Disord 6: 43.

14. McAlister FA, Stewart S, Ferrua S, McMurray JJ (2004) Multidisciplinary strategies for the management of heart failure patients at high risk for admission: a systematic review of randomized trials. J Am Coll Cardiol 44: 810-819.

15

Learning to Nurse in a Multicultural Society – The Experiences of Nursing Students in Sweden

Maria Jirwe[1*], Azita Emami[1] and Kate Gerrish[2]

[1]Department of Neurobiology, Care Sciences and Society, Division of Nursing, Karolinska Institutet, Sweden

[2]School of Nursing and Midwifery, University of Sheffield, UK

*Corresponding author: Maria Jirwe, Senior lecturer at Department of Neurobiology, Care Sciences and Society, Division of Nursing, Karolinska Institutet, Alfred Nobels Allé 23, 23 300, SE 141 83 Huddinge, Sweden, E-mail: maria.jirwe@ki.se

Abstract

Introduction: Transcultural nursing education is often neglected within nursing curricula and inclusion within curricula may be haphazard. Little is known about nursing students' views on transcultural nursing education. There is a lack of research examining how nursing students are prepared in university and practice settings for nursing in a multicultural society.

Objective: To examine nursing students' preparation for and experience of cross-cultural encounters.

Method: Semi-structured interviews were undertaken with a purposive sample of 10 final year students from one university in Sweden: 5 participants were from a Swedish background and 5 from an immigrant background. Interviews explored participant's experiences of preparation for and experience of nursing in a multi-cultural society. Interviews were audio recorded, transcribed and analysed using 'framework' approach.

Results: Three themes were identified in the analysis: experiential learning through life experience, educational preparation for practice, and learning in clinical education. Students from an immigrant background emphasized the importance of their life experiences while ethnic Swedish students emphasized education in equipping them to meet patients from another culture than their own. In clinical settings students used their skills of self-awareness to reflect upon their response to cross-cultural encounters as well as critical reflection on practice. In clinical placements, students were inadequately prepared to deal with negative attitudes, racism and discrimination towards patients and in some instances towards themselves.

Conclusion: Although nursing students felt nursing education had equipped them with the necessary self-awareness, knowledge and skills to face cross-cultural encounters, nursing education had failed in preparing students to deal with negative attitudes, racism and discrimination. Nurse educators need to place greater emphasis on preparing students deal with difficult situations arising from racism and discrimination that they may experience in clinical practice. Students need to understand why racism and discrimination may occur and also how to respond and act appropriately.

Keywords: Nursing students; Nursing education; Framework approach; Cross-cultural encounter; Multi-ethnic; Multi-cultural; Cultural competence; Racism; Discrimination

Introduction

According to the International Council of Nurses ethics code [1] nurses are not only responsible for promoting health, prevent illness, restoring health and relieving suffering but also for respecting human and cultural rights [1]. In order to meet these demands, nurses need to be self-aware and have the knowledge and skills to provide appropriate care for all patients. They need to provide nursing care unrestricted by considerations of age, colour, sexual orientation, nationality, politics, race or social status i.e. to be culturally competent [1]. Transcultural nursing is the field of study enabling nurses to provide culturally competent care [2]. Cultural competence is an important component to be included in nursing curricula [3]. Although it is often included, transcultural nursing education is frequently haphazard and lacks

integration [4,5], a view endorsed by an international project undertaken by a group of educators from five EU countries conducting a review of the nursing education at the eight institutions they were representing [6]. Furthermore, a study conducted by Momeni et al.[7] analysing the curricula in all 26 nursing programs in Sweden identified a lack of structure for students to become culturally competent [7]. A national study undertaken by Schüldt Håård et al. [8] found that only 41% of 1110 nursing students felt their education had equipped them with adequate understanding of people from other cultural backgrounds.

The need to prepare nursing students for international exchange programs has been acknowledged and described by several researchers [6,9-11]. However, the need for this preparation holds true for all nursing students due to the challenge many nurses face when caring for immigrant patients who are from a different cultural background to their own. According to the Institute of Medicine [12] cultural competence is essential for providing high quality care to diverse populations and for providing patient-centered care that identifies, respects and addresses differences in patients' values, preferences and expressed needs. This statement highlights the importance for nurse educators to develop nursing curricula and nursing education in a way that enables all nursing students to become culturally competent in order to provide nursing care to diverse populations.

Integrating cultural competence training into the nursing curricula in order to reach an effective outcome is challenging [13]. Different learning activities can be used to facilitate the development of cultural competence among nursing students [13,14]. International exchange programs that provide the opportunity for students to study in a different country are one successful learning activity (c.f. [9-11]. However not all nursing students have the opportunity to take part in an international exchange program and therefore other learning activities that enable similar learning opportunities are necessary. Simulation games e.g. Barnga [15,16], BaFá BaFá [15-18], Culture Copia [19] and High-fidelity patient simulation [13] are other forms of effective learning activities which can be used to enable students to develop culturally competence, either as a single method or in combination with other learning activities.

Little is known about nursing students view on transcultural nursing education. To date, the focus has mainly been on nursing students' experiences of specific learning activities such as exchange studies and simulation games. There is a lack of research examining how nursing students are prepared in university and practice settings for nursing in a multicultural society.

The Study

Aim

The aim of the study was to examine nursing students' preparation for and experience of cross-cultural encounters.

Method

An exploratory qualitative study was undertaken with semi-structured interviews using a purposive sample of 10 nursing students who were in the final year of a three year education programme in a Swedish University. The university was located in a city with a multicultural population drawn from over 180 countries so it was anticipated that students would gain experience of cross-cultural encounters during their clinical practice.

Participants

Five students with an ethnic Swedish background and five students from different immigrant backgrounds were recruited. Biographical details of the participants are provided in Table 1. All students with an immigrant background had migrated to Sweden during their childhood and were fluent in Swedish. All students had undertaken a 5 week course in transcultural nursing (Table 1).

Participant	Ethnic background	Age	Age when moving to Sweden	Years of experiences in the health care sector
3	Swedish	25	-	3
5	Swedish	29	-	0
6	Swedish	34	-	14
7	Swedish	26	-	0
8	Swedish	26	-	5
1	Finnish	40	7	0
2	Kurdish	36	16	1
4	Bosnian	21	8	0
9	Bangladeshi	21	1	0
10	Iranian	23	5	3

Table 1: Demographic characteristics of the participants

Data collection

The students received an interview guide in advance asking them to reflect upon how they had been prepared for cross-cultural encounters in clinical practice and to bring appropriate examples to the interview to discuss.

Interviews lasted between 20 to 45 minutes and were audio-recorded and transcribed verbatim. Interviews took place at a location convenient to the student. Six interviews were undertaken in the university and four by telephone.

Data analysis

The interviews were analysed using the five steps in the Framework approach developed by Lewis and Ritchie [20]. The steps involve:

- familiarisation with the richness, depth and diversity of the data.
- identification of a thematic framework
- indexing whereby the thematic framework is systematically applied to individual transcripts
- charting, whereby indexed data from different transcripts are grouped into common themes
- mapping and interpretation involves identifying the key characteristics of the data as a whole, and systematically examining the relationships between different themes.

The familiarization step began when transcribing the interviews as the researchers started to immerse themselves in the issues that participants raised. Each transcript was then read several times in order to become familiar with the data, gain an understanding of the breadth and depth of the data and identify key issues.

A thematic framework based on the key issues identified from the previous step was constructed. The thematic framework was used initially to code four transcripts and additional issues that were not included in the framework were identified. These additional issues were then incorporated into a revised thematic framework and codes identified for each theme and sub-themes: code 1 for the first theme (Educational preparation for practice), 1.1 for the first sub-theme (Nursing school), 1.2 for the next (Literature) and so on.

During the indexing step, the coding framework was systematically applied to individual transcripts. Summarized data from each participant's transcript were then brought together in order to chart the data as a whole. This involved constructing tables for each theme and sub-theme which included a summary of what each participant had said about the specific sub-theme, and specific quotes from the transcripts were also included. This process enabled the research team to gain an understanding of the extent to which different participants contributed data to the various themes and sub-themes.

The final step involved mapping the themes and sub-themes across the whole data set and interpreting the data in relation to nursing students' preparation for and experience of cross-cultural encounters. Interviews were analysed initially by one researcher and the interpretation validated by the other members of the research team.

Ethical considerations

Ethical approval was obtained from the Ethics Committee at the Karolinska Institutet (Dnr 03/550) and the study was conducted in accordance with the University's requirements. Potential participants were given information about the aims of the study and what their involvement would entail as part of the recruitment process. Verbal consent was obtained at the time of interview. Participants were assured that the information they provided would be treated confidentially and would not be disclosed to people outside the research team, and that their anonymity would be ensured in any publications arising from the study.

Findings

All students, irrespective of their ethnic background, referred to cross-cultural encounters in terms of their interaction with patients and relatives who were from an immigrant (i.e. non-ethnic Swedish) background. Interestingly, students who were themselves from an immigrant background did not conceptualise their interactions with ethnic Swedish patients as cross-cultural, rather they interpreted 'cross-cultural' in terms of encounters with other immigrant groups in Sweden.

Three themes relating to students' educational preparation to engage in cross-cultural encounters were identified, namely; (i) experiential learning through life experience, (ii) educational preparation for practice, and (iii) learning in clinical education. Each of these themes will be discussed in turn.

Experiential learning through life experience

Whereas all students had lived in a multi-cultural city in Sweden for a number of years, only students from an immigrant background saw life experience as meaningful in terms of their preparation to nurse in a multi-cultural society. Immigrant students drew attention to how their experiences of living in Sweden post-migration had shaped their understanding and receptiveness to cultural diversity.

Yes, I think it's due to immigration that I've developed as a person. You see and experience a lot during that time (P2)

Immigrant students perceived that their personal biography and their interactions with other immigrant communities in the neighborhoods where they grew up enabled them to be more attuned to the needs of patients and relatives from culturally diverse backgrounds.

I grew up in (suburb) and still live there. I speak some Somali, some Arabic, and some Turkish. I come from a Muslim family and I have Muslim relatives …. I've grown up in (suburb) where more than half the population is Muslim, so I understand Islam (P9).

Immigrant students also perceived that their life experiences of interacting with people from different immigrant communities enabled them to be confident in their interactions with patients from different cultural backgrounds. Rather than be concerned with potential cultural difference, they felt better able to focus on the needs of the individual patient.

I've had so many experiences in my past. It comes automatically in a way… you cross over a line, and finally you don't see cultural differences anymore, you see the person. It's the person that's important, not the culture, the religion or the background. I've reflected on whether it could be due to my background, my openness, that I am myself (P2).

In addition to influencing how students responded to cultural diversity, life experiences enabled immigrant students to develop skills and confidence in responding to racism.

I grew up in a neighbourhood where racism was common and I learnt how to confront it (P10)

By contrast, students with a Swedish background did not provide illustrations of how their life experiences had helped equip them to engage in cross-cultural encounters in nursing practice.

Educational preparation for practice

Students were generally positive about the contribution that formal education in the university had made to developing knowledge and skills to support cross-cultural encounters. Whereas immigrant students emphasized the contribution that life experiences made to helping them interact with patients from different cultural backgrounds, ethnic Swedish students placed more emphasis on the learning that had taken place within the university. The university provided a 5 week full-time course in transcultural nursing which introduced students to relevant theories from sociology and anthropology which helped inform their understanding of cultural diversity in relation to nursing practice and develop skills in intercultural communication.

The course in transcultural nursing increased my awareness about cultural differences, what is normal for me is not necessarily normal for others (P6)

Understanding the cultural practices of people from different cultural backgrounds enabled students to become more accepting of cultural difference and have greater confidence in their interactions with patients:

(It's about) how to encounter a person when it's normal for them but not for us. (P4)

Students perceived that their educational preparation had also enabled them to develop self-awareness in relation to cultural diversity. By developing greater awareness of their own cultural identity they felt better able to understand the patient's perspective.

You start to think about who you are and what cultural background others are from and what it is that affects their reactions… And then you look back on yourself. What is it that makes me react in the way I do or why do I handle the situation in the way I do? (P6)

You've learned how to put yourself in the situation, to handle cultural differences… to think in a different way (P8)

Teaching on communication in cross-cultural encounters had also aided students, for example:

I learned some words in Arabic. It came from what we have learned about cultural meetings, and I thought that this could help. I showed that I wanted to meet her, to understand (P1)

The opportunity to participate in overseas educational exchange visits was also seen by students to be beneficial in helping to raise their awareness of their own cultural identity.

Exchange studies helped further with the knowledge to know yourself... It feels more like I'm starting to understand who I am and beginning to accept that I cannot put myself in a box, I fit like a bit of everywhere. It is an advantage, not a disadvantage. (P9)

Whereas the majority of students were positive about the contribution that university-based education had made to equip them with the knowledge and skills for cross-cultural encounters, one student felt that the emphasis on cultural differences could result in stereotypical assumptions about different cultures developing.

I think in terms of cross-cultural care encounters, nursing education was rather problematic... to learn about this culture, read this book, it's a bit cookbook-like (P7).

In summary, students generally felt that their university-based education had developed their self-awareness and made them aware of cultural diversity in relation to patients they may encounter in clinical practice. Moreover, communication skills training had equipped them with techniques to facilitate communication across language barriers.

Learning in clinical education

The students' descriptions were quite similar when they shared their experiences about how clinical education in practice settings prepared them for their cross-cultural encounters. Students found themselves utilising their skills in self-awareness in order to reflect upon how they responded to cross-cultural encounters.

When you enter an unfamiliar situation, (you ask yourself) 'why is it like this?' 'what is it that stops me from acting properly?' (You think) 'well you are like this'... then you have a better understanding of why the patient acts in the way he does, if it is part of the culture or religion or whatever... (P6).

Critical reflection on practice was another means whereby students learnt in practice. One student recounted on how when faced with a potentially challenging cross-cultural encounter she had not engaged fully with the patient in ascertaining her needs but had made assumptions based on cultural stereotypes. Through reflection on practice she gained new insights into how stereotypical assumptions could influence her practice inappropriately.

It was really an eye-opener, I took for granted that she was very different, I probably became afraid of her and avoided her. Instead I could have just talked to her even if it would have been more demanding than if I'd have spoken to a Swedish woman (P7).

University-based education had provided students with a knowledge base to inform cross-cultural encounters. Although communicating with patients and relatives from different cultural backgrounds, especially where there were language barriers, was challenging students perceived that they could try different techniques to facilitate interaction.

It felt like it was another climate for communication (at the clinical placement). No one (the staff) assumed they would understand each other at once. It was almost as if they assumed there would be

problems communicating with each other but that you could solve it somehow (P8)

However, although students felt that they had had received some useful preparation for cross-cultural encounters, they experienced additional challenges in clinical practice for which they felt inadequately prepared. Several students were exposed to negative attitudes, racism and discrimination towards patients and in some instances towards themselves during their clinical placements which they found distressing and were inadequately prepared to deal with.

Some students reported instances where nursing staff had expressed prejudicial views towards specific patients. One student gave an example of a young immigrant female patient who had migrated to Sweden following an arranged marriage. The woman had subsequently felt socially isolated and was hospitalised following a suicide attempt. The student considered that both medical and nursing staff viewed arranged marriages as 'abnormal' and they did not want to understand the woman's situation.

The problem was that she (the patient) had problems with the staff who didn't take her seriously. They had some kind of prejudice towards her – 'you are so stupid to agree to get married'. They didn't want to understand her, but it was her culture and for her it was normal. They (the staff) looked upon it as unnatural; she (the patient) felt that she wasn't taken seriously... It didn't feel right with these prejudices that they (the staff) didn't even consider to think differently. (P10).

Other students provided illustrations of where they had observed other staff show unwillingness to engage fully with patients from a different culture to their own.

I don't know what causes it, but they'll go into a patient and come out again saying 'I have not been able to talk to him, it did not work, I can't, end of story.' (P2).

Alternatively, they found that staff expressed more general negative attitudes towards a specific culture. One student recalled that when she shared the focus of her final year project on cultural diversity, it promoted staff to voice their own prejudices.

When I said that I wrote about culture, the people (staff) individually began to say 'Yes, I think the worst cultures are Gypsies.' (P7).

Some students from an immigrant background had experienced disparaging attitudes in relation to their own ethnicity from patients and relatives.

A patient made some comments about not wanting dark skinned persons (looking after them), I am light brown (P9).

He says he doesn't want a 'wog'. Then he continued to call me 'wog', 'Negro', all kinds of things (P10).

Some students also interpreted patient or relatives behavior as disparaging, even when they could not fully understand the language.

I suspect that they were saying condescending things about me when I was in the room. I can't say it for sure (relatives were speaking in another language that the student did not understand) but it felt like it. I tried to be as professional as possible and do as a good job as possible (P1).

Immigrant students who had experienced prejudices suggested that if they were exposed to this directly they acted upon it but if it was second hand information they ignored it.

Nursing students emphasised that they had not learnt how to deal with racism during their university education. Whereas students from an immigrant background felt that their life experiences had helped them to deal with such situations, students from a Swedish background were less confident. Irrespective of ethnic background, students found their experiences of racism a cause of considerable distress and felt inadequately supported by other staff.

Several students expressed concern that if they witnessed racist comments from patients directed towards students from an immigrant background they experienced a lack of support from their clinical supervisors. The lack of active intervention meant that patients were able to continue their racist behaviours unchecked. A student from an Iranian background recounted a situation when a patient's behaviour was effectively condoned by a lack of intervention from a nursing assistant.

A man in his eighties came for a blood pressure check-up and he did not want me. He called me all sort of names. I told him that he can go somewhere else for a check-up and he says 'no I want someone else'. Then a nursing assistant came in and said 'I can take the blood pressure' and she did... I stayed in the room and watched and he was sitting there with a big smile looking at me. Afterwards I told the nursing assistant that I was disappointed at her and that she had allowed racism to continue due to her actions. She just said 'no, no, come on it wasn't like that, all old people are like that, it's normal' (P10)

Students also drew attention to instances where they would have valued the opportunity to observe and learn how more experienced staff dealt with difficult situations where patients expressed racist views.

I was in there by myself with the patient... It was good in one way but I think that I would have preferred to have someone with me a bit more often, and right then in this meeting I would have wanted my supervisor with me. I would have wanted to see how she would have handled the situation (P5)

In summary, it was evident that students were able to apply learning gained as part of formal university education in cross-cultural encounters in clinical practice, however they also experienced racism in clinical settings which they felt inadequately prepared to deal with.

Discussion

According to the literature (c.f. [21-23]) cultural awareness is an essential step towards developing cultural competence and thereby being able to provide cultural sensitive care to patients from diverse ethnic backgrounds. When it comes to developing cultural awareness, nursing students with an immigrant background appeared to be at an advantage compared to nursing students with an ethnic Swedish background, irrespective of whether nursing students with immigrant background came to Sweden at a very young age or as an older child closer to becoming an adult. It could be argued that their cultural awareness is due to the surrounding area in which they reside (usually living in multi-cultural suburbs since arriving in Sweden) as well as their own earlier experiences of not being able to communicate in Swedish. Not being able to understand others or being able to make oneself understood is an useful life experience to bring to cross-

cultural encounters [24]. The findings from this study indicate that immigrant students and ethnic Swedish students i.e. students from the majority population have different life experiences and perspective when entering nursing education and this may be why Swedish nursing students emphasized the importance of the theoretical university-based education to a greater extent than immigrant nursing students. Ethnic Swedish nursing students appear to have a greater need to develop cultural awareness through different educational activities such as exchange programs [9,25], simulation games [16] and immersion with specific cultural groups [26,27] compared to students with an immigrant background. The benefit of having an immigrant background was also identified in a Swedish study of health care workers in elderly care settings where first generation immigrants reported being more cultural aware than ethnic Swedes, even though the differences were not significant [28].

Transcultural nursing models highlight the importance of understanding cultural differences in order to be able to deliver cultural competent care (c.f. [2,29]). Cultural understanding was also emphasized by nursing students in this study. Nursing students highlighted that being able to understand cultural differences was something they had been prepared for during their nursing education. Whereas nursing students with an immigrant background emphasized the impact of the education, they also stressed that their experience as immigrants had enhanced their understanding of cultural difference. However, the education program had not prepared them to be able to handle negative attitudes, racism and discrimination, whether it was towards themselves, patients or other students/colleagues. Other research studies [28,30,31] have identified that minority ethnic healthcare staff perceive more discrimination than healthcare workers from the majority population. In this study, several nursing students were, in relation to ethnicity, exposed to prejudices, discrimination and racism or witnessed it from staff towards minority ethnic patients during their clinical placements. Nursing students emphasized that they were inadequately prepared during their nursing education to address prejudices, discrimination and/or racism, whether it was directed towards themselves or towards patients. Being able to address inequalities and discrimination is an important part of being culturally competent [4,21,29]. Students in this study had been taught how prejudices and racism occur, but not how to address it. Tilki, et al [32] emphasize that racism in nursing curricula is often neglected as nursing lecturers are not well equipped for this due to problems at both on an organisational level and an individual level. This may be the case in the present study. However, the failure to address racism and discrimination could also be related to the theoretical frameworks that Swedish nursing curricula usually draw upon. In Sweden, North American transcultural nursing models are often used and these models do not emphasise racism and discrimination to the same extent as transcultural nursing models from the United Kingdom and New Zealand [21].

Limitations

The findings from this study are based on interviews with ten nursing students who reflected on how their life experiences, their university education and their experiential learning in clinical education had prepared them for engaging in cross-cultural encounters. The small sample size which was drawn from one university in Sweden means that caution needs to be exercised in assuming that the findings are transferable. Nevertheless, the fact that some of the issues raised in this study are reflected in the wider literature suggests that the findings are relevant to other contexts. The study has also identified the different experiences of nursing students with ethnic Swedish and immigrant backgrounds. However, further research is required to ascertain where such differences exist more widely in Sweden and in other countries where people from immigrant backgrounds are recruited into nurse education. The findings in this study are based on interviews with nursing students reflecting over their experiences of cross-cultural encounters during clinical placements and their educational preparation for these encounters.

Conclusion

Although nursing education had equipped nursing students with the necessary tools, such as increased self-awareness, and the knowledge and skills, to manage cross-cultural encounters, it had failed to prepare students to deal with negative attitudes, racism and discrimination. Nurse educators need to place greater emphasis on preparing students deal with difficult situations arising from racism and discrimination that they may experience in clinical practice. Students need to understand why racism and discrimination may occur and also how to respond and act appropriately. Conclusively, this study provides important information about nursing students' experience of cross-cultural encounters that needs to be addressed in nursing education. Students need to be provided with educational opportunities to develop the necessary tools to care for patients from different cultural backgrounds as well as the tools to respond to negative attitudes, racism and discrimination. The findings from this study can therefore be used to inform the development of pre-registration programs and continuing professional development for registered nurses.

Acknowledgement

The authors would like to thank the Department of Neurobiology, Care Sciences and Society, the Division of Nursing at Karolinska Institutet for their support.

Source of funding

This research was supported by AMF pension.

References

1. International Council of Nurses (2012) The ICN Code of Ethics for Nurses, ed. I.C.o. Nurses. 2012, Geneva, Switzerland: International Council of Nurses. 10.

2. Giger, J.N, Davidhizar R.E (2004) Transcultural nursing : assessment & intervention. 4. ed. 2004, St. Louis, Mo. ; London: Mosby. 666.

3. Mareno N, Hart PL (2014) Cultural competency among nurses with undergraduate and graduate degrees: implications for nursing education. Nurs Educ Perspect 35: 83-88.

4. Gerrish K, Papadopoulos I (1999) Transcultural competence: the challenge for nurse education. Br J Nurs 8: 1453-1457.

5. Narayanasamy A, White E (2005) A review of transcultural nursing. Nurse Educ Today 25: 102-111.

6. Sairanen R, Richardson E, Kelly H, Bergknut E, Koskinen L, et al. (2013) Putting culture in the curriculum: a European project. Nurse Educ Pract 13: 118-124.

7. Momeni P, Jirwe M, Emami A (2008) Enabling nursing students to become culturally competent--a documentary analysis of curricula in all Swedish nursing programs. Scand J Caring Sci, 22: 499-506.

8. Schüldt Håård U, Ohlén J, Gustavsson PJ (2008) Generic and professional outcomes of a general nursing education program--a national study of higher education. Int J Nurs Educ Scholarsh 5: Article32.

9. Milne A, Cowie J (2013) Promoting culturally competent care: the Erasmus exchange programme. Nurs Stand 27: 42-46.

10. Koskinen L, Tossavainen K (2003) Characteristics [correction of charactersistics] of intercultural mentoring--a mentor perspective. Nurse Educ Today 23: 278-285.

11. Law K, Muir N (2006) The internationalisation of the nursing curriculum. Nurse Educ Pract 6: 149-155.

12. National Research Council (2003) Health Professions Education: A Bridge to Quality (2003), The National Academies Press: Washington, DC.

13. Roberts SG, Warda M, Garbutt S, Curry K (2014) The use of high-fidelity simulation to teach cultural competence in the nursing curriculum. J Prof Nurs 30: 259-265.

14. Gallagher RW, Polanin JR (2015) A meta-analysis of educational interventions designed to enhance cultural competence in professional nurses and nursing students. Nurse Educ Today 35: 333-340.

15. Graham I, Richardson E (2008) Experiential gaming to facilitate cultural awareness: its implication for developing emotional caring in nursing. Learning in Health and social Care 7: 37-45.

16. Koskinen L, Abdelhamid P, P Likitalo H (2008) The Simulation method for learning cultural awareness in nursing. Diversity in Health and Social Care 5: 55-63.

17. Hummel F, Peters D (1994) BaFá BaFá: A Cultural Awareness Game. Nurse Educator 19: 8.

18. O'Connor B, Rockney R, Alario A (2002)BaFá BaFá: a cross-cultural simulation experience for medical educators and trainees. Medical Education 36: 1102.

19. Farmer M., et al (2010) Development of an Extensible Game Architecture for Teaching Transcultural Nursing.

20. Lewis J, Ritchie J (2003) Qualitative research practice : a guide for social science students and researchers. London: SAGE. xv, 336 s.

21. Jirwe M., Gerrish K, Emami A (2006) The theoretical framework of cultural competence. Journal of Multicultural Nursing & Health 12: 6-16.

22. Balcazar FE, Suarez-Balcazar Y, Taylor-Ritzler T (2009) Cultural competence: development of a conceptual framework. Disabil Rehabil 31: 1153-1160.

23. Shen Z (2015) Cultural competence models and cultural competence assessment instruments in nursing: a literature review. J Transcult Nurs 26: 308-321.

24. Jirwe M, Gerrish K, Emami A (2010) Student nurses' experiences of communication in cross-cultural care encounters. Scand J Caring Sci 24: 436-444.

25. Koskinen L, Tossavainen K (2004) Study abroad as a process of learning intercultural competence in nursing. Int J Nurs Pract 10: 111-120.

26. Presley C (2013) Cultural awareness: Enhancing clinical experiences in rural Appalachia. Nurse Educ 38: 223-226.

27. Smit EM, Tremethick MJ (2013) Development of an international interdisciplinary course: a strategy to promote cultural competence and collaboration. Nurse Educ Pract 13: 132-136.

28. Olt, H, et al., (2014) Communication and equality in elderly care settings: perceptions of first- and secondgeneration immigrant and native Swedish healthcare workers. Diversity and Equality in Health and Care, 2014. 11: 99-111.

29. Jirwe M, Gerrish K, Keeney S, Emami A (2009) Identifying the core components of cultural competence: findings from a Delphi study. J Clin Nurs 18: 2622-2634.

30. Dreachslin JL, Hunt PL, Sprainer E (2000) Workforce diversity: implications for the effectiveness of health care delivery teams. Soc Sci Med 50: 1403-1414.

31. Khatutsky G, Wiener JM, Anderson WL (2010) Immigrant and non-immigrant certified nursing assistants in nursing homes: how do they differ? J Aging Soc Policy 22: 267-287.

32. Tilki M et al., (2007) Racism: the implications for nursing education. Diversity in Health and Social Care 4: 303-312.

16

Medical Error Reporting Attitudes of Healthcare Personnel, Barriers and Solutions

Aysun Ünal[1]* and Seyda Seren[2]

[1]Department of Pediatric Surgery, Dokuz Eylul University, Izmir, Turkey

[2]Department of Nursing Management, Dokuz Eylul University, Izmir, Turkey

*Corresponding author: Aysun Ünal, Department of Pediatric Surgery, Dokuz Eylul University Hospital, Izmir, Turkey, E-mail: aysun.unaldeu@gmail.com

Abstract

Introduction: Medical error reporting has been recognized as the cornerstone of patient safety practices; however, healthcare personnel often do not report errors. In order to increase the frequency of error reporting, it is important to understand both the healthcare workers' attitudes towards reporting, as well as what they perceive as barriers.

Aim: The aim of this literature review was to identify the medical error reporting attitudes of healthcare personnel worldwide, as well as the barriers they encounter and their suggestions to increase reporting.

Methods: The national and international databases were scanned to identify the studies performed on medical error attitudes and barriers. A total of 28 studies that fit the criteria were evaluated.

Results: According to the studies that were analyzed, the most commonly encountered reporting barrier was the fear of individual and legal accusations among healthcare personnel. The personnel most frequently suggested using anonymous reporting systems, modifying the "accusation" culture and encouraging timely reporting in order to eliminate the reporting barriers.

Conclusion: This review provides up-to-date information on medical error reporting barriers, solution suggestions directed towards these barriers, and suggestions from healthcare personnel for an effective reporting system. It will guide healthcare providers, quality and risk management unit employees, administrators, and institutions that are trying to develop an effective reporting system toward quality patient care.

Keywords: Nursing; Medical errors; Error reporting barriers; Attitudes

Introduction

Although significant efforts are made to prevent errors within any system, errors take place in every environment related to humans [1]. In the Institute of Medicine's (IOM) report Human Error, it was indicated that "medical care may not be safe" and it was estimated that, in US hospitals, between 44,000 and 98,000 individuals die annually from medical errors. This number is greater than the number of deaths due to traffic accidents, breast cancer, or AIDS. Furthermore, the cost of medical errors is estimated to be between 37.6 and 50 billion dollars [2,3]. Following this report, worldwide health systems began to collaborate over the concept of "Patient Safety" and took action; however, studies conducted recently show that there are still many practices that need to be applied. According to the IOM literature, an estimated number of 210,000 annual fatal medical errors (in an evidence based method) were related to preventable damages. The actual number of deaths related to preventable errors has been estimated to be 400,000 per year [4].

Patient safety requires careful organizational responsibility in order to prevent, identify, analyze and correct possible errors. All healthcare employees are responsible for preventing errors and identifying high risk situations, as well as reducing the dangers of high-risk situations and adverse events. In institutions where such an attitude exists, there also exists a patient safety culture [5,6].

Error reporting is generally accepted as a basic initiative in improving patient safety [7], and the main purpose of error reporting systems is to learn from experience. Often, health service institutions and employees do not share what they learn from errors; as a result, the same errors repeatedly occur in different environments, and patients constantly encounter preventable damage [8]. Although there is a high demand for reporting, it is never sufficient. For example, in England, simple errors are reported at a rate of 22%-39%, while more serious errors often go unreported [9].

There are many reasons for avoiding error reporting, including legal and institutional concerns, as well as personal guilt and regret. Other examples are damage to professional prestige, risk of job loss and fear of getting reprimanded or questioned [10,11]. These barriers substantially limit the monitoring of errors and improvement of patient safety [12]; therefore, it is difficult to establish an institutional or national error reporting system [13].

It has been emphasized that, in order to increase the efficiency of error reporting systems, these systems should be designed in such a way that they can be used by multiple healthcare personnel (doctors, nurses, pharmacists, etc.) [14]. For this reason, it is very important to identify the barriers presented in the literature, as well as the suggestions of healthcare personnel with regard to these barriers, in order for healthcare personnel to develop a positive attitude towards reporting. This positive attitude can then be used to develop an effective reporting system that can be used by all healthcare personnel.

Aim

The aim of this literature review was to identify the medical error reporting attitudes of the world's healthcare personnel, the barriers they encounter and their suggestions for increasing error reporting.

Literature review questions

- What are the medical error reporting attitudes among healthcare personnel?
- What are the medical error reporting barriers of healthcare personnel?

- What are the suggestions of healthcare personnel for increasing medical error reporting?

Methods

Search strategy

A systematic review of the literature relating to medical errors, error reporting, error reporting barriers, and reporting systems in all countries was conducted in February of 2014. Studies that were published between 1999 and 2013 were scanned using the following search engines: Google Scholar, EBSCOhost Online Research Databases, Medline/PubMed, Turkish Medline, and Health Source: Nursing/Academic Edition, Academic Google and the Cochrane Databases (Table 1). The search strategy included all languages and all types of trials and studies. The references from eligible articles were also hand-searched in order to identify additional relevant papers.

Databases	Keywords	Number of Titles Reviewed	Number of Abstracts Reviewed	Number of Studies Selected
PMC/PubMed	Medical Error/Error reporting barriers/attitude	1764	45	20
	Medical Error/Error reporting barriers/attitude	2887	11	10
http://deu.summon.serialssolutions.com/ (Wiley online library, EBSCOHOST)	Medical Error/Error reporting barriers/attitude	31	12	9
	Medical Error/Error reporting barriers/attitude	60	10	6
ProQuest Nursing and Allied Health Source	Medical Error/Error reporting barriers/attitude	53	40	16
	Medical Error/Error reporting barriers/attitude	8	7	2
Cochrane Database	Medical Error/Error reporting barriers/attitude	0	0	0
TOTAL		4803	128	28*

Table 1: Literature search and study selection, * A total of 28 articles were included to the review since studies were present in multiple databases.

Search terms

The following keywords were used as search terms: medical error(s), error reporting barrier(s), attitude(s), physician(s), pharmacist(s) and nurse(s) (in English). Each of these keywords were combined using "or" then combining it with "and."

Review procedure

Each of the studies was conducted in different countries using different definitions, different types of trials, and different methods to collect the data. Therefore, we did not try to analyze the data from a statistical point of view, but the results were summarized according to the error reporting barriers, medical error reporting attitudes of the healthcare personnel, and their suggestions for increasing reporting.

Article selection criteria

Inclusion/exclusion criteria

We included all types of studies, for example, randomized controlled trials, non-randomized controlled trials, longitudinal studies, cohort or case-control studies and descriptive and qualitative studies. Full-text studies conducted on healthcare personnel that included error reporting attitudes, barriers and healthcare personnel suggestions for medical error reporting were selected for the sample group. Studies that investigated medical error rates, whose samples included students or employees working in clinics or studies that were conducted outside clinics (e.g. radiation oncology, pharmacology, etc.), were excluded from the sample. In addition, we excluded reviews, letters, conference papers, opinions, reports and editorial papers.

Results

Features of the studies

A total of 4,806 studies were screened by their titles and 4,678 titles were excluded based on the fact that they were not related to the topic, or that they were letters, editorials or reports. Therefore, 128 article abstracts were considered, after the title evaluation; 61 articles were evaluated for full text suitability and 67 studies were excluded because the samples were students or employees working in clinical units or studies that were conducted outside the clinic (e.g. radiation oncology, pharmacology, etc.). After the evaluation, 28 studies were further analyzed, while the other 33 studies were not considered based on the exclusion criteria (Figure 1).

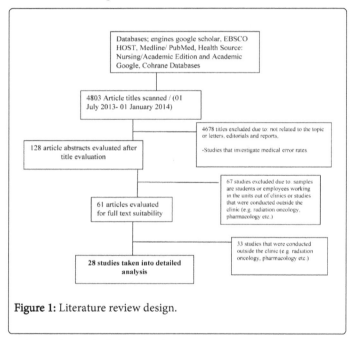

Figure 1: Literature review design.

The studies included in this literature review were those that were descriptive and qualitative and that investigated the medical error reporting attitudes and barriers of the healthcare personnel. When the methods of the studies were reviewed, 12 studies were descriptive, 4 studies were cross-sectional, 9 studies were qualitative and 3 studies were both qualitative and quantitative.

Medical error reporting attitudes among healthcare personnel

It was determined that, among all healthcare personnel, nurses reported more and knew more about the reporting system, when compared to the other healthcare personnel [15-17]. However, physicians were found to be the most reluctant when it came to reporting negative errors [16-19]. The employees tended to have the habit of instantly reporting falling, outcomes that required corrective treatment (such as medication errors), and errors that were witnessed. However, near-miss errors or errors that showed signs over time (Deep-vein thrombosis that developed due to insufficient prophylaxis, pressure ulcers, etc.) had a lower reporting rate. Since these errors occurred over time, they were considered to be complications due to prolonged hospitalization [16].

The type and severity of medical errors are perceived differently among healthcare professionals in those studies where the classifications of medical errors, according to their severity and outcomes, were examined. Nurses and pharmacists reported every type of error at a higher rate, regardless of the patient outcomes; whereas physicians reported errors with more serious outcomes at a higher rate [20]. Moreover, physicians were less likely to report near misses or less-serious patient outcomes, and a more limited proportion of their errors, when compared to the nurses [16,20]. However, the physicians classified the errors as errors at higher percentages when compared to the nurses [17]. In the literature, it was determined that more reporting was made when the outcomes of the errors were at the level of serious damage; in parallel, those errors with possible outcomes of no damage, or milder damage, were reported at a lower rate [15,21-24]. Although, the nurses did report errors that were committed by someone else in the team at a higher rate, when compared to the physicians (Table 2) [18].

References	Personnel involved/Setting	Method	Attitudes and Barriers to Medical Error Reporting
[25]	56 physicians and 66 nurses/University hospital	Qualitative; nominal group technique Quantitative; descriptive survey design	Barriers for physicians; not knowing the usefulness of the report, workload, the lack of information on how to report an error, thinking that reporting has little contribution for improvement of quality of care.Barriers for nurses; time involved in documenting an error, is not anonymous, extra work involved in reporting, hesitancy regarding "telling" on somebady else, it is unnecessary to report the error and fear of lawsuits.
[19]	315 participants were doctors, nurses, and midwives/three English NHS	Descriptive: survey design	Healthcare professionals are in general, reluctant to report behaviour. Doctors are less likely than nurses or midwives to report colleagues.
[26]	15 physicians/Acute hospital	Qualitative;semi-structured interviews	Take time to fill in reporting forms, lack of feedback and lack of training about error reporting.
[18]	74 doctors, 66 nurses/Children's Hospital	Descriptive; survey design,	Perception of whether the exact error events and blamed the concerns.

[27]	3 senior medical representatives and 25 specialist physicians District General Hospital	Qualitative semi-structured interviews	Blame culture, the most important barrier is reporting.
[28]	30 physicians/University Hospital	Descriptive; One group pre-post test study	Time constraints, the reporting process to disrupt work processes, extra paper work, worries about career and their personal reputations, is not sufficient incentives for reporting.
[14]	Eight physicians and six clinical assistant/University Hospital	Qualitative; focus group interviews	Long reporting process and personal factors (personal perceptions regarding the importance of error reporting) are determined barriers
[16]	186 doctors and 587 nurses/Various Hospitals	Descriptive; cross-sectional survey	For doctors were lack of feedback, the incident form taking too long to complete and a belief that the incident was unimportant. Major barriers to reporting for nurses were lack of feedback a belief that there was no point in reporting near misses and forgetting to make a report when the ward is busy.
[17]	40 physicians, 26 nurses, 35 emergency medical technicians/ Emergency clinics	Descriptive;cross-sectional study	Physicians were the least likely to report the error. For all groups and error types, identification, disclosure, and reporting increased with increasing severity.
[29]	597 nurses/University Hospital	Descriptive cross-sectional, correlational design	Reporting barriers in order of importance; fear of management and lack of sufficient time for reporting, documentation and interdisciplinary communications failure and concerned about colleagues.
[24]	799 nurses/Various hospitals	Comparative descriptive survey design	Exposure to disciplinary action and the fear of losing their jobs .
[29]	886 nurse/Training hospital	Descriptive; correlational study	Punitive culture and concerned about of errors is kept in their files
[30]	61 nurse/Medical Center	Descriptive; survey design	Descriptive indicated in barriers; fear of the reaction they would receive from the nurse manager and their peers
[15]	55 physicians and 82 nurses/Training Hospital	Descriptive; anonymous web-based questionnaire survey	Reporting take long and lack of time fear of legal action and discussion and reporting does not contribute to the quality of care is the idea that.
[31]	22 people consisting of doctors and nurses/teaching Hospitals	Qualitative; focus group interviews	Lack of a culture that encourages reporting and therefore, negative perception and attitudes towards reporting, lack of ability to report.
[20]	18 physicians, 22 nurses, 16 pharmacists/Third level referral hospital	Descriptive;a questionnaire using two different clinical scenarios	the type and severity of medication error influence healthcare professionals differently. Nurses and pharmacists were likely to report all medication errors, doctors were only likely to report an error that resulted in an adverse outcome.
[22]	37 nurses/Intensive care units	Qualitative; semi-structured questions with individual interviews	Lack of time, fear and lack of management feedback. When the patient wasn't harmed nurses dont prefer to do reporting.
[21]	430 nurses/Hospitals in various regions	Descriptive; A self-administered survey	Incidents were reported more frequently when the potential consequences were considered severe for the patient. when nurses and safety managers on wards discuss incidents and their root causes, nurses feel less afraid of incident reporting.
[32]	38 nurse/State hospital	Descriptive	Fear, manager of response, not know that the importance of reporting and the event is not perceived as an error.
[33]	62 nurses/University hospital	Descriptive; survey design	The most important factor in nursing management responses, another factor is the feeling of fear of legal action as a result of reporting.
[34]	Nine doctors, 14 nurses, seven pharmacists/Four community hospitals in Nova Scotia, Canada.	Qualitative; focus group interviews	Barriers to medication error reporting were thematised five categories: reporter workload, Professional identity, information gap, organisational factors and fear. Facilitators to encourage medication error reporting were classified three categories: reducing reporter workload, closing the communication gap and educating

[23]	733 nurses/University hospital	Descriptive; survey design	Blame and fear of punishment in addition nurses identified no need to report if no harm to patient.
[35]	1180 Nurse/Nursing Homes	Descriptive; cross sectional design	Risk of being harmed to confidence in the competencies and reporting is difficult for nurses
[36]	433 anesthesiologist/Various hospitals	Descriptive; self-administered, mailed survey	The barrier of being concerned about blame by colleagues.
[37]	115 nurse/University hospital	Qualitative; focus group interviews	Fear of legal procedures, threats of job, fear of losing respectability, lack of information, lack of skills to error management,unwillingness to accept responsibility for errors, and the manager's response is inappropriate.
[38]	30 nurse/Private and tertiary hospitals	Qualitative; (in-depth interviews) and descriptive survey design	barriers identified in the questionnaire; lack of training in reporting system, workload, lack of access to computers, the fear of being monitored, reporting of the form very detailed.

Table 2: Medical error reporting barriers and attitudes towards researches.

In the studies of the characteristics of professional groups, the educational backgrounds and cultural structures specific to their profession and existing complex organizations affected the attitudes toward reporting [16,18,19,34]. Accordingly, the nurses feared the administration more than the doctors [21,29], but the physicians' attitudes toward medical error reporting adversely affected that medical indemnity insurance for the hospital risk managers and lawyers. In addition, abstractions by colleagues' fears of criticism after making an error were also important factors, because their training to strive for an error-free practice and their cultures are not suitable for this [16,36], from the perspective of pharmacists with a better position to identify the causes of medication errors [34]. However, studies have been addressed with regard to all professionals, generally, and specific information regarding pharmacists was rarely encountered.

Medical error reporting barriers among healthcare personnel

The fear of individual and legal accusation has been determined to be the most frequently encountered reporting obstacle in the studies included in this literature review [15,18,20,23,24,29,30,32,33,35,36,39,40]. Particularly, in studies conducted on nurses, the fear of individual accusation and administrator reactions took the place at the top of the list of obstacles [23,29,32,33,35]. Other reporting barriers among nurses, in the order of significance, were found to be: being thought of as incompetent, patients' negative attitudes, the stigma of incompetence, unsupportive work environment, long reporting process, the idea that reporting errors that do not damage the patient is unnecessary, not knowing the importance of error reporting, and lack of education, lack of feedback on reporting and not perceiving the error as an error [22,23,29,32,37,38].

In those studies conducted with physicians only, the lengthy reporting process, as well as the additional workload associated with reporting errors, was found to be two of the leading error reporting barriers. Other barriers that were determined, in order of significance, were the lack of feedback and discipline procedures regarding the error [14,26,28]. In these three studies, it was accepted by the physicians that reporting was unnecessary, and that the errors were usually "inevitable". Moreover, according to two additional studies, medical error reporting was considered potentially unmanageable and "meaningless" [16,27]. In studies involving physicians and other healthcare personnel, the type of damage and severity of the error,

education level and occupation of the healthcare personnel, negative attitude towards reporting, lack of an encouraging culture in the institutions, and lack of reporting perception/education all affected the reporting rate (Table 2) [15,18,20,28,31].

Suggestions by healthcare personnel to increase medical error reporting

The factors that were analyzed in order to increase the medical error reporting rate of healthcare personnel were presented most often in the qualitative studies [14,37,34]. Increasing the nurses' knowledge, ability, undertaking, and accountability aspects, encouraging a scientific environment, an anonymous reporting system and lack of authority [37], clinicians and administrators learning from their mistakes, patient education, determining the basic ethical duties for reporting and encouraging the employees [14] were all leading motivational factors for error reporting.

In a study conducted with focus group interviews, the factors that facilitated error reporting were themed into three groups: preventing a communication gap after reporting, education for success, and decreasing the workload while reporting. The participants stated that they could report more often if they received sufficient education on reporting, timely feedback, and if the reporting process was simplified [34]. In a study in which the suggestions of the healthcare personnel were examined in order to increase the degree of reporting, it was determined that the necessity of education towards errors that should be reported, regular feedback about errors, and the development of an evidence based system change medical error reporting in an electronic environment [18]. In a study in which the simplifying factors for medication error reporting were investigated, the use of an anonymous reporting system, removal of a fear atmosphere from the institution, simplification of the reporting procedure, and the establishment of the perception that reporting is beneficial were recommended [23,31,41]. In Jee-In Hwang et al.'s study, the development of reward systems was the top priority implementation suggested by nurses to encourage error reporting [41].

In a study that determined the attempts to strengthen nurses reporting habits, the understanding and encouraging attitude of physicians and inspection authorities, identification of medication errors by the active participation of clinical nurses and clinical expert nurses, immediate reporting by the nursing administrator, sufficient time for reporting, and presence of nurse administrators to monitor the nurses who frequently commit errors with consistent disciplinary action were all specified [39].

Discussion

The reporting of medical errors is the focal point of the effort for reducing the incidence of these errors. The evaluation of the types and frequency of errors, and their effects on patients, have critical importance in the determination of the root causes of errors, and for the development of attempts toward the reduction and prevention of these errors [42,43]. Despite the critical importance of error reporting, healthcare professionals do not sufficiently report errors due to specific barriers.

It has been determined in studies that investigate the attitudes and perceptions towards medical error reporting that more reporting is done when the outcomes of the errors are at the level of severe damage; in parallel with this, less reporting is done when the potential outcome is harmless or only slightly harmful [21,22]. The types and severity of medical errors are perceived differently among healthcare professionals [17]. However, despite a common terminology related to the severity, types and outcomes of errors having been developed by international patient safety authorities, it was seen that this terminology is still not used and conceptualized as basic information by healthcare professionals.

When the error reporting barriers of healthcare personnel were investigated, the most commonly encountered obstacles were determined to be the fear of individual/legal accusation, and the fear of negative reactions from administrators and colleagues [15,20,23,24,32,33,35,36,39,40]. When the chronology of the studies was examined, a similar culture of fear seemed to be precedent in recent studies. Consequently, it was seen that, first of all, the fear obstacle toward medical error reporting remains and the strategies that have been developed are still insufficient.

The long duration of the reporting process, the belief that reporting errors that are not harmful to the patient is unnecessary and meaningless, the type of harm and severity of the error, lack of education, lack of feedback about reporting, the fact that the error is not perceived as an error, and lack of knowledge about the importance of error reporting were found to be other reporting barriers, determined in order of priority [16,23,27,29,32,37]. These determined barriers show the necessity for the development of health care personnel awareness about error types and severity, reportable errors and the importance of reporting.

Some suggestions have been offered to increase medical error reporting, in order to motivate and reinforce healthcare personnel in this direction. When these suggestions were evaluated in order of priority, education and the development of awareness about reporting, dissolution of the atmosphere of fear and potential risks as a consequence of reporting, delivery of constructive feedback in a reasonable amount of time, shortening of the reporting duration, and development of strategies to encourage reporting by administrators emerged [18,23,39,31,34]. Based on the results of these studies, the education of healthcare personnel with regard to error reporting has been proceeding, while the development of administrative strategies (positive feedback, absence of disciplinary action, etc.) is still required. The feedback of reporting has been seen as an important issue that requires emphasis. According to the results of this literature review, the identification of the feedback forms used in error reporting, and the best application suggestions in this field, including a safe feedback loop

in institutions, the use of effective feedback channels, supply of feedback about the analysis of reporting, and the results and corrective actions (in a timely manner), were considered to be the best applications. In this study, institutions were recommended to create forms and systems that included the best applications with regard to effective feedback [44].

In several studies, it was observed that the investigated preferences of healthcare personnel with regard to the type of error reporting system and their thoughts about the use of different systems were few. In one study, the thoughts and suggestions of the physicians and nurses about the features of the error reporting system were investigated. According to that study, the most important goal of the reporting system was to play an educational role for healthcare workers, administrators, and other health related institutions (i.e., pharmaceutical companies) and to be integrated in education [45]. The capability of the error reporting system to develop a resolution process, and to make suggestions for protection from errors, is important for the development of the best applications. For example, the corrective attempts and instruction of workers are the most important factors for the effectiveness of the error reporting system and for its adaptation by users [8]. Consequently, the basic aim of error reporting systems should be the initiation of education and corrective action.

Conclusion

Despite the fact that medical error reporting has been accepted as a basic attempt for the improvement of patient safety, error reporting barriers continue to be one of the most important healthcare problems worldwide. Since the reporting barriers determined by the literature review are similar, a common terminology that includes these barriers (similar to the classification of errors and their outcomes) could be developed. Via the development of measurement tools that include this terminology, worldwide standardization could be provided and could shed light on the attempts at proof-based reporting.

In many studies, no approaches or strategies were specified for the prevention of feelings of fear and accusation. In order to prevent a culture of fear, which is an important reporting obstacle, administrators should take charge of important responsibilities, attempts and approaches. In future studies, the reasons for a fear culture, and the suggestions of healthcare workers for changing a fear culture, could be investigated. Moreover, in light of the investigated suggestions, an improvement in reporting fear related approaches and an investigation of their results are important.

It was determined in the previously conducted studies that education provided to healthcare workers in the direction of medical error/error reporting, types and intensity of errors, and classification of errors according to patient outcomes is effective in improving the approach to error reporting. At present, technological methods present opportunities like distance training systems, simulation education, etc. and the use and investigation of these, and similar methods, is suggested to be effective on patient safety and error reporting education.

Implications for Practice and Future Research

This investigation presents up-to-date information about medical error reporting barriers, and the features of effective error reporting systems for nurse administrators, quality and risk management workers, institution administrators, and researchers. When evaluated within the scope of the investigated research questions, along with descriptive studies toward reporting barriers, more experimental studies are required. The constitution of error reporting systems, evaluation of its usage by healthcare workers, and sharing of the results will contribute to the literature in this field. Especially, studies that investigate the reporting barriers determined by the research and healthcare workers' suggestions, comprehensively, from a practical perspective, are thought to be beneficial.

By using the results of this review, nurse administrators could collaborate with system designers to develop effective, creative error reporting systems. At the same time, these results could contribute to the development of strategies that improve and encourage error reporting, with the aim of developing the awareness of error reporting and patient safety. The development of positive attitudes and behaviors of clinical nurses within a healthcare team, who have the potential and strength to be agents of change, would affect other team members. Accordingly, effective team cooperation, which is necessary for qualified patient care, will be provided, contributing to the leadership strength of nursing.

References

1. Marcus R (2006) Human factors in pediatric anesthesia incidents. Pediatr Anesth 16: 242–250.

2. Agency for Healthcare Research and Quality (2000) 20 Tips to help prevent medical errors 2101 East Jefferson Street. Rockville, MD.

3. Kohn LT, Corrigan JM, Donaldson MS (2000) To err is human: Building a safer health system. Institute of Medicine (US) Committee on Quality of Health Care in America, National Academies Press (US), Washington (DC).

4. John TAJ (2013) New, evidence-based estimate of patient harms associated with hospital care. J Patient Saf 9:122-128.

5. National Patient Safety Agency, National Reporting and Learning Service.

6. Page A (2004) Keeping patients safe: Transforming the work environment of nurses. The National Academies Press 500 Fifth Street, N.W. Washington, DC.

7. Pittet D, Donaldson L (2006) Challenging the world: Patient safety and health care-associated infection. Int J Qual Health Care 18: 4-8.

8. WHO (2005) Draft guidelines for adverse event reporting and learning systems from information to action. WHO/EIP/SPO/QPS/05.3 © World Health Organization.

9. Leigh E (2006) Great Britain Parliament House of Commons Committee of Public Accounts. A safer place for patients: Learning to improve patient safety. Fifty-first report of session 2005-06 report, together with formal minutes, oral and written evidence. London, UK: House of Commons Papers.

10. Walsh K, Burns C, Antony J (2010) Electronic adverse incident reporting in hospitals. Leadership in Health Services 23: 1751-1879.

11. Paterick ZR, Pateric JD (2009) The challenges to transparency in reporting medical errors. J Patient Saf 5: 205-209.

12. Noble DJ, Pronovost PJ (2010) Underreporting of patient safety incidents reduces health care's ability to quantify and accurately measure harm reduction. J Patient Saf 6: 247-50.

13. Karlsen KA, Hendrix TJ, O'Malley M (2009) Medical error reporting in America: A changing landscape. Qual Manag Health Care 18: 59-70.

14. Escoto KH, Karsh BT, Beasley JW (2006) Multiple user considerations and their implications in medical error reporting system design. human factors. The Journal of the Human Factors and Ergonomics Society 48: 48.

15. Kreckler S, Catchpole K, McCulloch P, Handa A (2009) Factors influencing incident reporting in surgical care. Quality Safety Health Care 18: 116–120.

16. Evans S, Berry JG, Smith BJ (2006) Attitudes and barriers to incident reporting: A collaborative hospital study. Quality Safety Health Care 15: 39-43.

17. Hobgood C, Weiner B, Tamayo-Sarver JH (2006) Medical error identification, disclosure and reporting: do emergency medicine provider groups differ? Acad Emerg Med 13: 443-451.

18. Taylor JA, Brownstein D, Christakis DA, Blackburn S, Strandjord TP, et al. (2004) Use of incident reports by physicians and nurses to document medical errors in pediatric patients. Pediatrics 114: 729-735.

19. Lawton R, Parker D (2002) Barriers to incident reporting in a healthcare system. Quality Safety Health Care 11: 15–18.

20. Sarvadikar A, Prescott G, Williams D (2010) Attitudes to reporting medication error among differing healthcare professionals. Eur J Clin Pharmacol 66: 843-53.

21. Okuyama A, Sasaki M, Kanda K (2010) The relationship between incident reporting by nurses and safety management in hospitals. Qual Manag Health Care 19: 164–172.

22. Espin S, Griffithsb AW, Wilson M, Lingardd L (2010) To report or not to report: A descriptive study exploring ICU nurses' perceptions of error and error reporting. Intensive and Critical Care Nursing 26: 1-9.

23. Bayazidi S, Zarezadeh Y, Zamanzadeh V, Parvan K (2012) Medication error reporting rate and its barriers and facilitators among nurses. J Caring Sci 1: 231-236.

24. Mrayyan MT, Shishani K, Al-Faouri I (2007) Rate, causes and reporting of medication errors in Jordan: Nurses' perspectives. J Nurs Manag 15: 659-670.

25. Uribe CL, Schweikhart SB, Pathak DS, Dow M, Marsh GB (2002) Perceived barriers to medical-error reporting: An exploratory investigation. J Healthc Manag 47: 263-279.

26. McArdle D, Burns N, Ireland A (2003) Attitudes and beliefs of doctors towards medication error reporting. Int J Health Care Qual Assur 16: 326-333.

27. Waring JJ (2005) Beyond blame: Cultural barriers to medical incident reporting. Social Science and Medicine 60: 1927-35.

28. Coyle YM, Mercer SQ, Murphy-Cullen CL, Schneider GW, Hynan LS (2005) Effectiveness of a graduate medical education program for improving medical event reporting attitude and behavior. Qualityand Safety Health Care 14: 383-388.

29. Chiang HY, Pepper GA (2006) Barriers to nurses' reporting of medication administration errors in Taiwan. J Nurs Scholarsh 38: 392-399.

30. Ulanimo VM, O'Leary-Kelley C, Connolly PM (2007) Nurses' perceptions of causes of medication errors and barriers to reporting. J Nurs Care Qual 22: 28-33.

31. Martowirono K, Jansma JD, Van Luijk SJ, Wagner CA. Bijnen AB (2012) Possible solutions for barriers in incident reporting by residents. J Eval Clin Pract 18: 76–81.

32. Petrova E, Baldacchino D, Camilleri M (2010) Nurses' perceptions of medication errors in Malta. Nursing Standard 24: 41-48.

33. Almutary HH, Lewis PA, Cert CC (2012) Nurses' willingness to report medication administration errors in Saudi Arabia. Qual Manag Health Care 21: 119–126.

34. Hartnell N, MacKinnon N, Sketris I, Fleming M (2012) Identifying, understanding and overcoming barriers to medication error reporting in hospitals: a focus group study. BMJ Qual Saf 21: 361-368.

35. Wagner LM, Damianakis T, Pho L, Tourangeau A (2013) Barriers and facilitators to communicating nursing errors in long-term care settings. J Patient Saf 9: 1-7.

36. Heard GC, Sanderson PM, Thomas RD (2012) Barriers to adverse event and error reporting in anesthesia. Anesthesia Analgesia 114: 604-614.

37. Hashemi F, Nasrabadi AN, Asghari F (2012) Factors associated with reporting nursing errors in Iran: a qualitative study. BMC Nurs 18: 11-20.

38. Lederman R, Dreyfus S, Matchan J, Knott JC, Milton SK (2013) Electronic error-reporting systems: A case study into the impact on nurse reporting of medical errors. Nurse Outlook 61: 417-426.

39. Ulanimo VM, O'Leary-Kelley C, Connolly PM (2007) Nurses' perceptions of causes of medication errors and barriers to reporting. J Nurs Care Qual 22: 28-33.

40. Kim J, An K, Kim MK, Yoon SH (2007) Nurses' perception of error reporting and patient safety culture in Korea. West J Nurs Res 29: 827-844.

41. Hwang JI, Lee SI, Park HA (2012) Barriers to the operation of patient safety incident reporting systems in Korean general hospitals. Healthc Inform Res 18: 279-286.

42. Ioannidis JP, Lau J (2001) Evidence on interventions to reduce medical errors: An overview and recommendations for future research. J Gen Intern Med 16: 325-334.

43. Milch CE, Salem DN, Pauker SG, Lundquist TG, Kumar S, Chen J (2006) Voluntary electronic reporting of medical errors and adverse events. An analysis of 92,547 reports from 26 acute care hospitals. J Gen Int Med 21: 165-170.

44. Benn J, Koutantji M, Wallace L, Spurgeon P, Rejman M, et al. (2009) Feedback from incident reporting: information and action to improve patient safety. Qual Saf Health Care 18: 11-21.

45. Karsh BT, Escoto KH, Beasley JW, Holden RJ (2006) Toward a theoretical approach to medical error reporting system research and design. Appl Ergon 37: 283–295.

17

Needle Stick and Sharp Injuries and Associated Factors among Nurses Working in Jimma University Specialized Hospital, South West Ethiopia

Jemal Beker* and Tesafa Bamlie

Department of Nursing, College of Public Health and Medical Sciences, Jimma University, Ethiopia

*Corresponding author: Jemal Beker, Nursing, College of Public Health and Medical Sciences, Jimma University, Ethiopia. E-mail: jemalbeker@yahoo.com

Abstract

Introduction: Needle Stick and Sharp Injuries (NSSIs) are the commonest rout by which blood borne infections such as HIV, HBV and HCV can transmit. Such infections serve as high occupational risks and threats to health professionals. The objective of this study was to assess the prevalence of Needle stick and sharp injuries and associated factors among nurses working in Jimma University Specialized Hospital, South West Ethiopia.

Methods: An institutional based cross sectional study design was employed among nurses with at least one year work experience in Jimma University Specialized Hospital from March 31 to April 04, 2014. A total of 173 study subjects were selected using simple random sampling technique from sampling frame using lottery method. Data was collected using pretested English version questionnaire through self-administered interview. To maintain the quality of data pretesting and supervision of data collection process was done. The collected data were checked for completeness, edited and entered into EpiData version 3.1 and exported to SPSS version 21.00 for analysis. To explain the study variables descriptive statistics was used. Association between dependent and independent variables was calculated using chi square test. P-value of less than 0.05 was considered as significant association.

Results: Out of the total 173 study subjects, 170 were included in the final analysis and giving a response rate of 98.3%. Majority of the study subjects 95 (55.88%) were female nurses. This study indicate that nurses' sex, monthly salary, marital status, work experience, working Unit/department/, training on IP and patent safety, presence of contaminated needle and sharps materials in the working area, job satisfaction, level of job stress on nurse respondents, use of personal protective and gloves during the practice work by needles/sharps and recapping of needles after use had significant association with the occurrence of sharp and needle stick injury in nurses. In general this study revealed that no single factor accounted for the occurrence of NSSIs.

Conclusion and recommendation: This study demonstrated a relatively high prevalence of NSSIs among nurses of JUSTH. The high prevalence of NSSIs highlights the need for developing effective preventing strategies. Training of nurses should be emphasized and essential in preventing high NSSIs risks in the hospital.

Keywords: Needles stick and sharp injuries; Nurses; Jimma University Specialized Hospital

Introduction

Needle stick and sharp injuries (NSSIs) are accidental skin penetrating wounds caused by sharp instruments in a health care setting. This occurs when health professionals perform their clinical activities in the health institutions such as hospitals, health centres and clinics. As a result of this, they are exposed to blood borne infections by pathogens such as blast mycosis, crypto mycosis, diphtheria, Ebola, gonorrhoea, hepatitis B, hepatitis C, HIV/AIDS, strep pyogens , tetanus , herpes, malaria, tuberculosis, syphilis, toxoplasmosis, leptospyrosis , rocky mountains, spotted fever\, scrub typhus, streptococcal infection, staphylococcal. Among these diseases Hepatitis B, Hepatitis C and HIV/AIDS are at most concern because they can cause significant morbidity or death [1].

According to the national institute of occupational safety and health study the design of device can increase the risk of injury such as devices with hollow bore needles, needle devices that need to be taken apart or manipulated by the health care worker like blood drawing devices that need to be detached after use, syringes that retain a exposed needle after use [2].

The activities that expose nurses to NSSIs includes recapping after use, handling specimens, collision between health care workers or sharps during clean up manipulating needles in patient line related work, passing handling devises or failure to dispose of the needle in puncture proof containers [3].

The World Health Organization (WHO) estimated that global disease burden from contaminated sharp injuries to nurses professional at the work place covered; occupation, environment, life style, diet, health practices and substance abuse. According to this report every year hundreds of thousands of HCWs are exposed to deadly viruses such as HBV, HCV, and HIV as a result of needle stick and sharp injuries. These preventable injuries expose workers to over twenty different blood borne pathogens and results in an estimated 1,000 infections per year, the most common being HBV, HCV and HIV [2].

NSSIs have significant indirect consequences in health care delivery for nurses especially in the developing countries, where already the qualified nurse professional are limited with respect to the disease burden in the population. These injuries not only potentiate health consequences but also cause emotional distresses which results in missed work days and directly affects the health care services and resources.

A study done by Lihan and Durkan showed that the percentage of nurses experiencing needle stick injuries during the year professionals' time was 79.7% and the incident of body fluid exposure in one year was 68.4%. Age less than 24 years, less than four years of nursing work experience, working in surgical intensive care unit and working for more than eight hours per day were the factors identified to increase needle stick injuries [4]. In developing country like Ethiopia where the basic rules of occupational safety and health is implemented poorly the prevalence NSSIs related infections among nurse professional increase dramatically.

Strategies are available to prevent infections due to NSSIs including education of nurses on the risks and precautions, reduction of invasive procedures, use of safer devices and management of exposures. In industrialized world occupational surveillances assess and monitor the health hazards related to blood borne pathogens and prevention measures which reduce the risk of transmission [5]. In contrast to this, in Ethiopia exposure and health impacts are rarely monitored and much remains to be done to protect nurses from such risks that cause infections, illnesses, disability and death that may intern impact on the quality of health care. This study would be the baseline for further related studies for nursing and other professions. Farther more, the result of the study will be helpful for Local health planners and Local health departments for improving the risk of infections due to NSSIs among nurses.

Methods and Subjects

The study setting

An institutional based cross sectional study was conducted among nurses who were worked in Jimma University Specialized Hospital, Jimma, Ethiopia. During the study period, there were 387 nurses who worked at JUSH. The data were collected over a period of 15 days (from March 31-April 15, 2014 G.C).

Population

All randomly selected nurses in Jimma University Specialized Hospital were included by considering both inclusive and exclusive criteria. Based on this staff nurses who were worked for at least one year in JUSTH were included in the study however those of Staff nurses who were critically ill during study period and Staff nurses who were under sick leave, delivery leave and annual leave during study period were excluded.

Sample size

The sample size for this study was calculated using the single population proportion formula:

$$ni = \frac{((z\alpha/2)^2 \times p(1-p))}{d^2}$$

Where n=Sample size (the desired sample size)

Z α/2=Standard normal deviation, set at 1.96, to correspond to the 95%confidence interval

p=Prevalence of NSSIs among health care workers was 22% (30).

q=1.0-p

d=Margin of error/an absolute precision=5%=0.05

$$ni = \frac{((1.96)^2 \times 0.22(1-0.22)}{(0.05)^2}$$

ni=264

For population less than 10,000 populations we use the following correction formula.

nf=ni/1+(ni/N)=264/1+264/387=157

Where, nf=the desired sample size when the population is <10,000.

ni=the desired sample size when the population is >10,000.

N=the estimate of the population size who are worked for at least one year (387).

- By considering 10% non-response rate; the total final sample size was 173.

Sampling technique

The sample size was selected using simple random sampling technique from sampling frame using lottery method.

Data collection technique

Data was collected from the study individuals using self-administered questionnaire which consists of description on socio-demographic characteristics, behavioral characteristics, and environmental characteristics of the respondents. Data was collected by four trained B.Sc. Nurses.

Data quality control

Five percent of the questionnaires were pre- tested in Bedelle Hospital to assess the reliability, clarity, sequence, consistency and understandability and the total time it takes to finish the questionnaire before the actual data collection. Then after, the necessary comments and feedbacks were incorporated in the final tool.

Data analysis and presentation

Data were checked for completeness, edited and entered into EpiData version 3.1 and exported to SPSS version 21.00 for analysis. Chi-squared test was done to see the association between important baseline variables and outcome variable. P-value of less than 0.05 was considered as significant association.

Ethical considerations

Ethical clearance and approval to conduct the research was obtained from Jimma University College of health science, Ethical Review Board. Then a letter was secured from the university to respective hospital management to gain support for the study. Prior to administering the questionnaires, the aims and objectives of the study were explained to the participants and personal consent was also being obtained from study participant after explaining the objective of study.

They were also told that participation is voluntarily and confidentiality and anonymity will be ensured throughout the execution of the study as participants are not required to disclose personal information on the questionnaire.

Result

A total of 173 study subjects participated in the study. Three of them were excluded due to the incomplete filling of the questionnaires. Thus, 170 study subjects were included in the final analyses giving a response rate of 98.3%.

From the total respondents 95 (55.88%) were female nurses while 75 (44.12%) were male nurses and 56 (32.94%) were between age of 25-29 with the mean age of 29.56 years (SD 8.1 years). Seventy two (42.4%) were Orthodox Christians followed by Protestant which accounts 51 (30%). In the context of ethnicity 105 (61.70%) were Oromo followed by Amhara which accounts 32 (18.82%). In the marital status condition of nurse, 95 (53.53%) were single followed by married which accounts 66 (38.82). One hundred fifteen (67.65%) nurses have work experience of 1-5 years with the mean work experience of 5 year (SD 6.6 years). Majority to the study subjects 99 (58.23 %) were clinical nurses by profession.

Working environment characteristics

Out of the total nurses working in JUSTH, majority 48 (28.24%) were working in surgical/OR unit and 26 (15.29%) worked in medical units followed by pediatric/neonatology unit which accounts 23 (13.53%) (Figure 1).

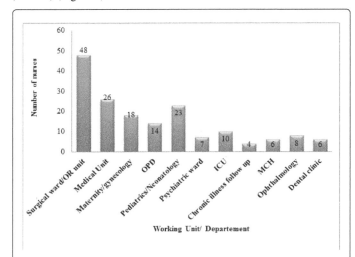

Figure 1: Distribution of nurses by working unit/department in JUSTH, Jimma, South west Ethiopia, March 31 to April 04, 2014.

From the total respondents, one hundred fifty (88.24%) had night shift work in the hospital, 122 (71.76%) had got information about health and safety information access, only 39 (22.94%) had got training on infection prevention and patient safety in the last one year prior to the study and 90 (52.94%) had been supervised by the concerned body on the application of infection prevention. 123 (72.35%) have safety box in their working rooms to dispose infectious wastes including needle stick and sharp materials and 75 (44.12%) of

the respondents had reported that there are contaminated needle stick and sharp materials around their working area (Table 1).

Variable	Response	Frequency	Percent
Night shift work	Yes	150	88.24
	No	20	11.76
Health and safety information access	Yes	122	71.76
	No	48	28.24
Training on IP and patent safety	Yes	39	22.94
	No	131	77.06
Supervision by others in working room	Yes	90	52.94
	No	80	47.06
Presence of contaminated needle and sharps materials in the working area	Yes	75	44.12
	No	95	55.88
Presence of safety box in the room for used needles	Yes	123	72.35
	No	47	27.65
Condition of safety box in the working unit	Over filled	53	43.09
	Turnout	42	34.15
	Empty	28	22.76
	Total	123	100

Table 1: Showing working environment of nurses working in JUSTH, Jimma, South west Ethiopia, March 31-April 04, 2014.

Nurses behavior related attributes

From the total respondents, 28 (16.47%) chew khat, 11 (6.47%) smoke cigarettes, 69 (40.59%) have a problem of sleeping disturbance during work time. 93 (54.71%) of the workers were satisfied by their job and 91 (53.53%) have job related stresses. Majority of them 147 (86.47%) believe that needle stick and sharp injury is a preventable problem and they believes that nurses have high risk to NSSIs 96 (56.47%) (Table 2).

Variable	Category	Frequency	Percent
Chat chewing	Yes	28	16.47
	No	142	83.53
	Total	170	100
Cigarette smoking	Yes	11	6.47
	No	159	93.53
	Total	170	100
Sleeping disturbance	Yes	69	40.59
	No	101	59.41
	Total	170	100

Needle Stick and Sharp Injuries and Associated Factors among Nurses Working in Jimma University...

101

Belief on preventability of Needle stick/sharp injuries	Yes	147	86.47
	No	23	13.53
	Total	170	100
Belief on risky nature of nurses to needle stick/sharp injuries	High risk	96	56.47
	Moderate risk	46	27.06
	Low risk	28	16.47
	Total	170	100
Job satisfaction level of nurse respondents	Dissatisfied	77	45.29
	Satisfied	93	54.71

Level of job stress on nurse respondents	Total	170	100
	Not stressed	79	46.47
	Stressed	91	53.53
	Total	170	100

Table 2: Showing behavior related attributes of nurses working in JUSPH Jimma South west Ethiopia March 31-April 04, 2014.

Related to PPE usage, 65 (38.24%) of the study subjects used most of the time, 55 (32%) sometimes, 39 (23%) all of the time and 11 (7%) never used PPE (Figure 2).

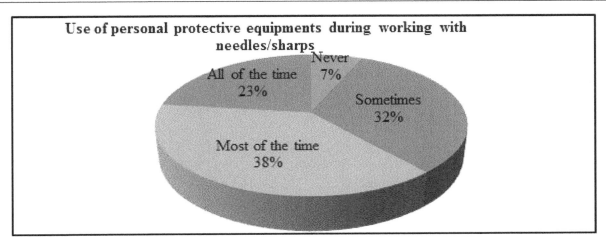

Figure 2: Distribution of nurses by use of personal protective equipments during working with needles/sharps in JUSTH, Jimma, South west Ethiopia, March 31-Aril 04, 2014.

On recapping of needles after use, 61 (35.88%) of the respondents recap needles sometimes, 49 (28.83%) never recap, 33 (19.41%) recap most of the time and 27 (15.88%) recap all of the time (Figure 3).

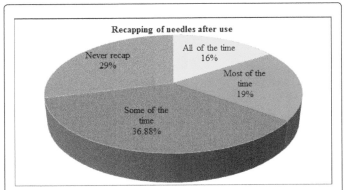

Figure 3: Distribution of nurses by recapping of needles after use in JUSTH, Jimma, South west Ethiopia, March 31-Aril 04, 2014.

Prevalence of needle stick and sharp injury

The prevalence (occurrence) of needle stick and sharp injury to nurses in JUSTH was 61.76% (105) (Figure 4).

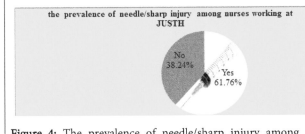

Figure 4: The prevalence of needle/sharp injury among nurses working at JUSTH, Jimma, South west Ethiopia, March 31-April 04, 2014.

The frequency of needle stick and sharp injury 1-2 times was 53 (50.48%), 3-4 times was (30.48%). Concerning the condition of needles/sharps during injury 61 (58.09%) nurse respond that they were injured by dirty needles/sharps. The types of injury sustained were superficial 47 (39.49%) and slight skin penetration 40 (33.62%). In the health status of source clients/patients in relation to blood borne pathogens 47 (44.76%) were unknown status followed by clinically suspected HIV/AIDS cases which accounts 21 (20.19%). Almost all nurses 167 (98.24%) were not vaccinated against Hepatitis B virus because not available in the hospital 150 (88.24%). One hundred sixty (94.12%) respondents knew the presence of prophylaxis service to HIV after injury by needle /sharp in the hospital (Table 3).

Variable	Category	Frequency	Percent
The frequency of injury occurred on respondents	1-2 times	53	50.48
	3-4times	32	30.48
	>5times	20	19.04
	Total	105	100
The condition of the needles sharps during injury	Dirty needle/sharps	61	58.09
	Sterile needle/sharp	20	19.05
	Both sterile and dirty needle/sharps	24	22.86
	Total	105	100
Type of injury sustained	Deep	32	26.89
	Slight skin penetration	40	33.62
	Superficial	47	39.49
	Total	119	100
Health status of clients in relation to blood borne pathogens	Known HIV/AIDS positive	19	18.27
	Clinically suspected HIV/AIDS case	21	20.19
	Jaundiced and clinically diagnosed hepatitis patient	10	9.5
	Unknown states	47	44.7
	Total	105	100
Report to concerning body	Yes	84	80
	No	21	20
	Total	105	100
Measures they take after exposure	Washing with soap and water	41	19.62
	Wash with alcohol, iodine, chlorine	66	31.58
	Take TAT	11	5.26
	Visiting VCT	63	30.14
	Seek Post Exposure Prophylaxis	19	9.09

	Squeezing to extract more blood	9	4.31
	Total	209	100
Vaccination against hepatitis B virus	Yes	3	1.76
	No	167	98.24
	Total	170	100
Reasons why not vaccinated	High cost	17	10.18
	Not aware	3	1.79
	Not available	147	88.02
	Total	167	100
Transmission of diseases by dirty needles/sharps	Yes	158	92.94
	No	12	7.06
	Total	170	100
Diseases that can be transmitted through dirty needles/sharps	Hepatitis B	140	33.18
	Hepatitis C	121	28.67
	HIV	161	38.15
	Total	422	100
Program should initiate to protect staff nurses from risk of Needle stick and sharp injuries	Improved facilities for needle/sharps	153	27.42
	Enforced AIDS testing of all patients before admission to hospital	141	25.27
	Education talks on risky behaviors	53	9.49
	Improved reporting procedures for injuries	123	22.04
	Increased punishment for staffs who don't properly dispose needles/sharps, therefore place other staffs at risk	88	15.77
	Total	558	100

Table 3: Needle stick and sharp injury related attributes among nurses working in JUSTH, Jimma, southwest Ethiopia, March 31-Aril 04, 2014.

The major types of needles/sharps that cause injury to nurses were IV needle 32 (25.6%) followed by surgical blade 29 (23.2%) and IM needles 26 (20.8%) (Figure 5).

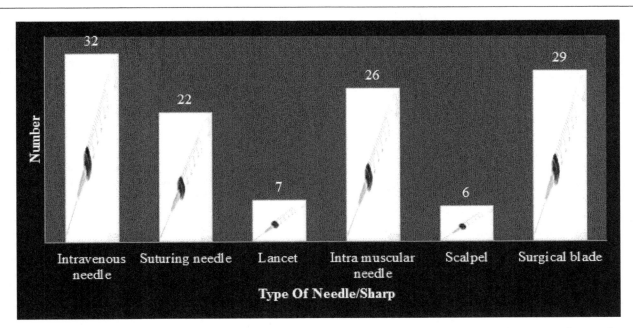

Figure 5: Distribution of nurses by type of needle/sharp that causes the injury in JUSTH, Jimma, South west Ethiopia, March 31-Aril 04, 2014.

Recapping needle after use and suturing/injection, 36 (24.16%) and 37 (24.83%) were the major activities that lead to NSSIs, respectively. The least activities that lead to NSSIs were immunization, patient aggressiveness and negligence which account 1 (0.01%) 6 (0.04%) and10 (0.07%), respectively (Figure 6).

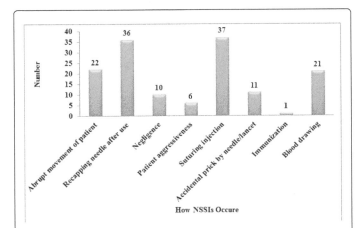

Figure 6: Distribution of nurses how NSSIs are occurred among nurses working in JUSTH, Jimma, South west Ethiopia, March 31-April 04, 2014.

Association between independent variable with NSSIs

Among the socio demographic variables sex, monthly salary, marital status and work experience had shown association with the occurrence of needle stick and sharp injury at p<0.05.

Working environment related variable working Unit/department/, training on IP and patent safety and presence of contaminated needle and sharps materials in the working area had showed significant association at p<0.05.

Among the worker behavior related factors job satisfaction, Level of job stress on nurse respondents, Use of personal protective and gloves during the practice work by needles/sharps and Recapping of needles after use had showed a significant association at p<0.0 (Table 4).

Variable	Category	NSSIs		Values	
		Yes	No	x^2	P
Sex	Male	56	19	9.46	0.002
	Female	49	46		
Marital status	Single	70	21	19.1	0.001
	Married	29	37		
	Divorced	6	7		
	Widowed	-	-		
Monthly salary in ETB	<1500	22	33	16.3	0.001
	>1500	83	32		
Year of service	5-Jan	73	42	6.6	0.037
	10-Jun	13	17		
	>10	19	6		
Working Unit/ department/	Surgical wards	38	10	8.23	0.001
	Medical wards	19	7		
	Maternity/Gynecology	10	8		
	OPD	9	5		

	Pediatrics/ Neonatology	10	13		
	Psychiatric ward	6	1		
	ICU	8	2		
	Chronic Illness	0	4		
	MCH	1	5		
	Ophthalmology	2	6		
	Dental clinic	2	4		
Training on IP and patent safety	Yes	10	29	28	0.001
	No	95	36		
Presence of contaminated needle and sharps materials in the working area	Yes	54	21	5.95	0.015
	No	51	44		
level of job satisfaction	Satisfied	32	45	24.3	0.001
	Dissatisfied	73	20		
Level of job stress on nurses'	Not stressed	37	42	13.9	0.001
	Stressed	68	23		
Use of personal protective equipment during handling needles/ sharps	Never	7	4	7.93	0.047
	Sometimes	41	14		
	Most of the time	39	26		
	All of the time	18	21		
Recapping of needles after use	All of the time	22	5	50.4	0.001
	Most of the time	27	6		
	Some of the time	46	15		
	Never	10	39		

Table 4: showing the association between independent variables with NSSIs among nurses working in JUSTH, Jimma, South west Ethiopia, March 31-April 04, 2014.

Discussion

This study revealed that the one year prevalence of needle stick and sharp injury was 44.12%. The study conducted on one year prevalence of needle stick and sharp injury in East Gojjam Zone Health Institutions, Sidama Zone and North western Ethiopia had showed 22%, 32%and 31% respectively [6]. There is big difference with current study this difference might be related to the fact that the above studies were conducted by mixing all types of health professionals from hospitals, health centers and clinics so that the number of screening, diagnostic, follow up and other intervention procedures that use needles and medical sharp materials were less in health centers. The other possible reason might be related to work load.

In this study the major types of needles/sharps that cause the injury to nurses were IV needle 25.6%, surgical blade 23.2% and IM needles 20.8%. Hollow bore needles are responsible for the occurrence of 46.4% of NSSIs. This result is lower than study done by National surveillance for health care workers (NASH) of USA show that 59% of all sharp injuries were caused by hollow bore needles and study conducted in India showed that 71% the needles involved in the NSSIs injury were hollow bore needles [7,8]. This variation might be due to the use of hollow bore needles by nurses in this hospital may be less than the above countries.

Concerning the condition of needles/sharps during injury this study showed that 61 (58.09%) nurse were injured by dirty needles/sharps. This result is lower than Study conducted in Saud Arabia, showed that 89.3% of the sharp items involved in the injuries are contaminated. But this study result is higher than a result of a study done in Japan showed that 22% NSSIS involved device that had been used on a patient prior to the NSSIS (contaminated devices) [9].

Recapping needle after use 24.16%, suturing/injection 24.83% and blood withdrawal 14.09% were the major clinical activities that lead to NSSIs in this study. Study conducted in Saud Arabia, showed that most of the injuries occur during suturing/injections 31.8% and drawing of venous blood samples 17.2% [9]. And study conducted in India showed that the commonest clinical activities to cause NSSIS in that study were, 55% blood withdrawal, 20.3% suturing, 11.7% vaccination and recapping needles after use was 66.3% and according to a study done in Malaysia hospitals nurses 27.2% NSSIs causes were recapping of syringes after use [10].

One hundred sixty (94.12%) respondents knew the presence of prophylaxis service to HIV after injury by needle /sharp in the hospital in this study. This result is more and greater than a result of study conducted in India which showed that only about 40% health care workers knew the availability of post exposure prophylaxis services in the studied hospital [10]. This may be due to there is good awareness about post exposure prophylaxis of nurses in JUSH. Almost all nurses 98.24% were not vaccinated against Hepatitis B. This result is lower than a study done in Addis Ababa hospitals showed that 11.6% of the study subjects were vaccinated for hepatitis B vaccine. This variation may be due to the absence of the vaccine in JUSH [11].

Working Unit/department/, training on IP and patent safety and presence of contaminated needle and sharps materials in the working area had significant association with the occurrence of sharp and needle stick injury in nurses. Among the worker behavior related factors, job satisfaction, level of job stress on nurse respondents, use of personal protective and gloves during the practice work by needles/ sharps and recapping of needles after use showed a significant association with the occurrence of needle stick and sharp injuries (p<0.05). This result is almost similar with study conducted in East Gojjam Zone Health Institutions health care workers which showed the following results: sex of the worker, monthly salary of worker, infection prevention and safety information access, getting training on infection prevention and, sleeping disturbance problem, job satisfaction and job stress showed a significant association with the occurrence of needle stick and sharp injuries in health care workers [12]. This similarity may be related to similarity of the setups they use (standard precaution guidelines).

Conclusion

This study revealed that the lifelong and one year prevalence of needle stick and sharp injuries among nurses in this hospital was 61.76% and 44.12% respectively. In general, this study findings indicate a relatively high prevalence of needle stick and sharps injuries among nurses.

In general this study revealed that no single factor accounted for the occurrence of NSSIs. So nurses' sex, monthly salary, marital status, work experience, working Unit/department/, training on IP and patent safety, presence of contaminated needle and sharps materials in the working area, job satisfaction, level of job stress on nurse respondents, use of personal protective and gloves during the practice work by needles/sharps and recapping of needles after use; had significant association with the occurrence of sharp and needle stick injury in nurses.

Recommendation

Based on the findings of this study the following recommendations were forwarded to reduce the occurrence of NSSIs and the consequences of NSSIs among nurses working in JUSTH:

- Hospital administrates, nursing service directors and different nongovernmental organizations should strengthened regular provision of information on infection prevention and safety to nurses at all levels.
- The hospital administrator should work hard with other stakeholders to avail Vaccination against hepatitis B virus for the staff nurses.
- Hospital administrates, nursing service director and supervisors should strengthen mechanisms to improve nurses' job satisfaction.
- All stakeholders including staff nurses' should work together to reduce job stressors.
- Nurses' should practice proper use of safety box and personal protective equipment during handing needle and sharps.
- Special attention should be given for nurses with low monthly salary.

References

1. Chalupa S, Markkanen PK, Galligan CJ, Quinn MM (2008). Needles stick and sharps injury prevention: are we reaching out goals? AACN View point retrieved.

2. NIOSH (1999) Preventing needle stick injuries in health care settings. Washington DC, National Institute for occupational safety and health 2000-2108.

3. Wilburn SQ (2004) Needlestick and sharps injury prevention. Online J Issues Nurs 9: 5.

4. Ilhan MN, Durukan E, Aras E, Türkçüoğlu S (2006) Long working hours increase the risk of sharp and needlestick injury in nurses: The need for new policy implication. J Adv Nurs 56: 563-568.

5. Berhanu EF (2013) Prevalence and determinant factors for sharp injuries Among Addis Ababa Hospitals Health professionals Science of public Health 1: 189-193.

6. Hanrahan A, Reutter L (1997) A critical review of the literature on sharps injuries: Epidemiology, management of exposures and prevention. J Adv Nurs 25: 144-154.

7. Alysia Giany (2012) EPInet TM Report: needle sticks injury Incidents, Are High SAFE.6.

8. Sumati M, Kumar S, Mesenakshi M, Manju B (2013) Needle sticks injuries among health care worker in tertiary care hospital of India; Global journal of Medical research 13: 41-50.

9. Alam M (2002) Knowledge, attitude and practices among health care workers on needle-stick injuries. Ann Saudi Med 22: 396-399.

10. Smith DR, Mihashi M, Adachi Y, Nakashima Y, Ishitake T (2006) Epidemiology of needlestick and sharps injuries among nurses in a Japanese teaching hospital. J Hosp Infect 64: 44-49.

11. Hofmann F, Kralj N, Beie M (2002) Needle stick injuries in health care - frequency, causes und preventive strategies. Gesundheitswesen 64: 259-266.

12. Zewdie A (2013) Assessment on Magnitude Needle stick and sharp injuries and associated factors among health care workers in east Gojjam zone health Institutions; Global Journal of medical research 13.

18

Nurses Challenges of Supporting Hospitalized Patients Regarding Sexual-Health Issues

Anette C Ekstrom[1]*, Lena Nilsson[1], Caroline Apell[2], David Palmius[3], Lena B Martensson[1]

[1]*School of Health and Education, University of Skovde, P.O. Box 408, SE-54128 Skovde, Sweden*

[2]*The Municipality of Alingsas, SE-44181 Alingsas, Sweden*

[3]*Skaraborg Hospital Skovde, SE-54182 Skovde, Sweden*

***Corresponding author:** Anette C Ekstrom, School of Health and Education, University of Skövde, P.O. Box 408, SE-54128 Skövde, Sweden, E-mail: anette.ekstrom@his.se

Abstract

Background: The approach to nursing should be characterized by a holistic view of the human being which includes sexual health. From a nursing perspective, it is therefore of most importance to have a dialogue about factors associated with sexual health also among hospitalized patients. However, to our knowledge there is a lack of qualitative studies regarding nurses attitudes about dialogue with patients about sexual health.

Objective: To investigate nurses attitudes towards dialogue with hospitalized patients about sexual health.

Methods: A qualitative method was used and interviews were conducted which then were analyzed using a qualitative content analysis. Eleven registered nurses were included, the inclusion criteria was: at least one year of experience as a nurse and working on a medical or surgical ward in a hospital in the southwest of Sweden. The participants were in the ages 25-65 and had worked as nurses between 2 and 30 years. Nine of the participants were women. The data were collected during 2011.

Results: The nurses experiences of and reflections on dialogue with patients about sexual health were presented as a single main theme: Nurses challenges to support hospitalized patients with sexual health issues. This theme had three categories: Feeling uncomfortable, Feeling inadequate and Task-oriented care with related subcategories respectively.

Conclusions: Nurses attitudes towards their dialogues about sexual health with hospitalized patients were less challenging if they were initiated by the patients or if the patients were men with medical causes related to sexual health. Lack of knowledge and support from colleagues became reasons why nurses felt inadequate about discussing sexual health with their patients.

Keywords: Sexual health; Nursing care; Qualitative analysis; Dialogue

Introduction

Sexual health is present throughout life, regardless of the individuals age, [1,2]. According to the definition by the World Health Organization, sexual health is "... a central aspect of being human throughout life... and sexual health is ... a state of physical, emotional, mental and social well-being in relation to sexual health" [3] and "...is influenced by the interaction of biological, psychological, social, economic, political, cultural, legal, historical, religious and spiritual factors." [3]. From a nursing perspective, it is therefore of great importance to be aware of factors associated with sexual health also among older people [4]. Higgins et al., [5] describe sexual health as an important aspect of good quality of life and even more important when sexual health is threatened by disease. There are a lot of aspects which have an impact on sexual health. For instance, in relation to type 2 diabetes [6], stroke [7], and prostatectomy [8] sexual health may be affected. Further psychotropic medication could have an impact on sexual health [9], for example after hysterectomy [10]. However, sexual health does not only include somatic function or dysfunction but also the psychological and existential aspect of a human being [3]. Briggs [11] states that sexual health is not only limited by the physical impact of disease but also by anxiety and self-experienced ill-health.

On the one hand, it is the nurses responsibility to talk about sexual health in an informative and responsive manner [5], on the other hand, it has been reported that nurses avoid illuminating sexual health with patients even if they are aware of their responsibility regarding this issue [12,13]. Education is an important aspect to overcome nurses perceived barriers of social and personal perceptions in relation to supporting patients sexual health [14]. It has been stated that nurses also lack the confidence to bring up the subject with the patient [15,16]; they do not feel comfortable enough [13] and they are reluctant to initiate a conversation related to sexual health and therefore await the patients initiative [5,17]. Further, there are also other barriers such as appropriate customized environments in the ward [18,19] and insufficient time to discuss these matters with the patient [13] and therefore it is challenging for nurses to create a private dialogue about sexual health with the patients. Nurses experience conflicting feelings when talking to patients about sexual health;

however, the ones who actually talk about sexual health have a strong desire to help their patients [20]. Important when offering support are non-judgmental attitudes [21] as well as an understanding of unique support needs and knowledge of the specific supportive situation [21-25]. The professional provider may also hesitate to offer support from fear of inflicting harm [26]. Attitudes are based on feelings for and a varying degree of knowledge about a specific phenomenon [27] and could be described as the individuals disposition to act or respond in a positive or a negative way in relation to this phenomenon [28]. Although sexual-health care is often not prioritized in practice, nurses are in a prime position to promote sexual health and well-being for patients. In summary, to our knowledge there is a lack of qualitative studies regarding nurses attitudes and dialogue with patients about sexual health. It is therefore important to increase knowledge about the nurses views about their insufficient dialogue and documentation regarding patient's sexual health. Therefore, this study aims to investigate nurses attitudes towards dialogue with hospitalized patients about sexual health.

Methods

Design

A qualitative design with content analysis [29] was chosen for this study. It was decided that the most suitable data collection method was individual interviews since the direct voices of the nurses can provide information about meaningful values and life experiences [30]. This data collection method aimed to elucidate the participants perception [31] of dialogue about sexual health with hospitalized patients.

Participants

To ensure variation, a purposive sampling strategy was adopted [32,33] regarding age, gender, and years of experience as a nurse. Eleven registered nurses who fulfilled criteria of at least one year of experience as a nurse and working on a medical or surgical ward or in a hospital in the southwest of Sweden participated in the study. They were between 25 and 65 years of age and they had worked as nurses between 2 and 30 years. Nine of the participants were women and two were men. In their daily work, the participants met patients with different medical and surgical illnesses which could have an impact on sexual health.

Data collection procedure

Access to the informants was gained through the head of the medical or surgical ward. Information about the study was given during workplace meetings. Thereafter, the head of each ward asked the nurses if they were willing to participate. None of the nurses had any previous relationship with the researchers responsible for the study. The nurses who met the inclusion criteria and who fulfilled the purposive sampling criteria were approached by this head of the ward. The nurses were informed about the study and asked to give their consent to participate in the study. Thereafter, the interviews were conducted by two of the authors, CA and DP, who alternated during the interview with the exception of one interview which was conducted by CA alone. The interviews were held at the ward in a secluded room or in an office were the interview could be in private [34]. The average length of the interviews was 30 minutes, starting with an interview guide containing themes about age, gender, and years of experience as a nurse. The interviews were digitally recorded and all the recorded

interviews were transcribed verbatim before an analysis was made. The data were collected during 2011.

The nurses were asked to talk about their experiences of dialogue with patients about sexual health. The interview started with an open question "Can you tell us about your experiences talking with patients about sexual health?" This open question was followed by questions aiming to encourage the nurses to freely elaborate on the description of their experiences. Probing questions such as "Could you explain more?" were used to create a deeper understanding of the nurses answers.

The audio-taped interviews with the nurses were transcribed verbatim and analysed separately using latent content analysis [29]. Data collection and analysis were carried out simultaneously, in part to follow up the issues that were emerging but also to decide when saturation of the topics and the respondents had been reached [35].

Data analysis

Content analysis is a stepwise process of categorization based on the expression of thoughts, feelings, and actions described throughout the text [29]. The intentions of the analytical process are to remain close to the words of the text and to bring out the contextual meanings. The material was analyzed according to a model described by Graneheim and Lundman [29]. In the first phase, the material was read several times to create comprehension of the material. The authors initially read the material separately and then together. When the authors were familiar with the material, the analysis moved on to the second phase. In that phase, units which emphasized a meaning were detected with focus on differences and similarities. The questions the authors had in mind during this process were in line with what was said in the text, how it was said and the meaning of what was said. The authors highlighted meaning units and placed similar parts into subcategories. In the third phase, the units were put together and the material became presentable with focus now on the new comprehension that emerged from the material [29]. Subcategories were formed according to similarities and differences in the nurses perceptions. All subcategories of a similar kind were put together and formed new main categories. In order to achieve trustworthiness in the data analysis, the concepts credibility, dependability, and transferability were taken into account. We made certain that the analysis agreed with the purpose; the entire material was analyzed simultaneously and all authors read through the text material to ensure that the material was categorized appropriately. Moreover, the context and the participants were described as clearly as possible to facilitate the transferability of the results [36]. In the final step, data were analyzed by reading across the categories, searching for new associations and meanings and in this process the theme was identified.

Ethical considerations

Permission to carry out this study was given by the head nurse at each ward. The procedure followed the principles of the Declaration of Helsinki [37]. The participants received written and oral information including participation being voluntary and that they could withdraw their participation at any time without explanation. According to Swedish law [38], no ethical approval is required when the study does not include patients.

Results

The nurses experiences of and reflections on dialogue with patients about sexual health were presented as a single main theme: Nurses challenges to support hospitalized patients with sexual-health issues. This theme had three categories: Feeling uncomfortable, Feeling inadequate and Task-oriented care with related subcategories respectively (Table 1). Each category and their subcategories were presented using direct quotations in a conversational format. A code number for each respondent is included after the quotation here below (Nurse: N1-N11).

Subcategories	Categories	Theme
Taboo		
Prejudices include gender	Feeling uncomfortable	
Patients´ initiative and responsibility		Nurses challenges of supporting hospitalized patients with sexual-health issues
Lack of knowledge		
Education	Feeling inadequate	
The working groups influence		
Medical problems was easier to relate to sexual health	Task-oriented care	
Sexual health has low priority during the acute phase of a disease		

Table 1: Categories with subcategories and theme identified from interviews with nurses.

Feeling uncomfortable

The nurses described feeling uncomfortable when discussing sexual health with patients. They highlighted that discussions about sexual health sometimes felt taboo and therefore was often avoided because of their own prejudices. However, the nurses thought that it was easier to discuss sexual health when the patients initiated the dialogue although they did not feel comfortable enough to initiate a dialogue themselves. They also thought that the patients were not comfortable discussing sexual health with the nurses.

Taboo

A perceived overall taboo was sometimes the main reason for the nurses not to initiate dialogue about sexual health with the patients. They emphasized that sexual health was not discussed neither with patients nor colleagues and was therefore a subject which was not focused on. The taboo did not only include the staff and the nurses in the study, but it was also presumed that patients considered sexual health to be something that was private and taboo.

... I do not talk about sexuality, with anyone... (N11)

Prejudices included gender

One barrier for the nurses to initiate a dialogue about sexual health was their own prejudices which made them uncomfortable. The prejudices included gender age and the relationship status of the patient. The nurses mentioned that the dialogue about sexual health was often focused on men who had medical treatment or had had surgery which could have an impact on their sexual health. They believed that women´s sexual health was not affected in the same way and that women were not considered as sexual beings to the same extent as men. The informants were also affected by the patients relationship status because of the nurses prejudice that patients who were not in a relationship did not have a sexual life.

One expects maybe that if you live in a relationship and you also have an intimacy together. Ehm ... I do not think about that you have a life together in the same way when you are single, but of course one has a sexual life anyway. (N5)

The informants stressed that it was important to be aware of their own attitudes to be able to have a dialogue about sexual health for patients.

Sexuality keeps you on course for many years, many younger people believe that people stop just because you are 40 or older. But here they are older than that, so that´s a topic we need to address, it is important! (N7)

Patients initiative and responsibility

The nurses mentioned that a dialogue about sexual health was held on the patients terms. A majority of the informants expressed the opinion that it was easier to discuss sexual health if it was on the patients initiative. They felt that the patient should initiate the dialogue if they had problems, which meant that the nurses disclaimed any responsibility for the patients sexual health. However, some of the nurses highlight that it was important to raise the issue to show the patients that it was essential to discuss the subject, if the patients wanted this.

But it's more that you raise the question, many times I can feel that it's enough to just open up, so they feel it's okay to talk about it. (N6).

Feeling inadequate

The nurses stated that they had a feeling of being inadequate when it came to starting a dialogue about sexual health with patients. They were afraid of talking about issues they could not help the patient with and they described their knowledge as limited. Further, all of the respondents expressed how sexual-health was absent in their training to become a nurse. Some of them had participated in theme days about sexual health, but they experienced this as insufficient. Knowledge and experiences about sexual health were not shared between colleagues which increased their feeling inadequate.

Lack of knowledge and education

The informants felt that they lacked education and knowledge about sexual health in their training to become a nurse which made initiating a dialogue about sexual health more difficult. The nurses were worried that they could not provide sufficient support regarding sexual health. Therefore they too often avoided the topic.

For the patient it is about to continue living. So really, you should bring this up more. But I do not really feel that I have the tools to do it in a good way. (N4)

Education was as an important factor for the nurses. It gave them better knowledge and tools to provide support and to have a dialogue with the patients. The informants highlighted that their own private experiences influenced their dialogue with the patients, which made it difficult to offer good support.

I think we need education and perhaps guidance in discussing this type of topics, in a comfortable and secure way for both ourselves and the patient. (N5).

The working group´s influence

The colleagues support was of great importance for the nurses in their work. Sharing knowledge and discussing the approach to various issues were of great importance. However, they perceived it as unfortunate that the patients sexual health was an issue being discussed only to a very limited extent. Furthermore, it was stressed that it was important to talk about sexual health within the working group.

… It would be good to discuss this in the staff group between us nurses. Why is it difficult to talk and advise each other about this, we are doing it in many other subjects? (N5)

The nurses pointed out that they had had theme days when the topic was discussed, although without continuing the discussion afterwards. This reinforced their feeling that the topic was not relevant to discuss with the patients and colleagues.

Task-oriented care

The results show that it was obvious that the care of the patient is task-oriented. The nursing care is much too often focused on practical issues and the nurses state it is easily the case that priority is not given to dialogue about sexual health if the issue is not of a medical character.

Medical problems were easier to relate to than sexual health

The nurses stated that it was not easy to give priority to a dialogue with the patients about sexual health if the issue was not of medical causes. Medical causes, for example, could be erectile dysfunction caused by blood-pressure treatment where it was possible to prescribe drugs for erectile dysfunction.

If the patient gets any side effect associated with the diseases or the medication you may bring it up trying to get help, otherwise I don´t think it is common to bring it up… [11]

Sexual health has low priority during the acute phase of a disease

It became clear that sexual health had low priority, especially during the acute phase of a disease. The nurses described how the focus for the patient was to regain health and therefore sexual health had no place during hospitalization. However, they pointed out that the patients maybe had questions about sexual health when they were discharged from the hospital.

Thus, it has not the highest priority soon after an acute event…/…It is probably something that could be an issue later… [13]

Nurses challenges of supporting hospitalized patients with sexual-health issues

The main theme showed that nurses had challenges of supporting hospitalized patients with sexual-health issues, something which often was a result of the nurses own uncertainty and priority given to medical causes. They highlighted that sexual health much too often was taboo and therefore they avoided this issue in their professional support. The dialogue about sexual health was usually focused on men while women were not considered as sexual beings to the same extent. The informants said that it was easier to discuss sexual health if it was on the patients initiative. Lack of knowledge and lack of support from colleagues was a major reason why nurses felt inadequate to discuss sexual health with patients. Education was an important factor that would give the nurses tools and knowledge in order to perform dialogues about sexual health.

Discussion

As mentioned above, the results showed that nurses felt challenges when supporting hospitalized patients with sexual-health issues which often was affected by uncertainty and a priority to medical causes. The respondents felt uncomfortable initiating a dialogue about sexual health with patients. On the other hand, if it was the patient´s initiative, they did not have this feeling. This attitude puts the responsibility on the patient and the nurses meant that it was the patient´s responsibility to initiate the dialogue if a problem existed. This is something also described by Higgins, Barker and Begley [5], and Guthrie [17] who mention that nurses largely await the patient´s initiative. A clearly distinguishable category of feeling uncomfortable was based on sexual health as private and experienced by the nurses as a taboo subject. It became clear that sexual health was not something that was openly discussed among colleagues and thus also hampered the dialogue with the patient. Research shows that the professional support provider may also hesitate to offer support from fear of inflicting harm [26] and it is important when offering support to express non-judgmental attitudes [21] as well as an understanding of unique support needs and knowledge of the specific supportive situation [22-24].

Age was another factor of the prevailing prejudices about sexual health as described by the nurses. Although the nurses stressed that age should not be a deciding factor in the initiation of dialogue about sexual health, they anyway described how their prejudices about an elderly patient´s sexual health prevented them from bringing this up.

Peate [1] emphasizes that sexual health has no age limit, something which is supported by Skoog [39] who highlights that old people continue to be sexually active, a view that is in line with the definition by the World Health Organization [3]. Another noticeable prejudice was that individuals not in relationships were not sexually active, which was based on the idea that only those who live in a relationship were expected to have a sexual relation. This prejudice could be reasons the nurses did not initiate a dialogue with a patient who were not in a relationship.

The result showed that the nurses had a feeling of being inadequate when it came to starting a dialogue with patients about sexual health due to limited knowledge. Further, all of the respondents meant that sexual health was absent in their training to become a nurse and theme days. In addition, knowledge and experiences about sexual health were not shared between colleagues who increased their feelings of being inadequate. This pattern of feeling inadequate is confirmed by Price [15] who highlights that most of the nurses do not feel confident enough to start a dialogue about sexual health. According to Higgins et al [5], the nurses themselves need to admit sexual health as something important for human beings as well as becoming aware that patients have a desire for nurses to bring this topic up.

Another significant result is that the nurses described their work as task-oriented which meant that if they wanted to initiate a dialogue about sexual health, it required that the problem had medical causes. This was exemplified by the prescription of drugs for problems of erectile dysfunction. Further, dialogue about sexual health often focused on eliminating physical barriers to be able to be sexually active. Briggs [11] and Peate [1] describe how the nurses role is to advise the patient about possible side effects of the drugs and that they should be able to give the patient advice and support when side effects occur. The informants also highlighted the problem that they felt it was of major importance to give priority to more urgent problems of the patient and that it was likely that the patient did not always feel that it was relevant to discuss sexual health. There is an underlying mix of sexual function and sexual health, which are not the same concepts although they are inter-related, something that needs to be discussed. Professionals dialogue with patients about sexual health therefore had low priority.

In addition, safe care requires proper documentation; however, documentation is inadequate, much too often due to lack of time and knowledge [40,41]. A patient´s medical record has many different functions and should reflect the contents of the main components of care [42]. VIPS is a model for nursing documentation and consists of keywords in a person´s nursing history, status, and measures of nursing work [42]. Sexual health is one of the keywords, but too often documentation under the keyword sexual health is missing.

However, a minority of the informants stated that even during hospitalization, it might be necessary to open up discussions about sexual health for the patient to feel comfortable to return to this issue at a later stage. Health is a combination of physical and mental wellbeing in a holistic perspective [3]. The dialogue should therefore not only focus on knowledge provision but also aim to provide support and confirmation. This is a challenge for the nurses who need good training and support in order to promote sexual health throughout life.

Limitations

Throughout the study, various steps were considered and taken in order to enhance the trustworthiness of the study. In qualitative research; credibility, dependability, confirmability, and transferability build trustworthiness [43]. Individual interviews were chosen as the data-collection method; interviews made it possible to grasp the individuals narratives which could provide information about meaningful values, experiences, and reflections [30]. To ensure variation, a purposive sampling strategy was adopted [32,33] regarding age, gender, and years of experience as a nurse. The interviews were performed by two of the authors. One of the authors conducted the interview and the other observed. This was a positive strategy for the interview technique, which provides dependability. The study is limited by its small sample size, but the context and the participants are described as clearly as possible to facilitate the transferability of the results [30]. Data collection and analysis were carried out simultaneously, in part to follow up the issues that were emerging but also to decide when saturation of the topics and the respondents had been reached [35]. Thus, it is our estimation that the content of the interviews was adequate, especially since in the interviews analysed at the latest stage, no new conclusions emerged. In order to strengthen the credibility of the present study, the analysis process was performed individually as well as jointly discussed between the authors. The confirmability quotations are presented in the results, which enables validation of the relevance of the nurses attitudes. Nurses who met the inclusion criteria were strategically included to enable as many variations of perceptions as possible. We have described the setting and data collection procedure as clearly as possible in order to promote the transferability of design and findings.

Conclusions

Nurses attitudes towards their dialogues about sexual health with hospitalized patients were less challenging if they were initiated by the patients or if the patients were men with medical causes related to sexual health. Lack of knowledge and support from colleagues became reasons why nurses felt inadequate about discussing sexual health with their patients.

Relevance to Clinical Practice

To offer adequate professional support for patients sexual health, education is an important factor. Education gives the nurses tools to reflect on their own attitudes and hence to facilitate their dialogue about sexual health with the hospitalized patients, especially with women.

Acknowledgements

We want to express our appreciation to all the nurses who participated in this study.

What does this paper contribute to the wider global clinical community?

On the topic of dialogue about sexual health with hospitalized patients, this study contributes the following:

- Knowledge about nurses having feelings of being uncomfortable and that their challenges of talking about sexual health are affected by their own uncertainty and a priority given to medical issues.
- Education is an important factor that gives the nurses tools to reflect on their own attitudes and hence to facilitate their dialogues about sexual health with the hospitalized patients, especially women.

Funding

The study was funded by the University of Skovde, Sweden.

References

1. Peate I (2004) Sexuality and sexual health promotion for the older person. Br J Nurs 13: 188-193.

2. Mercer CH, Tanton C, Prah P, Erens B, Sonnenberg P, et al. (2013) Changes in sexual attitudes and lifestyles in Britain through the life course and over time: findings from the National Surveys of Sexual Attitudes and Lifestyles (Natsal). Lancet 382: 1781-94.

3. World Health Organization. Sexual and reproductive health 2006.

4. Killinger KA, Boura JA, Diokno AC (2014) Exploring factors associated with sexual activity in community-dwelling older adults. Res Gerontol Nurs 7: 256-263.

5. Higgins A, Barker P, Begley CM (2006) Sexuality: the challenge to espoused holistic care. Int J Nurs Pract 12: 345-351.

6. Tamas V, Kempler P (2014) Sexual dysfunction in diabetes. Handb Clin Neurol 126: 223-232.

7. Korpelainen JT, Kauhanen ML, Kemola H, Malinen U, Myllylä VV (1998) Sexual dysfunction in stroke patients. Acta Neurol Scand 98: 400-405.

8. Benson CR, Serefoglu EC, Hellstrom WJ (2012) Sexual dysfunction following radical prostatectomy. J Androl 33: 1143-1154.

9. Higgins A (2007) Impact of psychotropic medication on sexuality: literature review. Br J Nurs 16: 545-550.

10. Vomvolaki E, Kalmantis K, Kioses E, Antsaklis A (2006) The effect of hysterectomy on sexuality and psychological changes. The European journal of contraception & reproductive health care: the official journal of the European Society of Contraception 11: 23-7.

11. Briggs LM (1994) Sexual healing: caring for patients recovering from myocardial infarction. Br J Nurs 3: 837-842.

12. Jaarsma T, Stromberg A, Fridlund B, De Geest S, Martensson J, et al. (2010) Sexual counselling of cardiac patients: nurses' perception of practice, responsibility and confidence. European journal of cardiovascular nursing : journal of the Working Group on Cardiovascular Nursing of the European Society of Cardiology 9: 24-9.

13. Saunamaki N, Andersson M, Engström M (2010) Discussing sexuality with patients: nurses' attitudes and beliefs. J Adv Nurs 66: 1308-1316.

14. East L, Hutchinson M (2013) Moving beyond the therapeutic relationship: a selective review of intimacy in the sexual health encounter in nursing practice. J Clin Nurs 22: 3568-3576.

15. Price B (2010) Sexuality: raising the issue with patients. Cancer Nursing practice 9: 29-35.

16. Shuman NA, Bohachick P (1987) Nurses' attitudes towards sexual counseling. Dimens Crit Care Nurs 6: 75-81.

17. Guthrie C (1999) Nurses' perceptions of sexuality relating to patient care. J Clin Nurs 8: 313-321.

18. Kim S, Kang HS, Kim JH (2011) A sexual health care attitude scale for nurses: development and psychometric evaluation. Int J Nurs Stud 48: 1522-1532.

19. Nakopoulou E, Papaharitou S, Hatzichristou D (2009) Patients' sexual health: a qualitative research approach on Greek nurses' perceptions. J Sex Med 6: 2124-2132.

20. Saunamaki N, Engström M (2014) Registered nurses' reflections on discussing sexuality with patients: responsibilities, doubts and fears. J Clin Nurs 23: 531-540.

21. Oakely A. Giving support in pregnancy; the role of research midwives in a randomized controlled trial. Midwives, Research and Childbirth. 3. London: Chapman & Hall.; 1994. p. 30-63.

22. Langford CP, Bowsher J, Maloney JP, Lillis PP (1997) Social support: a conceptual analysis. J Adv Nurs 25: 95-100.

23. Oakley A (1994) Giving support in pregnancy; the role of research midwives in a randomized controlled trial, Midwives, Research and Childbirth. 3. London: Chapman & Hall 30-63.

24. Hupcey JE (1998) Clarifying the social support theory-research linkage. J Adv Nurs 27: 1231-1241.

25. Langford CP, Bowsher J, Maloney JP, Lillis PP (1997) Social support: a conceptual analysis. J Adv Nurs 25: 95-100.

26. Schumaker S, Brownell A (1984) Towards a theory of social support: closing conceptual gaps. Journal of social issues 4: 11-36.

27. Zanna M, Rempel J (1986) Attitudes, a new look at an old concept. The social psychology of knowledge, University Press, Camebridge.

28. Ajzen I (2005) Attitudes, personality and behavior. 2nd ed. Maidenhead, Berkshire: Open University Press.

29. Graneheim UH, Lundman B (2004) Qualitative content analysis in nursing research: concepts, procedures and measures to achieve trustworthiness. Nurse Educ Today 24: 105-112.

30. Kvale S (1996) Interviews: an Introduction to Qualitative Research Interviewing. California.: Sage Publications.

31. Drennan J (2003) Cognitive interviewing: verbal data in the design and pretesting of questionnaires. J Adv Nurs 42: 57-63.

32. Patton M (2002) Qualitative research and evaluation methods. 3 ed. California: Sage; 2002.

33. Polit D, Beck C (2004) Nursing research principles and methods. 7 ed. Philadelphia: Lippincott Williams & Wilkins.

34. Kvale S (1997) Den kvalitativaforskningsintervjun [The qualitative research interview]: Studentlitteratur.

35. Mayan M (2001) An introduction to qualitative methods: A training module for students and professionals.: University of Alberta: International Institute for Methodology.

36. Morse J, Barrett M, Mayan M, Olson K, Spiers J (2002) Verification Strategies for Establishing Reliability and Validity in Qualitative Research. International Journal of Qualitative Methods.

37. Declaration of Helsinki (2002) World Medical Association Declaration ethical principles for medical research involving human subjects. J Postgrad Med 48: 206-8.

38. Law for ethical review of research involving humans 2003: 460.

39. Skoog I (1996) Sex and Swedish 85-year olds. N Engl J Med 334: 1140-1141.

40. Ehrenberg A (2001) Nurses perceptions concerning patient records in Swedish nursing homes. Nordic Journal of Nursing Research 21: 9-14.

41. Nordström G, Gardulf A (1996) Nursing documentation in patient records. Scand J Caring Sci 10: 27-33.

42. Ehnfors M, Thorell-Ekstrand I, Ehrenberg A (1991) Towards basic nursing information in patient records. Vard Nord Utveckl Forsk 11: 12-31.

43. Lincon Y, Guba E (1985) Naturalistic Inguiry. London: Sage Publications Inc.

19

Nursing as a Profession in Brazil: Sociological Contributions

Adriana Lima Pimenta, Maria de Lourdes de Souza* and Flavia Regina de Souza Ramos

Federal University of Santa, Brazil

*Corresponding author: Maria de Lourdes Souza, Nursing, Rua Delfino Conti s/n, Bairro Trindade, Florianópolis, Santa Catarina 88040.370, Brazil; E-mail: repensul@uol.com.br

Abstract

Aim: The objective was to analyze the content of Nursing Professional Practice Law and compare it to the content of papers addressing professional identity published in Revista Brasileira de Enfermagem.

Methods: Bibliographic and documental searches were conducted using qualitative analysis grounded on Eliot Freidson's Sociology of Professions. The corpus consisted of texts published between 1983 and 2012, and Brazilian Legal Documents.

Results: The thematic category "Contradictions of the nursing profession" emerged. A weakness of the professional project was identified, which is based on the fragmentation of work. This reductionist approach legitimizes the maintenance of nursing divided into professional and non-professional workers, restricting the practice of nurses.

Conclusion: The complexity of care requires social responsibility to construct a professional project that provides scientific, ethical, philosophical and political foundations to workers to support their practice.

Keywords: Nursing; Sociology; Laws; Nurse's role; Nursing care

Introduction

Nursing in Brazil is a discipline from the field of health, knowledge that is produced and reproduced in undergraduate and graduate programs and specialization programs, which make up the foundation of the work of professionals called nurses. The core identity of nursing is care [1-5]. Nursing is represented by an occupational group in the health field that is composed of workers with an undergraduate degree (nurses), those with a technical/vocational certificate (nursing technicians and auxiliaries) and also individuals with no specific education (nursing aides) [6]. Nursing is one of the 14 professions that compose the health field (CNS, 1998), comprising 60% of the total workers in the field, a figure that includes all multi-disciplinary team members. These data reveal the social importance of this occupational group to ensuring care is delivered to the population. The Federal Council of Nursing was created in 1973 to regulate professional practice [7] and in 1986, the regulation of professional practice (LEP) was the content of Law 7,498/86, which excluded all workers without specific qualification and established that nursing practice would be exclusively performed by nurses, nursing technicians and auxiliaries, in addition to midwives, according to their respective levels of qualification.

The scientific studies authored by Brazilian nurses address various problems faced in nursing practice, referred to as "contradictions of the profession," such as a lack of distinction between the tasks performed by nursing technicians and auxiliaries [8], a blurred definition of the scope of nurses' competencies [9], and the distancing of nurses from their core identity, coupled with a lack of appreciation for the profession on the part of society [10]. Most of these contradictions

have not being resolved by how LEP defined the profession and assigned responsibilities, with contributes to undermining the identity of nursing professionals.

In Brazil, according to the Federal Constitution, lawmaking concerning the organization of professions is a responsibility exclusive to the federal government. The Brazilian State, based on the 1988's Constitution, Article 22, Section XVI, spells out the commitment in which health is established as a fundamental right of citizens. In this constitutional context, health actions and services gained relevance to public interest. This "new order" establishes that the training and competence of healthcare professionals meet parameters that ensure the fundamental rights of the population do not remain at the market's mercy [11,12].

Considering that constitutional interests provide that health is a fundamental right of citizens, professional regulation becomes an integrating part of a larger project aimed to guarantee constitutional rights. Hence, discussing the potential contradictions of nursing's LEP is relevant to analyzing the current status and ensuring the right to health. The theoretical framework provided by the Sociology of Professions is one of the foundations that can ground this type of discussion.

Given the previous discussion, this study's objective was: to analyze the content of the Law of Nursing Professional Practice and compare it to the scientific studies published in *Revista Brasileira de Enfermagem* (Reben) [13] concerning the professional identify of Nursing, considering the theoretical propositions provided by the Sociology of Professions by Eliot Freidson.

This context was chosen according to certain theoretical assumptions, such as: that LEP and complementary acts that regulate the professional practice of different Nursing professionals in Brazil (the most in the health field), created in the 1980s, has left many gaps and do not respond to current issues; the years that followed the establishment of LEP witnessed profound changes in public health policies when health became a right of every citizen and a duty of the State to ensure it; that professionalization requires self-regulation mechanisms and mechanisms to produce/disseminate knowledge; and that Reben is the oldest (1932) and one of the most qualified scientific journals for Brazilian Nursing, also responsible for disseminating the political thought of the Brazilian Association of Nursing, Brazil's first such entity (1926). Laws are supposed to express the will of the collective, resulting in a social agreement that harmonizes conflicts of interests and protects the fundamental, political, social and economic rights of citizens and institutions. The regulation of professions is a topic specific to economic and social regulation. Hence, laws regulating professional practice, among other purposes, serve as guidelines and boundaries of professional jurisdictions and responsibilities [12]. Therefore, a relationship of mutual influence is established between the law of professional nursing practice, in its specificity, and the configuration of professional identity.

Method

This qualitative study was preceded by bibliographic and documental research. The study's *corpus* was composed of scientific studies published by Reben between 1983 and 2012, and Legal Documents that regulate the professional practice of Nursing, Law 7,498 [14] from June 25th 1986, Decree 94,406 [15] from June 8th 1987 and Law 8,967 [16] from December 28th 1994.

Papers were collected from 1983 to 2012 because 1983 was the year in which the journal adopted standards for the publication of papers with mandatory abstracts. Having the abstracts and establishing this period of time was appropriate to create favorable conditions to deepen the analysis. The following inclusion criteria were used to select the papers: scientific papers addressing the topic; full texts; published from 1983 and 2012. Editorials and sections titled Student Page, Readers' letters, Abstracts of Theses and Dissertations, Book Reviews, and the publication of documents were excluded.

The papers were selected according to the relevance of the topics presented in the abstracts to the study question. This criterion was established while skimming the texts and after verifying that merely searching for the terms of legislation, professional regulation, professional practice, identity, professional identity, professional role, and professionalization, in the titles, abstracts and keywords, was insufficient, because papers that were relevant to the topic were being overlooked.

A total of 89 papers were selected and printed between May and September 2013. After reading, 34 papers were excluded for not being relevant to the study so that a total of 55 papers composed the study *corpus* (Figure 1).

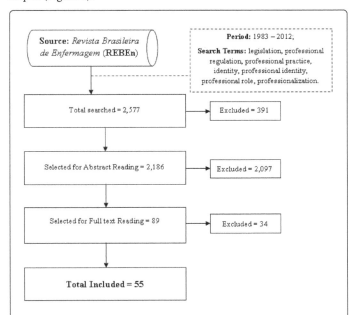

Figure 1: Flow chart showing the process of identification and screening

The periodical's full texts are available online on Scielo (Scientific Electronic Library Online) only beginning with 2003. Therefore, the physical collection available at the library at the Federal University of Santa Catarina was used to access the abstracts of papers published from 1983 to 2012. The texts were organized and systematized using content analysis, understood as a "set of techniques to analyze communication using systematic procedures and objectives of description of the content of messages". Thematic content analysis was chosen because it "seeks the core meanings that compose communication" [17].

The thematic analysis was developed in three phases. Pre-analysis, the first phase, includes skimming the text, composition of the *corpus*, and establishment of objectives. In the second phase, we explored the material, which was categorized according to "core meanings". The third phase included treatment and interpretation of results in light of Freidson's concept of professional identity and five concepts denoted here are thematic axes, which served as a "conducting wire" to understand and categorize the papers (Table 1).

Professional identity according to Eliot Freidson	
Thematic axes	Undergraduate program: accreditation via university degree
	Technical autonomy: the essence of work is established; specific expertise is instituted and controlled
	Socioeconomic autonomy: ability to provide social and economic organization of work
	Professional regulation: the State acknowledges professional jurisdictions

	Market shelters: monopoly of specific areas in the labor market

Table 1: Professional identity and its thematic axes, Source: Author's based on Reben [13] (1983 to 2012).

After the analysis of texts, we analyzed Law 7,498 [14] from June 25, 1986, Decree 94,406 [15] from June 8, 1987, and Law 8, 967 [16] from December 28, 1994. Finally, we compared the results from the analysis of the papers published in Reben with the legal framework that regulates professional nursing practice. This study used secondary data available from public domain sources.

Results and Discussion

The analysis of the texts published in Reben using the theoretical support of thematic axes based on the understanding of professional identity proposed by Eliot Freidson, resulted in the identification of the thematic category "Nursing Contradictions", and three subcategories are shown in Table 2.

	Category: Nursing Contradictions	
Subcategories	1. Naturalization of nursing organization.	
	2. Work's identity core is not defined	a. Object of knowledge is not defined;
		b. The core identity of the work of nurses is not defined: care delivery or services administration and team management?
		c. The statement that Nursing is "essentially" divided between manual and intellectual labor, hindering understanding of its object.
	3. Systematization of the Nursing process as a strategy to legitimate market shelters.	

Table 2: Nursing contradictions identified in the papers published in Reben – 1983 to 2012, Source: Author's based on Reben [13] (1983 to 2012).

These results were compared to the content of Law 7,498 [14], Decree 94,406 [15] and Law 8,967 [16], which constitute the Legal Documents regulating the professional practice of nursing in Brazil, shown in the discussion that follows.

1. Naturalization of the nursing organization

We present a synthesis of the content provided in Law 7,498 [14], from June 25, 1986, which regulates the professional practice of Nursing, describes its organization and lists the workers belonging to the profession, to facilitate understanding of our analytical approach and legally establish to whom we refer when we use the term "Nursing".

According to LEP, Law 7,498 [14] from June 25, 1986, Nursing workers (or the Nursing staff) include nurses, Nursing technicians, Nursing auxiliaries, and midwives. There are also nursing aides, workers without specific qualification, described in legal texts as "an individual, without specific education regulated by law, who performs Nursing tasks due to a lack of human resources with technical education in the field" [14]. Later, Law 8,967 [16] ensured that Nursing aides, hired before the enactment of this Law, had the right to perform elementary Nursing tasks as long as supervised by a nurse. Hence, after the enactment of the Law, no workers could be hired under this condition who has only in-service training. Nursing technicians and Nursing auxiliaries are professionals with technical/vocational training; that is, they met technical training requirements (either completed High School or Middle School) for receiving accreditation for their practice.

Nursing leadership and those in the federal and state governments have proposed organizing and providing alternatives to train individuals already working in the field who lack formal education. Regardless, they are in fact legally authorized to work in the field without any "accreditation". The law was enacted more than 20 years ago and this period of time should have been sufficient to extinguish this condition, either because old workers would have retired or acquired education in order to ascend to the condition of Nursing technician or auxiliary. In practice, however, nursing aides are still hired under new denominations, especially in private health services, as a way to circumvent Law 8,967 [16], which prohibits the hiring of this category of workers [18,19].

The focus of this study lies on Nursing, thereby there is a need to recognize there is a hierarchy grounded on differentiated qualification for performing the work, which is led by nurses, the only professional within the team who meets the professional requirements and has decision-making autonomy in regard to Nursing acts. Hence, in the Brazilian context, when one refers to Nursing as a profession, one refers to a heterogeneous group composed of professional and non-professional categories of workers; the latter exist only by the force of historical controversies and because individuals without professional qualification are still hired, despite standards regulating professional practice.

According to Freidson's Sociology of Professions, the first contradiction in the Nursing profession was exposed here. As stated by Freidson, in agreement with the theoretical theories on professions, these are occupations that necessarily require a college degree [20,21]. According to Freidson, the heterogeneous organization of Nursing workers consolidated by the law, weakens the professional project: "Decisive for the analysis of the success or failure of an occupation in achieving and maintaining its protections is the analysis of its internal stratification and segmentation [...]" [20].

The fragmented organization of Nursing is also identified in the texts published in Reben as a contradictory element; however, at the same time, the authors considered it necessary in the performance of the Nursing work. The content expressed in the papers and confirmed by law, was identified as the first subcategory – "naturalization of Nursing organization". The division of the Nursing work between professionals and non-professionals, seen as "natural" or even "typical" in this occupational group, neglects the Nursing professional project and impedes a more critical position regarding its historical circumstances and propositions for the future.

2. The profession's core identity is not defined

The second category identified in the manuscripts published in Reben, "the profession's core identity is not defined", includes: object of knowledge has not been defined; the nursing professional's core identity has not been defined: care delivery or administration of services and team management?; the statement that Nursing practice is "essentially" divided between manual and intellectual labor hinders understanding of its object.

The content of Law 7,498 [14] does not confirm what would be, from Freidson's perspective, the specific quality of Nursing expertise. Rather, it confirms a lack of definition of what the object of knowledge or what the profession's core identity is, as shown in the publications under study. The nucleus of professional competence, or the very quality that prohibits others from developing or performing it, is the core of the profession. This property is grounded on highly qualified knowledge and on social acknowledgment [20]. Law 7,498 [14], however, and confirmed by Decree 94,406 [15], states that the exercise of Nursing, "respecting degrees of habilitation", is exclusive to nurses, nursing technicians and auxiliaries, in addition to midwives. That is, Nursing actions are shared by all the team members, but not all members have Nursing expertise, which is attributed by a college degree. This condition raises controversies in regard to the complexity of its object of knowledge.

Law 7.498 [14] acknowledges that some actions are exclusive to nurses only, such as: leading, organizing, planning, supervising Nursing services and issuing reports, in addition to giving consultations, prescribing Nursing care, directly providing care to critical patients at the risk of death and under care of high technical complexity that requires scientific expertise, and the ability to make immediate decisions. If, on one hand, the fact that planning actions and supervision are considered to be exclusive to nurses corroborates professional power that derives from expertise itself [20], on the other hand, it reveals another contradiction, as other members of the Nursing team also provide care though they are not professional colleagues.

The description of acts exclusive to nurses expresses the division of Nursing practice between manual and intellectual work. This proposition may refer to a symbolic boundary established by medieval universities in regard to the intellectual specificity of the nature of academic work [22], but which, in the publications analyzed, gains further meanings that refer to the technical division of work. This division corresponds to the qualification of its workers' actions according to the rank they occupy in the team's hierarchy. Intellectual work is the responsibility of nurses who hold knowledge that is identified with "scientific management" and "complex care", while manual labor is to be performed by the remaining workers; that is, most care actions that are "expropriated of the most valued knowledge". Based on this understanding, fragmented care is legitimated by the law and the practice of care, and is often restricted to small tasks with little or no complexity.

Is it, however, feasible to accept Nursing work grounded on this fragmentation? How should we determine what "less complex" care actions dispenses with the need for the presence of a professional? What determines "greater technical competence"? How do we avoid a reductionist analysis that confounds "basic" action, in the sense of human condition, with "simple" action, that is, from fundamental to rudimentary? "El cuidado se encuentra en la raíz primera del ser humano y representa un modo-de-ser esencial, presente, irreductible, constituyente y base posibilitadora de la existencia humana" [23]. Nursing care, historically and ontologically, emerges as a basic condition to reestablishing human health or comfort [24].

Fully establishing social acknowledgment of this quality of Nursing care demands constituting authority of Nursing knowledge as a complex action, considering the totality of its acts, because the basic, in it's fundamental nature, is closer to complex than simple. Hence, grounded in the Sociology of professions' propositions, we state that it is the professional condition that infers authority and social acknowledgment to Nursing care as a complex action that should be necessarily performed in accordance with scientific, technical, philosophical and ethical foundations. Recognition of care and its valorization simultaneously converge in the legitimacy of Nursing as a profession and affirms the value of human life and citizenship, because Nursing care has a "political-social dimension that reverberates in the lives of citizens", so that, it is not "a merely instrumental and operational issue of labor, but rather a recognition of its purpose for human life" [4].

Nursing care in the 21st century cannot be learned in manuals or performed in static routines. It demands scientific and philosophically grounded training to respond to a working routine in which decision-making is urgent.

The law that regulates the professional practice of Nursing in Brazil seems insufficient to identify the allegedly distinct nature of the role played by Nursing technicians and auxiliaries [14].

Instead of a clear distinction of actions performed during care delivery, only hierarchical organization prevails, making use of a criterion that enables technicians to help nurses, also helping to supervise auxiliaries. In the legal text, the use of the adjectives "simple" and "repetitive" applied to hygiene care and comfort care is intended to qualify the type of care actions auxiliaries can perform, summarizing the alleged differentiation of tasks. But what qualifies as simple and repetitive? Considering the value of human life, are hygiene and comfort care actions devoid of complexity?

Relating hygiene to simple, repetitive, and valueless care actions compromises the meanings of right, beauty, and prevention. Representations of clean and dirty and hygiene practices are socially constructed and have complex meanings that even assign boundaries of social distances between individuals [25]. Anthropological theories support understanding regarding symbolic elements that serve as an amalgam of society and culture. Hence, the human being seems to be the only animal who is horrified at his/her own blood, vomit, sexual secretions, and who feels cruelly affected by them because s/he is the only one to have Culture" [26]. Symbolically, hygiene care ranks the lowest among care actions, as do those who perform them. Aware of this fact, we identify another controversy in the content of the Law and papers published in Reben in regard to the assignment of hygiene care to Nursing auxiliaries, which could be seen as an affirmation of power of the professional elite – nurses – to avoid a symbolic identification with not-so-noble tasks.

This controversy is in agreement with Freidson's studies on paramedic professions in the United States in the 1970s. The fact that American nurses distanced themselves from patients' beds was the result of a search for professional legitimacy. By taking management positions within the hospital administration, nurses found a prominent position in the division of labor in order to achieve professional autonomy, "eradicating their relationship of dependency with Medicine" [27]. Therefore, similar to American nurses, Brazilian nurses distanced themselves from direct care provided to patients in order to become engaged with leadership [28]. This achievement, however, may come at a price, weakening the profession's core identity and devaluating care.

The content of Decree 94,406 [15] from June 8, 1987, which regulated Law 7,498 [14], adds a more detailed description concerning the responsibilities of each team member, as shown below:

Art. 10. Nursing Technicians perform auxiliary activities, technical level tasks assigned to the nursing team, such as: I – assisting Nurses: a) planning, programing, orienting and supervising nursing care activities; b) providing direct nursing care to patients in severe conditions; c) preventing and controlling transmissible diseases in general in epidemiological surveillance programs; d) preventing and systematically controlling hospital infection; e) preventing and systematically controlling physical harm that may be caused to patients during care delivery; f) implementing the programs referred to in letter i and item II of Article 8; II – performing nursing activities except those exclusive to nurses, and those reported in article 9 of this Decree; III – integrate the health team.

Art. 11. Nursing Auxiliaries perform auxiliary activities, technical level tasks assigned to the Nursing team, such as: I – preparing patients for consultations, exams and treatments; II - observing, recognizing and describing signs and symptoms according to their level of qualification; III – performing specific prescribed or routine treatments, in addition to other nursing tasks like: a) ministering oral or parenteral medications; b) maintaining hydric control; c) applying dressings; d) applying oxygen therapy, nebulizer, enteroclysis, enema and heat or cold; e) performing tasks regarding the conservation and application of vaccines; f) controlling patients and communicants in transmissible diseases; g) implementing and reading tests to support diagnosis; h) collecting material for laboratory exams; i) providing nursing care before and after surgery; j) circulating in surgery rooms and, if necessary, instrumenting; l) working on disinfection and sterilization; IV – providing hygiene and comfort care to patients and taking care of their safety including: a) feeding or helping patients to feed themselves; b) cleaning and organizing material, equipment, and the health unit premises; V – integrating the health team; VI – participating of health education actions, including: a) orienting patients after consultations on how to follow nursing and medical prescriptions; b) helping Nurses and Nursing technicians to implement health education programs; VII – performing routine tasks related to patients' discharge; VIII – participating of post-death procedures.

This text shows an exacerbation of the contradiction underlying the fragmentation of the functions of Nursing work. Item II of Article 11, for instance, describes observation, recognition and description of signs and symptoms according to "one's level of qualification". Identifying the signs and symptoms that typify a pathological state or other characteristics that may occur in order to establish a morbid process requires technical and scientific competence, thus, requires training. How should the addition to the text "according to one's level of qualification" be understood? What signs and symptoms, which are not at the level of a nursing auxiliary's qualification, will not be identified? Or, is this Nursing worker exempt from responsibility in case s/he is not able to identify signs and symptoms that are beyond his/her level of qualification? What is the situation of individuals/patients/recipients of care, especially those in a large number of healthcare facilities that have a reduced number of nurses, and, for this reason, only occasionally participate in the direct delivery of care? [28,29]. Nurses depend on information provided by their auxiliaries to diagnose and plan care actions, but how is this information collected if these auxiliaries are not properly qualified to make observations that would support a Nursing diagnosis? These contradictions are appointed in the routine of Nursing practice and identified in the papers published in Reben, as well as by the content of LEP.

Item III of Article 11 also includes in the actions of auxiliaries "specifically prescribed treatments" or "routine treatments," in the sense that such treatments are already known or habitual. Note there is a textual effort to discriminate the activities of the team's auxiliary members as less qualified, activities that would demand less thorough theoretical knowledge or minimum learning, no decision-making ability or judgment to take actions, only compliance with prescriptions or following a manual. One should take into account that a less-qualified education provided by technical/vocational middle schools, in comparison to undergraduate programs, represents fewer costs. The economic interests of specific groups, however, should not trump the interests of the population and disregard their constitutional rights, promoting distortions in relation to the educational needs of healthcare professionals. The training and competence of these workers should meet quality parameters to ensure the fundamental rights of the population and cannot be at the mercy of the market [12].

The descriptions of some actions, which according to the law, are of a less-qualified or routine nature, make contradictions even more explicit. As in any sort of work intended to be professional, Nursing care is based on judgment and decision-making ability when in face of its object of knowledge. That is, the "authority of knowledge is decisive to define a profession" [20]. Therefore, in the professional organization of Nursing practice there is no justification for workers who lack the qualification to be responsible for performing such activities without the risk of harming those under their care. Even though LEP considers the decision-making ability of Nursing auxiliaries to be limited and subordinated, their field of work, as expressed in the tasks described, is broad and implies the existence of formal knowledge constructed by Nursing but which was not provided to them. It reveals disqualification of care as the object of knowledge and inadequate organization of Nursing's occupational group to achieve its social purpose.

The State, through its definitions spelled out in Law 7,498 [14], reaffirms the contradiction concerning a lack of definition of the profession's core identity identified in the papers published in Reben, a contradiction that weakens the professional project, posing a risk to the quality of care provided to the population and to the credibility of the authority of Nursing and the very government making the laws.

3. Adopting the systematization of the nursing process as a strategy to legitimate market protections

In the systematization of the Nursing process, nurses organize teamwork, planning care delivery to achieve desired results. The stages of Nursing care include: data collection, Nursing diagnosis, Nursing planning, implementation, and assessment [30]. Therefore, the systematization of the Nursing process should not be confounded with care delivery just because it is a tool that provides logical structure to the nurse's work [31].

Article 8 from Decree 94,406 [15], June 8, 1987, which regulates the exclusive acts of nurse, includes, among others: consultation and Nursing care prescription, based on care planning. The legitimacy of nurses regarding their professional competence "to establish a problem and propose a solution for it" is acknowledged; that is, nurses are responsible for establishing care. It confers professional status consistent with the power of authority of "authorized knowledge" and justifies nurses' prerogatives regarding the monopoly of professional Nursing services.

Therefore, the adoption of the systematization of the Nursing process as a strategy to legitimate market shelters is revealed as an important resource for the professional apparatus of Nursing to the extent it proposes the construction of an organizational plot in the context of the workspace. On the other hand, the papers published in Reben show the expression of ambivalent meanings regarding the efficacy of the functioning of this organizational structure. Conflicts are exposed regarding the prestige and power that the systematization of the Nursing process confers on nurses working as an exclusionary strategy, not integrating the team as a whole. What should be an organizational resource is revealed in the texts as the focus of contradictions to the extent to which it exposes a structure of inequalities upon which the organization of the Nursing team is based.

Additionally, content indicate that nurses are responsible for "providing tools" to the remaining members of the team, that is, creating conditions for the team to execute nursing prescriptions. But, how can nurses ensure that Nursing work is performed in accordance to the parameters learned within highly specialized university education when the remaining members of the Nursing team did not acquire the same training, knowledge, and education? As a consequence, conflict can erupt inside the Nursing team. According to content identified in the texts, the response to such conflicts would be to unify Nursing workers into one single category of professionals, understood here as a representative unit of workers, that is, unifying this class of workers via a labor union.

Thus, professional autonomy is constructed, among other aspects, based on the definition and construction of an identity that makes clear characteristics that are inherent to the profession. We observe there is a role assigned to class representativeness as a potential substitute for the power of expertise, which is the authority of professional power to ensure market reserve, in addition to an attempt to dilute inter-occupational conflicts and unequal education in Nursing through a proposition to equalize its unequal structure via the labor union struggle and by identifying Nursing workers as workers of a dominated class.

Therefore, the systematization of the Nursing process to legitimate market shelters is also revealed to be a contradiction of the profession and in the profession because it is based on reinforcing the structure of inequalities existing within the team and on the fact that nurses distanced themselves from directly providing care to patients, rather delegating care actions.

Final Considerations

The Brazilian Nursing elite, composed in this study by the authors of papers published in Reben, as well as the State, represented by the Law on Professional Nursing Practice, has assumed the fragmentation of the nursing work to be "natural to the profession". The weight of the historical construction of Nursing allied with a reductionist view of care delivery underlying the content of papers, contributes to reinforcing this lack of definition regarding the identity core of the Nursing profession.

Reducing or simplifying care to legitimate fragmented care and less-qualified education reveals a lack of knowledge concerning the unstable and subjective nature of phenomena that occur during the delivery of care. This rationale supports the maintenance of divided Nursing, preventing Nursing professionals from applying their rich cognitive and interpretative capacity to judge, replacing it with technical regulations justified by academic rhetoric.

The fragmentation of Nursing work also reflects what sociologists identify as a structure of inequalities where the professional elite controls "the best opportunities in the market". Considering Freidson's propositions, we understand that internal disputes within the professional group itself are phenomena that move the organization of the profession, oscillating reorganization and transformation. he problem occurs when the structure of inequalities is established and weakens the professional project itself, as seems to be the case in Nursing.

Professional regulation, that is, the regulation of professions, is not static. It should follow the dynamic of social demands, as well as enlarged and more complex knowledge and practice of professions to respond to such demands. For Brazilian society to become the democratic and inclusive society it aims to become, it needs to participate in and deepen the debate regarding the parameters used to qualify our healthcare professionals.

It is essential that the Nursing profession construct its own professional project grounded on expertise acquired by all the team members in higher educational institutions, considering the responsibility of these workers with human care. The complexity of care requires social responsibility when constructing a professional project that confers to its workers scientific, ethical, philosophical, and political qualification and legislation that, in fact, substantiates the practice.

References

1. Bueno FM, Queiroz Mde S (2006) The nurse and the construction of professional autonomy in the care process. Rev Bras Enferm 59: 222-227.

2. Carvalho V (2013) Sobre a identidade profissional na enfermagem: reconsiderações pontuais em visão filosófica, Revista Brasileira de Enfermagem 66: 24-32.

3. Leopardi MT, Gelbcke FL, Ramos FRS (2001) Cuidado: objeto de trabalho ou objeto epistemológico da enfermagem, Texto e Contexto Enfermagem 10: 32-49.

4. Souza ML, Sartor VVB, Padilha MICS, Prado ML (2005) O cuidado em enfermagem: uma aproximação teórica. Texto e Contexto Enfermagem 14: 266-270.

5.   Vale EG, Pagliuca LM (2011) Construction of a nursing care concept: contribution for undergraduate nursing education. Rev Bras Enferm 64: 106-113.

6.   Kletemberg DF, Siqueira MT, Mantovani Mde F, Padilha MI, Amante LN, et al. (2010) The nursing process and the law of professional exercise. Rev Bras Enferm 63: 26-32.

7.   Velloso ISC, Ceci C (2015) Power and practices: Questions concerning the legislation of health professions in Brazil. Nursing Philosophy 16: 153-160.

8.   Peduzzi M, Anselmi ML (2004) Nursing auxiliaries and nursing technicians: Different professional categories and equivalent jobs. Rev Bras Enferm 57: 425-429.

9.   Borges MS Silva HCP (2010) Cuidar ou tratar? busca do campo de competência e identidade profissional da enfermagem. Revista Brasileira de Enfermagem 63: 26-32.

10. Da Silva AL, Padilha MI, Borenstein MS (2002) Professional image and identity in the building of nursing knowledge. Rev Lat Am Enfermagem 10: 586-595.

11. Constituição (1988) Constituição [da] Republica Federativa do Brasil. Brasília (DF), Senado Federal.

12. Girardi SN, Seixas PH (2002) Dilemas da regulação profissional na área de saúde: questões para um governo democrático e inclusionista. Formação 5: 30-43.

13. Reben (Revista Brasileira de Enfermagem) (2003-2013) ABEn, Brasília (DF).

14. Brasil (1986) Lei n. 7.498, de 25 de junho de 1986. Dispõe sobre a Regulamentação do Exercício da Enfermagem e dá outras providências. DOU, Brasília (DF): 9.273.

15. Brasil (1987) Decreto n. 94.406, de 8 de junho de 1987. Regulamenta a Lei n° 7.498, de 25 de junho de 1986, que dispõe sobre o exercício da Enfermagem, e dá outras providências. DOU, Brasília (DF), seção I: 8.853-5.

16. Brasil (1994) Lei n° 8.967, de 28 de dezembro de 1994. Altera a redação do parágrafo único do Art. 23 da Lei n.° 7.498, de 25 de junho de 1986, que dispõe sobre a regulamentação do exercício da enfermagem e dá outras providências. DOU, Brasília DF.

17. Aguiar Neto Z, Soares CB (2004) The qualification of nursing attendants: transformations in work and life. Rev Lat Am Enfermagem 12: 614-622.

18. Bardin L (2011) Análise de conteúdo. Setenta, São Paulo.

19. Freidson E (1998) O renascimento do profissionalismo. Edusp, São Paulo (SP).

20. Diniz M (2001) Os donos do saber: profissões e monopólios profissionais. Revan, Rio de Janeiro (RJ).

21. Göttems LBD, Alves ED, Sena RR (2007) A enfermagem brasileira e a profissionalização de nível técnico: análise em retrospectiva. Revista Latino-Americana de Enfermagem 15: 9.

22. Le Goff J (2013) Para uma outra idade média: tempo, trabalho e cultura no ocidente. Vozes, Rio de Janeiro (RJ).

23. Malvarez S (2011) Editorial. Texto e Contexto Enfermagem 20: 23-24.

24. De Oliveira Mde F, Carraro TE (2011) Care in Heidegger: an ontological possibility for nursing. Rev Bras Enferm 64: 376-380.

25. Sacramento MH (2009) Higiene e representação social: o sujo e o limpo na percepção de futuros professores de Ciências [Tese]. Programa de Pós-Graduação em Educação, Faculdade de Educação, Universidade de Brasília (UNb). Brasília.

26. Rodrigues JC (2006) Tabu do corpo. Fiocruz, Rio de Janeiro (RJ).

27. Pereira MJ, Fortuna CM, Mishima SM, de Almeida MC, Matumoto S (2009) Nursing in Brazil in the context of the work force of the health: profile and legislation. Rev Bras Enferm 62: 771-777.

28. Lucena Ade F, Paskulin LM, de Souza MF, de Gutiérrez MG (2006) Health care models and the building of nursing knowledge and practice. Rev Esc Enferm USP 40: 292-298.

29. Peduzzi M, Anselmi ML (2002) The nursing work process: the gap between planning and care delivery. Rev Bras Enferm 55: 392-398.

30. COFEN - Conselho Federal de Enfermagem (2012) [homepage] Cofen, Brasília (DF).

31. Argenta MI (2011) Congruência entre o ensino da sistematização da assistência de enfermagem e o processo de trabalho do enfermeiro [Tese]. Programa de Pós-Graduação em Enfermagem, Universidade Federal de Santa Catarina, Florianópolis.

20

Nursing Clinical Instructor Needs Assessment

Donna M. Glynn, PhD, ANP-BC*; **Kelsey W. ILL, MS; Margaret Taylor, MSN, FNP-BC; Athena Lynch, MSN, FNP-BC; and Jodi DeLibertis, BA.**

Assistant Professor of Practice, Simmons College, School of Nursing and Health Sciences, USA.

*Corresponding author : Donna M. Glynn, PhD, ANP-BC, Assistant Professor of Practice, Simmons College, School of Nursing and Health Sciences, Boston, MA USA, E-mail: donna.glynn@simmons.edu

Abstract

Introduction: To date there is limited research related to the perceived learning needs of adjunct clinical nursing instructors and the development of an effective clinical instructor certificate program. The purpose of this study is to identify the perceived learning needs of clinical instructors teaching in a variety of clinical settings.

Methods: A qualitative survey is designed and administered to 230 adjunct clinical instructors at a small urban college in the Northeast using an Internet-based survey. The central aim of the survey is to identify the level of support for a formal orientation program and the "Nurse of the Future Core Competencies" that are of most value.

Results: 80% of respondents reported that a structured orientation program would be of value. Legal and ethical issues, reflective practice and informatics were identified as priority topics to be incorporated into the program. The study also identified concerns related to aging clinical nursing faculty and the institutional support necessary to foster the development of clinical nursing instructors.

Conclusion: As critical stakeholders in the development of nursing students, this study supports the need for a structured orientation program in order to improve nursing clinical education and retain qualified nursing clinical faculty members. The information gained from this study could serve as a basis for a future structured orientation program that may result in a successful model of well-prepared clinical faculty.

Keywords: Nursing clinical instruction; Aging faculty; Theory-practice gap; Structured orientation; Instructor evaluation; Core competencies

Introduction

The theory-practice gap in nursing education has been discussed, debated, and documented for several decades [1,2]. The nursing literature identified multiple issues that contribute to this theory-practice gap; including underutilization of core competencies, faculty shortages, limited clinical experiences and skills acquisition, emerging technology, and inconsistencies in the preparation of clinical faculty [3-6]. The Joint Commission on the Accreditation of Healthcare Organizations (2002) described a "continental divide" (p. 30) related to nursing education and practice, and recommended nursing educational reform to include competency-based education in an effort to merge theory and practice. With the development of the "Nurse of the Future Core Competencies" (2010), adjunct clinical instructors are faced with the challenge of incorporating consensus competencies to transition nurses into their practice settings.

Many of the identified core competencies do not lend themselves to instruction in the classroom. Rather, the acknowledged skills require the clinical experience for students to successfully transition to the nursing role [7]. Adjunct clinical instructors have reported the need and desire to participate in a formal preparation program or receive informal mentoring by educationally prepared peers or academic faculty [8]. The Oregon Consortium for Nursing Education found that an educational curriculum based on course competencies reduced the strain of clinical education and improved student transition to the professional role [9].

Adjunct clinical instructors play a critical role in the success of undergraduate nursing programs. Adjunct clinical instructors have the challenge of merging theory and practice to prepare the nurses of the future. The availability of qualified clinical instructors, training, and retention are major obstacles for nursing programs. Many programs rely on part-time clinical instructors to teach students at clinical sites [5,6]. Nursing programs report that shortages in the clinical areas were three times greater than in the classroom. In an effort to fill these clinical needs, preparing and mentoring staff nurses for the role of clinical nurse educators were inconsistent and limited [10]. Expert clinicians were enlisted without satisfactory orientation prior to clinical teaching assignments and they reported limited ongoing support from the academic institution. The need to provide adjunct clinical instructors a formal orientation program has been recognized in nursing literature for many years [11]. To date, however, there is limited research related to the perceived learning needs of adjunct clinical instructors and the development of an effective clinical instructor certificate program [10].

As documented in the "Project Leonardo" (2010), patient care can be improved with the development of a strong partnership between health professionals. Through the development and implementation of structured guidelines and collaboration, the study reported high satisfaction ratings from the health care team and a positive impact on patient health and patient care delivery [12].

The purpose of this Nursing Clinical Instructor Needs Assessment project was to identify the demographics of clinical instructors participating in a variety of clinical sites and the perceived learning needs and instructional support identified as success factors by adjunct clinical instructors. As critical stakeholders in the educational development of nursing students, the results of this study serve as a starting point in the development of a formal orientation program for clinical instructors.

Methods

A one-time survey of clinical adjunct nursing faculty was developed and administered at a small urban college in the Northeast. Eligible participants included the 230 clinical adjunct nursing instructors who taught within the past calendar year, which consisted of three semesters. The clinical instructors taught a variety of courses including medical surgical nursing, pediatrics, obstetrics, community health, and psychiatric nursing. The survey collected faculty demographics, such as years in the nursing profession, level of education, and teaching history. Guidance and support received from the course coordinators was assessed. Lastly, participants were asked if a faculty orientation program would be of value. Survey participants were asked to rank the "Nurse of the Future Competencies" from most to least important in terms of their value in being incorporated in a future faculty orientation program using a rating scale.

Survey design was qualitative, using Likert scales, rating scales, and participants were allowed to provide open-ended responses to several of the questions. Survey design was reviewed by a statistician.

IRB approval was obtained prior to survey administration. The participants were made aware of the purpose of the study and the expected duration of the survey. Participation was voluntary. Informed consent was obtained from all participants. The survey was administered via the Internet using *SurveyMonkey* and a direct link was presented to all 230 eligible participants by email. A reminder email was sent one week following the initial email. The window of time for responses was three weeks. Participants were able to skip questions and continue answering the survey as desired. Contact information of the survey designers was provided to participants in case of any questions regarding survey. No personal identifiers were collected. Anonymity and confidentiality were maintained.

Survey results were analyzed using SPSS statistical software. A biostatistician was also consulted in data analysis.

Limitations of the study include qualitative design, open-ended response questions, and lack of formal validity/reliability testing prior to administration.

Results

A total of 61 adjunct clinical faculty members participated in the survey, a response rate of 27%. The majority of the respondents were female and masters prepared. The age of the participants was evaluated and 76.7% were over the age of 40, with 20% over the age of 61. Only 5% of the respondents reported an age of less than 30. A total of 70.5% reported more than 20 years of experience as a professional nurse with 39.3% stating more than 30 years of experience. A total of 85% reported teaching in the clinical setting for 1-3 schools of nursing over their career. The majority of the clinical faculty adjuncts participated in medical surgical nursing courses.

On the subject of perceived support from the academic institution, findings showed that 56.1% acknowledged full support in their efforts and 81% reported multiple contacts during the semester with course coordinators.

The lack of clinical instructor evaluations was noted by many respondents, with 79.2% of the participants reporting that they did not receive an evaluation of their performance at the completion of the clinical session. Respondents stated the importance of feedback from the course coordinators related to their clinical teaching and the need for constructive measures to improve the clinical experience for their students.

The participants overwhelmingly acknowledged the perceived benefits of a clinical faculty orientation program. Eighty percent of the respondents believed that a structured orientation program would be of value and improve the role of adjunct clinical nursing instructor. The respondents identified legal and ethical issues, reflective practice, and informatics as priority topics. Teaching and learning theory, core competencies, and grading assignments received the lowest rating for incorporation into a clinical faculty orientation program.

Discussion

Aging clinical instructors

The results of the study are consistent with the expected decline in the availability of qualified clinical instructors due to advancing age in the near future. In 2009, U.S. nursing programs turned away 54,991 qualified student applicants due to faculty shortages [10] and it has been reported that the faculty shortage is three times greater in the clinical areas than in the classroom [5,6]. Nationally, 60% of nurses are over age 50 (US Department of Health & Human Services HRSA); this was mirrored in the clinical faculty survey in which exactly 60% of respondents reported being 50 years of age or older. Respondents over aged 50 were almost twice as likely to have a master's degree or higher than those 49 years and younger. Given the educational requirements as well as the required years of clinical practice for clinical instructors, this age disparity may have a profound impact on the school's ability to hire qualified instructors.

Taking into account the average retirement age of nurse educators (62.5 years old) and the age of 60% of the survey respondents (aged 50 or older), the next decade will bring worsening faculty shortage unless action is taken to recruit and retain younger clinical nurse instructors. An orientation program, which provides new entrants into nursing clinical education the skills and knowledge for success, may be a competitive advantage in attracting younger instructors, retention rates, and merging theory and practice. Younger clinical instructors, particularly those without advanced degrees or a nursing education background, will need an orientation program focused on clinical instruction, which may contribute to student success related to the clinical expectations.

Support of the clinical faculty

The ability to contact the course coordinator, help dealing with difficult students, peer support, and clear written instructions on how to conduct and manage a clinical group were key factors in perceived clinical instructor support.

Several respondents reported that the course coordinator did not visit the site during the semester, and perceived this as lack of support. Also, clinical instructors felt their questions were not answered by the course coordinator in a timely fashion. Respondents reported that improved contact with the course coordinator would help to bridge the classroom-clinical chasm. Many new clinical faculty members reported that the lack of a formal orientation course made the first clinical rotations more difficult. Eighty percent of respondents felt a formal orientation course would be of benefit, which further supports the need for the development of a clinical faculty orientation program.

Evaluation of clinical instructors

The findings of this survey support the need for consistent formal evaluations of clinical instructors. There is a lack of a formal evaluation process in the clinical setting today. Timely, thoughtful feedback regarding clinical instructors' performance is critical in advancing the clinical faculty member's skills and knowledge. It is common for clinical nursing instructors to receive feedback from only the disgruntled students who may have struggled; however, the positive feedback is highly valuable as well. It is also imperative for the clinical instructors to receive feedback from both students and the course coordinator.

Recommendations for future research include designing a reliable tool to evaluate clinical faculty in a variety of clinical settings. The evaluation must incorporate both positive and constructive feedback from several sources, including students, the facility or agency, and course coordinators' site visits.

Development of a clinical faculty orientation program

The results of this study document the perceived benefits of a formal orientation program for adjunct clinical instructors. This result is consistent with the findings in "Project Leonardo" [12] which reported that structured support and guidelines create improved partnerships that will ultimately improve patient care. Adjunct clinical nursing instructors who participated in the survey reported the need for a program which incorporates legal and ethical issues, diversity, reflective practice, and informatics in order to reach the educational goals at the clinical sites. Core competencies, a leading initiative in nursing, ensure consistency in nursing education and will be an essential component of an orientation program for adjunct clinical instructors [13]. Providing clinical adjunct instructors with a structured orientation program based on the perceived needs and core competencies may lead to a successful model of well-prepared clinical faculty. Well-prepared clinical instructors may strengthen the student experience and increase clinical faculty job satisfaction and retention [14,15].

Conclusion

The renewed focus on theory-practice gap in nursing education and the recommendations to unite nursing education and practice are critical to the success of clinical education and the student's transition to professional practice. This project identified the concerns related to aging clinical nursing instructors, areas to improve professional partnerships, and the need for a formalized evaluation of clinical instructors. The results support the development of a formal orientation program for clinical instructors to merge the academic preparation with the clinical experience and assimilate core competencies throughout the educational preparation of nursing students. Because clinical instructors are a critical piece in the educational development of nursing students, it is essential that the curriculum design includes and incorporates the learning needs and instructional support required for improved job satisfaction, improved clinical education, and retention of qualified clinical faculty members.

References

1. Corlett J (2000) The perceptions of nurse teachers, student nurses and preceptors of the theory- practice gap in nurse education. Nursing Education Today 20: 499-505.

2. Dale AE (1994) The theory-theory gap: the challenge for nurse teachers. J Adv Nurs 20: 521-524.

3. Scully NJ (2011) The theory-practice gap and skill acquisition: an issue for nursing education. Collegian 18: 93-98.

4. Hutchinson PJ, Tate MA, Torbeck JM, Smith E (2011) "Know worries!" a clinical faculty orientation model. Nurse Educ 36: 59-61.

5. Kowalski K, Homer M, Carroll K, Center D, Foss K, et al. (2007) Nursing clinical faculty revisited: the benefits of developing staff nurses as clinical scholars. J Contin Educ Nurs 38: 69-75.

6. Kowalski K, Horner MD, Houser J (2011) Evaluation of a model for preparing staff nurses to teach clinical groups of nursing students. J Contin Educ Nurs 42: 233-240.

7. Connolly MA, Wilson CJ (2008) Revitalizing academic-service partnerships to resolve nursing faculty shortages. AACN Adv Crit Care 19: 85-97.

8. Kelly RE (2006) Engaging baccalaureate clinical faculty. Int J Nurs Educ Scholarsh 3: Article 14.

9. Tanner CA, Gubrud-Howe P, Shores L (2008) The Oregon Consortium for Nursing Education: a response to the nursing shortage. Policy Polit Nurs Pract 9: 203-209.

10. American Association of Colleges of Nursing (2010) Nursing Faculty Shortage Fact Sheet.

11. Blauvelt MJ, Spath ML (2008) Passing the torch: a faculty mentoring program at one school of nursing. Nurs Educ Perspect 29: 29-33.

12. Ciccone MM, Aquilino A, Cortese F, Scicchitano P, Sassara M, et al. (2010) Feasibility and effectiveness of a disease and care management model in the primary health care system for patients with heart failure and diabetes (Project Leonardo). Vasc Health Risk Manag 6: 297-305.

13. Joint Commission Report (2002) Health Care at the Crossroads: Strategies for Addressing the Evolving Nursing Crisis.

14. Oermann MH (1998) How to assess critical thinking in clinical practice. Dimens Crit Care Nurs 17: 322-327.

15. Pierangeli L (2006) Developing a clinical teaching handbook and reference manual for part-time clinical faculty. Nurse Educ 31: 183-185.

21

Perception and Core Competencies of Disaster Nursing in South Korea

Ji Young Noh[1], Eui Geum Oh[2]*, Won Hee Lee[2] and Mona Choi[2]

[1]Severance Hospital, Yonsei University, Korea

[2]College of Nursing, Yonsei University, Korea

*Corresponding author: Eui Geum Oh, 50 Yonsei-ro, Seodaemun-gu, Seoul, Korea 03722, E-mail: euigeum@yuhs.ac

Abstract

Background: A descriptive correlational study was conducted to investigate the disaster-related experience, perception, and core competency of nurses in South Korea.

Methods: Data were collected through a self-administered questionnaire given to 163 nurses working in tertiary hospitals in Seoul, Korea. The questionnaire was developed based on the frame of Disaster Nursing Competencies by International Council of Nurses (ICN) and Emergency Preparedness Questionnaire (EPIQ).

Results: In a 5-point scale, the awareness of nurses for disaster events, and the importance of education for disaster nursing were 3.93 ± 0.91 and 3.63 ± 0.93, respectively. Among ICN core competencies on perceived importance in disaster nursing, "Risk reduction, disease prevention and health promotion and psychological care" was scored highest, whereas "Policy development and planning, communication and information sharing" was the lowest. The higher level of awareness of a disaster was related to the higher level of perceived importance of education.

Conclusion: The results support that the level of awareness of a disaster is a factor affecting the importance of education in disaster nursing. Thus, educational programs focusing on practical topics in disaster nursing should be developed for continuous training to increase the core competency and the understanding of disaster nursing.

Keywords: Disaster nursing; Perception; Core competencies; Korea

Introduction

Numerous countries around the world are experiencing various types of unexpected disasters such as tsunamis and earthquakes. Extreme weather events such as the effects of global warming and environmental destruction due to rapid industrialization have caused natural disasters, as well as various man-made disasters. Furthermore, there has recently been an increase in the tendency for South Korea to experience numerous large-scale disasters in social and anthropogenic terms leading to mass casualties and large property losses [1]. Recent events such as the Sewol Ferry sinking incident, as well as the Middle East Respiratory Syndrome pandemic has elevated government and public awareness in the importance of disaster preparedness. A disaster is an event that harms people's lives, and causes physical and financial damages at individual and national level; in a large-scale disaster, it can generate demands exceeding available resources. Furthermore, from a medical and health sciences perspective, a disaster, especially large-scale disaster signifies an event that generates numerous patients that exceed medical resources available for treatment [2,3]. In relation to these various contemporary changes, it is predicted that the possibility and frequency regarding the occurrence of various disasters will continue to increase. Although there is urgent need for the health and medical professions to prepare for such events, a systematic health care system in response to various disasters has still not been established. Temporary measures such as experiences learned from participation in medical field support or emergency teams cannot meet the complex needs of nursing that are required in these new disaster situations.

Nurses in disaster situations must be able to assess a wide range of nursing needs and to establish plans within situational context of disasters, which differs from the health care that they normally provide in the clinics or to the local community. They also must be able to maintain a comprehensive and collaborative cooperation system, understand the special environments, and serve to ensure safety [4]. Up to now, nurses were assigned to disaster sites in relation to their department positions or personal experiences. However, systematic education and training in preparation for disaster nursing is needed. In accordance to 'Disaster Nursing Competencies' published by the International Council of Nurses (ICN) in 2009, as a guide on training and education development to promote disaster nursing competency, the ability required to perform disaster nursing involves an integrated and mutually supportive attitude, and nurses must be equipped with knowledge and capabilities to provide disaster nursing services; and this can be strengthened by demonstrating their leadership qualities. During a disaster, nurses must monitor the changes in the environment and organizational activities, reduce the threats to health, assess the health care needs of targets, as well as bear the legal and ethical responsibility in accordance with the medical laws. Furthermore, as facilitator for appropriate resource utilization, they must be able to act within the cooperative systems and be responsible for the corresponding role. To achieve this task, nurses must first be equipped with the ability to protect themselves from the disaster, and acquire professional development in preparation and training for disaster events [5]. Korean Nurses Association [6] has also stated that the role of nurses during disaster events has the contextual features distinct from everyday clinical settings or health care services in the local community; in terms of the principles or basic techniques of nursing, it has mentioned that disaster events demand further requirements in physical, social, emotional, spiritual, and management aspects of nursing, which contain the features of core competencies published by ICN. Therefore, disaster nursing education must be based on the core competency requirements as described above, such as definition of disaster, philosophy of disaster nursing (e.g., causes, impacts, disaster phases, survival strategies, etc.), mass casualty care, communication, systematization, coordination issues, triage process, psychological issues pertinent in disaster situations, overall role of nurses, role of leadership, assessment of health needs, utilization of personnel and resources and evaluation of provided nursing care and services [7,8]. Numerous studies have mentioned the need for education and training regarding the nurse's own field to care for patients during disaster events that are rarely encountered in the usual practice [9-12] and countries that have experienced disasters such as the United States and India recognized the severity of the problem and organized discussions and workshops regarding nurse education [13-15]. Meanwhile, researches in South Korea are mainly focused on the field of emergency medicine in the response phase during the occurrence of a disaster, and the administrative approach for the maintenance of a disaster management system [16-18]. In nursing, research has been limited to developing and promoting the disaster nursing curriculum for students, such as family recovery support system [19], social support [20] or research on disaster experience and disaster preparedness of college students in a certain region [21]. There are insufficient research works done on disaster preparedness and response capacity building for nurses [22]. The purpose of this study is to find out the level of disaster awareness of nurses, importance of disaster nursing education, and core competencies, and to identify the relationship between the variables.

Materials and Methods

Study design and participants

The authors conducted a descriptive and cross-sectional survey to identify the level of disaster awareness of nurses, importance of disaster nursing education, and core competencies of Korean nurses on disaster nursing. Convenience sampling was conducted in three general hospitals with over 500 beds located in Seoul, Korea. Participants were selected using the G*power 3 program [23], which is a sample size calculation program based on Cohen's sampling formula, and a sample size of 120 was calculated at the 5% significance level and 80% statistical power with effect size of 0.25 when using the t-tests. Total of 200 samples were used considering drop out and incomplete responses of the survey.

Measurement tools

A structured questionnaire was used as the tool for data collection, and the questionnaire consisted of 11 general questions regarding the participants, 13 questions on experience with disaster, disaster nursing, and perception, and 15 questions on disaster nursing core competencies, for a total of 39 questions.

Perception and experience on disaster and disaster nursing

After reviewing the literature, 13 questions were created to measure the level of general experience and perception of nurses regarding disaster and disaster nursing. Out of the 13 questions, 11 questions on the characteristics of disaster-related experience and the perception of

disaster were measured through nominal scale, while the other 2 questions on the awareness about seriousness of disaster and about importance of disaster nursing education were measured on a 5-point Likert scale: a higher score indicates higher perception level on disaster. Developed questions were modified and refined after being reviewed for inadequate phrases or contents, and the face validity of the questions were verified through sample survey conducted by three nursing school professors and three nurses with disaster experiences.

Measuring tools for core competencies on disaster nursing

A total of 15 questions were developed based on the 44 Emergency Preparedness Questionnaire (EPIQ) [24] developed by the Wisconsin Health Alert Network in 2003, and 10 Frames of Disaster Nursing Competencies published by the International Council of Nurses (ICN) in 2009 [5]. Each question item selected was scored using a 5-point Likert scale that ranged from 5 points 'strongly agree', 4 points 'agree', 3 points 'neither agree nor disagree', 2 points 'disagree', and 1 point 'strongly disagree.' The total sum of the points ranged from 15 points to 75 points, and a higher score indicates a higher level of core competencies on the ability to perform regarding disaster nursing. The face validity of the questionnaire was verified by three nursing school professors and three nurses with disaster experiences, and a preliminary examination was conducted to modify and refine any inadequate contents or phrases of the questionnaire. The Cronbach's alpha coefficient regarding the measurement tools for disaster nursing competencies in this study was 0.94.

General characteristics of the nurses

A total of 11 questions were developed consisting of demographic characteristics such as gender, age, education, and religion, as well as job-related characteristics (e.g. position within the department, type of work, total clinical nursing experience, and hospital department they are currently working).

Data collection

The data for this study were collected from May 1 through May 30, 2010 after being approved by the Research Ethics Committee of the College of Nursing at Yonsei University. Data were collected by visiting three general hospitals in Seoul, Korea. Participants were extracted using convenience sampling and by obtaining informed consent to participate in the study. The researcher visited the corresponding sites to distribute the questionnaires and to communicate general information and details regarding the questionnaire. The participants themselves filled out the questionnaire, and a contact number of the researcher was provided on the cover of the questionnaire in case the participants had hard time understanding the questionnaire or had any questions about the research. A total of 200 copies were distributed; of which 25 copies (12.5%) were not returned, and 12 copies (6%) with inadequate responses were excluded from the collection, resulting in a total of 163 samples (81.5%) being used in the analysis.

Statistical analysis

For data analysis, SPSS/WIN version 12.0 was used. Participant's general and job characteristics, as well as characteristics on disaster-related experience were expressed using descriptive statistics using numbers, percentage, as well as means and standard deviation. Descriptive statistics were also used to analyze participant's level of awareness and importance of education about disaster nursing and the self-rating core competency scores, each expressed in frequency, percentage, as well as means and standard deviation. Independent t-tests were conducted for an analysis on the level of disaster awareness and core competencies related to disaster nursing based on the characteristics of the participants. Pearson correlation was used to analyze the relationship between the levels of disaster awareness and importance of education. Cronbach's alpha coefficient was used to calculate the internal reliability of the tool.

Results

General characteristics of the participants

The general characteristics of the participants are shown in Table 1. The average age of the participants was 28.3 years old, and 96.3% of the

participants were female. Among work related characteristics, the participants' average clinical experience from their respective hospitals was 2.9 years, ranging from a minimum of 2 months to a maximum of 21 years, with the highest percentage (38%) for the group of 2 to 4 years. Eleven respondents (6.7%) said they had personally experienced or witnessed a disaster, which indicates that majority of nurses had no experience with disasters. Only 57 participants (35%) had learning experience in disaster-related education, and 126 participants (77.3%) expressed willingness to participate in an educational program on disaster nursing if provided.

Category		N (%)	M (SD)
Age (year)			28.3 (± 5.2)
Sex	Male	6 (3.7)	
	Female	157 (96.3)	
Level of Education	Diploma graduates	67 (41.1)	
	Bachelor degree	78 (47.8)	
	Master's degree or over	18 (11.1)	
Experience in Nursing (year)	<2	35 (21.5)	
	2-4	62 (38)	
	5-7	34 (20.9)	2.9 (± 1.6)
	8-10	10 (6.1)	
	10<	22 (13.5)	
Clinical Area	Medical/Surgical Unit	40 (24.5)	
	Critical Care Unit	38 (23.3)	
	Emergency Room	28 (17.2)	
	Operation Room	36 (22.1)	
	Outpatient/Lab, etc.	21 (12.9)	
Experience of education on disaster nursing	Yes	57 (35)	
	No	106 (65)	
Need on disaster nursing education	Yes	126 (77.3)	
	No	37 (22.7)	
Nurses who have witnessed or experienced disaster	Yes	11 (6.7)	
	No	152 (93.3)	

The level of perception and core competencies of nurses on disasters

The average score for the level of disaster awareness was 3.93 (± 0.91). Over 55% of the participants (97 nurses) answered that disaster

can happen, indicating seriousness of disasters. And 65 participants (37.4%) expressed their awareness of the importance of disaster nursing education by answering that such education is 'necessary', which resulted in an average score of 3.63 (± 0.93) (Table 2).

Category	M (SD)
Disaster awareness	3.93 (± 0.91)
Importance of disaster nursing education	3.63 (± 0.93)

Table 2: The level of perception of nurses on disasters.

As for the self-assessment scores on the level of core competencies on disaster nursing, the total average was 40.82 (± 9.77) out of 75 points, and the average scores for each item was 2.73 (± 0.27) out of 5 points, indicating that the participants' level of core competencies on disaster nursing were moderate. However, given that this was a self-reporting questionnaire, it should be noted that there can be a difference between this result and the actual competencies. The highest average of 3.14 (± 0.79) among the core competency category was reported in the item "Aware of duties medical staffs have to perform under disaster", whereas the lowest average of 2.14 (± 0.83) was reported in the item "Aware of procedure to record nursing in documents" (Table 3).

ICN Frame	Category	M (SD)
Care of the community, Communication and information sharing	Aware of procedure to record nursing documents.	2.14 (± 0.83)
	Aware of procedure to transfer information of important targets to other medical staffs and those concerned.	2.35 (± 0.89)
Policy development and planning	Able to inspect, monitor, and report on patients as nurses.	2.54 (± 0.87)
Care of the community and accountability	Aware of medical system of local community and perform nurses' roles.	2.56 (± 0.83)
Communication and information sharing	Able to collect necessary information and share it with heath managers effectively.	2.59 (± 0.92)
Ethical and legal practice, and accountability	Aware of disaster-related guidelines of current respective organization.	2.63 (± 0.93)
Care of individuals and families	Able to provide proper nursing care according to triage.	2.72 (± 0.97)
Long term care and evaluation	Health consulting/training can be provided to targets on long-term impact by disaster.	2.73 (± 0.85)
Ethical and legal practice, and accountability	Missions can be shared together with main partners who are concerned in disaster prevention.	2.81 (± 0.93)
Care of individuals and families	Backgrounds and conditions of different targets can be understood and inspected.	2.85 (± 0.87)
Education and Preparedness	Aware of role and general response to disaster situation	2.89 (± 0.77)
Care of vulnerable populations	Sensitive and weak targets (seniors, pregnant women, the disabled, etc.) can be provided with proper nursing care during disaster.	2.89 (± 0.89)
Psychological care	Proper psychological support can be provided to all people concerned in disaster occurrence.	2.90 (± 0.91)
Risk reduction, disease prevention and health promotion	Able to provide emergency first-aid to victims of disaster	3.09 (± 0.81)
Education and Preparedness	Aware of duties medical staffs have to perform under disaster.	3.14 (± 0.79)
	Subtotal	2.73 (± 0.27) [1]
	Overall	40.82 (± 9.77) [2]

Table 3: The level of core competencies on disaster nursing, N=163; 1) Range: 1~5, 2) Range:15~75 (5 points × 15 items).

The level of disaster awareness and core competencies in accordance to participant's characteristics

Group with over 3 years of clinical nursing experience had higher levels of disaster awareness when compared to the group with less than 3 years of experience and the difference was statistically significant (t=2.414, p=0.017). Among job-related characteristics, nurses with over 3 years of work experience reported a higher core competency value of 41.83 (± 9.69) points, however, work experience and core competencies were not statistically significant (t=1.287, p=0.200). Furthermore, in terms of disaster-related experience characteristics, nurses that recently experienced or witnessed a disaster had the highest core competency level of 45.46 (± 10.10) points, but also was not statistically significant (t=1.726, p=0.107).

Relationship between disaster awareness and importance of education

The awareness level regarding the seriousness of disasters and the level of perceived importance regarding education on disaster nursing present a significant quantitative correlation, indicating that the more seriously the participants perceive disasters, the higher awareness they have regarding the necessity for disaster nursing education (r=0.583, p<0.001).

Discussion

In this study, the level of seriousness felt towards disaster nursing and the importance felt towards the need for disaster nursing education scored 14.82 out of 25 points, which is a similar result with previous studies that were conducted with an emphasis on the importance of disaster nursing education [9,25-27]. In many of the countries, there is a growing trend to establish disaster focused department, to provide education for providers to manage disaster prevention, response, and recovery phases in an integrated manner and to exhibit their leadership in preparation for disasters [28-30]. However, disaster nursing education in South Korea is limited to creating workforces in the prevention-oriented sectors, which is important. But additionally, training approaches to an integrated management of each disaster phase led by capable disaster managers are required. In response to these needs, South Korean researchers have studied the development of a 2 year curriculum associated with a bachelor degree in disaster management, as well as related research and evaluation [31]. To achieve this goal, a viable learning environment such as lectures, hands-on training, simulations, and seminars with case studies needs to be provided by connecting undergraduate courses with graduate courses, hospitals, local communities, and government organizations [32]. In addition, sustainable programs must be created for the skilled practitioners to have the capability as a manager, leader, and educator to facilitate an integrated disaster management.

The results for the level of core competencies on disaster nursing indicated that the highest average value was "aware of duties medical staffs have to do under disaster" at 3.14 (± 0.79) out of 5 points, followed by "able to provide emergency first-aid to victims of disaster" at 3.09 (± 0.81), whereas the lowest average value was "aware of procedure to record nursing in documents" at 2.14 (± 0.83) points. Preceding research by Ablah et al. [33], which used the 44 question EPIQ developed by the Wisconsin Health Alert Network in 2003, also indicated a similar result with the highest average of 3.15 points in the basic emergency responses, followed by the ability to identify and respond to general tasks related to disasters with a high score of 2.85 points. The category with the lowest value in this study was the section about recording documents on nursing provided during the disaster to communicate with other disaster managers. Furthermore, psychological care scored 2.90 (± 0.91) low points among core competencies. Because the perceived performance competency scores were low, this suggests that competency enhancement of nurses in the event of a disaster should be directed more to the bridging role between the hospital and the local community through continuous data collection and management, and towards psychological support interventions immediately after the disaster. When examining studies related to disaster and stress, Kato et al. [34] reported that disaster damage, self-efficacy, and social support were factors that affected psychological stress of the disaster patient after a volcanic eruption event. Math et al. [35] reported that prevalence of mental health problems in disaster affected population is found to be higher by two to three times than that of the general population. In a systemic review study, it was found that 11%-38% distressed individuals presenting for evaluation at shelters and family assistance centers have stress-related and adjustment disorders, and up to 40% of distressed individuals had pre-existing disorders [36]. A strategy for the psychological care such as emotional support is necessary and must not be overlooked considering that the relocation of victims' lives due to natural disasters causes environmental, social, and psychosocial stress.

This study indicates an increase in the level of awareness in relation to an increase in work experience. This result indicates that this group is the most motivated group of learners that could be the best candidate for developing expert and specialized disaster care providers.

In the United States, disaster-related health services are managed and directed by professional nurses, and disaster-related health services training programs are established and operated as supplemental education programs for nurses. As new aspects of health and medical problems are expected to emerge due to frequently occurring disasters, preparing professional workforces responsible for the activities in disaster events is needed along with the development of a process for educational preparation, and the need for the development of task protocols for providing disaster-related health services. However, increased work experience and previous disaster experience did not show statistically significant result when compared to core competencies. This means that experience alone cannot fulfil nursing competencies in disaster management. To achieve core competencies in disaster nursing, structured and integrated curriculum developed is important.

The results of this study indicate high relationship between disaster nursing awareness and importance of education. Nurses without any disaster-related event experience, information on disaster events are gained through the media, and there is a tendency of growing awareness in disaster in South Korea due to increased media reports related to the increasing disaster events occurring around the world.

There are several limitations to this study. First, the data were collected 6 years ago, but it still represents valuable information. Until now, there hasn't been any research in analyzing the perception of nurses in disaster field in Korea, and these data forms the baseline for current ongoing and future research in this field. Data from this study can be used as a comparison in the changes that may occur to the providers of disaster care, where disaster continues to occur locally and regionally. Second, this study was based on an analysis of nurses selected through convenience sampling. Therefore, features such as work environment or organizational culture of each hospital could not be controlled and thus, one must be cautious to generalize the findings. Furthermore, the perception and experience related to disasters, as well as the level of core competencies on disaster nursing of local community nurses, nurses in local hospitals besides Seoul, and nurses of small and medium hospitals with less than 500 beds were not reflected in the study. Also, because a self-administered questionnaire method was used for the data collection process, there can be individual variations in accordance to the characteristics of the research participant. This may not accurately reflect the level of core competencies in this study and thus requires cautious interpretation.

Conclusion

This study investigated the level of perception and core competencies of nurses on disasters to achieve better understanding, and to confirm actual conditions of disaster preparedness for nurses. Level of disaster awareness was high for the group with higher total work experience, and the level of core competencies on disaster nursing remained in the average range. In the case of the perceived awareness of disasters and the perceived importance of education on disaster nursing, the more serious feeling towards disaster, there was higher level of need for disaster nursing education. Since disaster events continuously occur in Korea, the large workforce of nurses must be trained and prepared in disaster response. We must be proactive in developing and providing education and training for disaster responses and pay more attention towards disaster nursing field. The results of this study conclude that a structured educational program for disaster nursing at the individual level must be developed to improve the quality of disaster nursing services. Furthermore, this study could be the basis for future development of programs in an organizational level.

References

1. National Emergency Management Agency (2014) Disasters Annual Report, National Disaster Information Center, Seoul.

2. National Law Information Center (2014) Framework Act on the Management of Disaster and Safety. Ministry of Public Safety and Security, National Law Information Center.

3. American Medical Association (2012) Basic disaster life support: Provider manual (ver 3.0): American Medical Association.

4. Powers R, Daily E (2008) Nursing issues in disaster health. Prehosp Disaster Med 23: 1-2.

5. International Council of Nurses (2015) ICN Framework of disaster Nursing Competencies.

6. Korean Nurses Association (2015) Code of ethics for Korean nurses.

7. Silenas R, Akins R, Parrish AR, Edwards JC (2008) Developing disaster preparedness competence: an experiential learning exercise for multiprofessional education. Teach Learn Med 20: 62-68.

8. Williams J, Nocera M, Casteel C (2008) The effectiveness of disaster training for health care workers: A systematic review. Ann Emerg Med 52: 211-222.

9. Fung WM, Lai KY, Loke AY (2009) Nurses' perception of disaster: implications for disaster nursing curriculum. J Clin Nurs 18: 3165-3171.

10. Öztekin SD, Larson EE, Altun Uğraş G, Yüksel S, Savaşer S (2015) Nursing educators' perceptions about disaster preparedness and response in Istanbul and Miyazaki. Jpn J Nurs Sci 12: 99-112.

11. Kuntz SW, Frable P, Qureshi K, Strong LL, Association of Community Health Nursing Educators (2008) Association of Community Health Nursing Educators: Disaster preparedness white paper for community/public health nursing educators. Public Health Nurs 25: 362-369.

12. Pattillo MM, O'Day TM (2009) Disaster response: the University of Texas School of Nursing experience. Nurs Health Sci 11: 378-381.

13. Danna D, Bernard M, Schaubhut R, Mathews P (2010) Experiences of nurse leaders surviving Hurricane Katrina, New Orleans, Louisiana, USA. Nurs Health Sci 12: 9-13.

14. Asia Pacific Emergency and Disaster Nursing Network (APEDNN) Workshop (2013). Aus Nurs J, 20: 38-39.

15. Subbian N (2005) Workshop on "Role of Nurses in Disaster Preparedness and Management". Nurs J India 96: 151-152.

16. Ahn ME, Hwang SO, Lim KS, Kang SJ (1993) Analysis of Korean Disaster plan with the review of three cases of disasters. J Korean Soc Eme Med 4: 27-39.

17. Jang B, Cho J, Kim J, Lim Y, Lee G, et al. (2013) Disaster Medical Responses to the Shelling of Yeonpyeong Island. J Korean Soc Eme Med 24: 439-445.

18. Kim J, Kim T (2002) The Normative Structure of the National Disaster Management System. Fire Science and Engineering 16: 8-17.

19. Lee O (2000) Development of a Restoration Protocol for the Flood Victims. Seoul: The Graduate School Yonsei University.

20. Lee O, Ahn E, Jeon M (2000) Social Support and Stress in Flood Victims. J Red Cross Nur 23: 153-167.

21. Kang KH, Uhm DC, Nam ES (2012) A Study on Disaster Experience and Preparedness of University Students. J Korean Acad Nurs 18: 424-435.

22. Lee O, Wang SJ (2008) Exploration on Disaster Nursing Education in Korea. J Korean Soc Disaster Inf 4: 94-104.

23. Faul F, Erdfelder E, Lang AG, Buchner A (2007) G*Power 3: A flexible statistical power analysis program for the social, behavioral, and biomedical sciences. Behavior Res Med 39: 175-191.

24. Hu G, Rao K, Sun Z (2008) Development and testing of a preparedness and response capacity questionnaire in public health emergency for Chinese provincial and municipal governments. J Cent South Univ T 33: 1142-1147.

25. Pesiridis T, Kalokairinou A, Sourtzi P (2013) Nursing student's perceptions of disaster nursing: implications for curricula development. Nur Care and Res 35: 63-74.

26. Wickramasinghe KK, Ishara MH, Liyanage P, Karunathilake IM, Samarasekera D (2007) Outcome-based approach in development of a disaster management course for healthcare workers. Ann Acad Med Singapore 36: 765-769.

27. Loke AY, Fung OW (2014) Nurses' competencies in disaster nursing: Implications for curriculum development and public health. Int J Environ Res Public Health 11: 3289-3303.

28. Scott LA, Smith C, Jones EM, Manaker LW, Seymore AC, et al. (2013) Regional approach to competency-based patient care provider disaster training: The Center for Health Professional Training and Emergency Response. South Med J 106: 43-48.

29. Nolting FW (2008) Disaster training enters the 21st century. Northwest Dentistry 87: 21-23.

30. Shover H (2007) Understanding the chain of communication during a disaster. J Korean Acad Nurs 43: 4-14.

31. Kang Y, Lee O, Lee G (1998) A curriculum development on the disaster management. J Korean Acad Nurs 28: 210-220.

32. Chan SS, Chan WS, Cheng Y, Fung OW, Lai TK, et al. (2010) Development and evaluation of an undergraduate training course for developing International Council of Nurses disaster nursing competencies in China. J Nurs Scholarsh 42(4): 405-413.

33. Ablah E, Tinius AM, Horn L, Williams C, Gebbie KM (2008) Community health centers and emergency preparedness: An assessment of competencies and training needs. J Community Health 33: 241-247.

34. Kato H, Miyai H, Uchiumi C, Fujii S, Osawa T (2009) Psychological effects and intervention following a traffic disaster involving a large number of victims. Seishin Shinkeigaku Zasshi 111: 411-416.

35. Math SB, Nirmala MC, Moirangthem S, Kumar NC (2015) Disaster management: Mental health perspective. Indian J Psychol Med 37: 261-271.

36. North CS, Pfefferbaum B (2013) Mental health response to community disasters: A systematic review. JAMA 310: 507-518.

22

Professional Ambivalence: Understanding of the Eminence of Advanced Clinical Nursing Specialization in the Philippines

Marica Guevarra Estrada[1,2]* and Crestita Tan[1,2]

[1]*The Graduate School University of Santo Tomas, Philippines*

[2]*University of Santo Tomas College of Nursing, Philippines*

***Corresponding author:** Marica Guevarra Estrada, RN, MAN, University of Santo Tomas College of Nursing, Manila, Philippines, E-mail: estradamarica@yahoo.com

Abstract

As the practice of nursing continuously evolves, the registered nurses' role has expanded from basic practice to advanced nursing practice over the last 100 years. Following the demands of healthcare organizations worldwide, Philippines adopted the Nursing Specialty Program that aims to promote presence of clinical nurse specialists in the country.

Cognizant of this challenging role, this phenomenological inquiry has eidetically captured their collective experiences as clinical nurse specialists. A series of semi-structured, in-depth, one on one interview was conducted. Driven by the central question, "What describes the acceptance and utilization of CNS in the health care institution?" Field text were transcribed and subjected to phenomenological reduction via cool and warm analyses.

Four clusters of themes delineated the participant's collective experiences namely: (a) Inspired to perform a new role (b) Blinded acceptance of embodied role (c) Narrowed opportunities to practice area of specialization and (d) Divided to one's own achievements. An experience of "professional ambivalence" greatly characterized the narrowed response of the community and healthcare professionals that led to the feelings of ambivalence to one's own achievements, from being fulfilled to frustrated, dissatisfied and uncertain to practice confidently and independently.

The Filipino clinical nurse specialists are initially motivated to improve one's practice and the nation's health but, unfortunately enjoy sparingly the eminence and appreciation as foreign nurse specialists do. To be able to empower more Filipino nurses to struggle for professional growth and for advanced nursing practice in the Philippines to continue to flourish, it is imperative that nursing leaders must begin to organize a unified vision of advanced nursing practice by amending the existing law, delineating the scope of their practice, reviewing the existing requirements for certification to meet global standards and making the healthcare community mindful of the existence and value of such professionals.

Keywords: Clinical nurse specialists; Acceptance; Utilization; Professional ambivalence; Philippines

Introduction

Advanced Nursing Practice has totally transformed the direction and future of the nursing profession. The intense demand to address the need for health promotion, disease prevention, and to provide for evidence- based care to the underserved populations of the world led to the development and expansion of this advanced nursing role. Though it has grown scale in other countries especially in developed countries like the United States, Australia and United Kingdom, Advanced Nursing Practice in the Asia Pacific region especially in the Philippines, has received diminutive attention.

The growth and development of nursing specialties has, from its earliest inception, been an interesting and challenging journey. Early in the 20th century, nurse midwives and nurse anesthetists' laid the formative foundations for what we now know as advanced practice nursing [1,2].Four distinct advanced practice nursing roles evolved from the early beginnings- the nurse midwife (CNM), the nurse anesthetists (CRNA), the clinical nurse specialists (CNS), and the nurse practitioner (NP). New roles continue to emerge or morph into new configuration.

A number of authors have noted patterns in the evolution of nursing specialties to an advanced practice level [1,3].Initially, it was driven by the changes in patient needs, new technology, and changing opportunities within the workforce and insufficient physician supply. In the second stage, the specialty required organized training for nurses. This specialty training programs were institution-specific and essentially consisted of a paid apprenticeship with some organized classes. These "certificate programs" were not standardized, and quality was uneven [1]. The third stage is characterized by pressures for standardization of education and skills involved in the specialty both as a means of increasing standardization and to raise the status of the specialty to an advanced practice level. There is growing recognition of the additional knowledge and skills needed for increasingly complex practice in the specialty [1].

Certification, as defined by the American Board of Nursing Specialties [4], is the formal recognition of specialized knowledge, skills and experience demonstrated by achievement of standards identified by a nursing specialty to promote optimal health outcomes. It is an accepted method to validate that nurses have knowledge, skills and abilities that are fundamental to accomplishing their job functions as advanced nurse practitioners. While basic nursing licensure indicates a minimal professional practice standard, certification denotes a high level of knowledge and practice, with the intent to protect the public. The purpose of certification is to assure members of the public that an individual has mastered a body of knowledge and acquired skills in a particular specialty [5].

Internationally, the current processes for CNSs entry into practice are: (1) to graduate from an accredited master's or doctoral level program that prepares the student for practice as a CNS with a specialty and (2) to secure employment.5 According to the National Association of Clinical Nurse Specialists, this is the most appropriate pathway because this recognizes the value of the additional credentials earned through advanced education preparation. Some states have additional requirements such as: (3) to pass the national certification examination in the specialty; (4) to apply for licensure or authorization to practice in a state where title protection is in place; (5) to apply for credentialing and privileging process if necessary or if required by the facility in which the CNS works. More recently, certification at the advanced practice level has been used as a quasi-regulatory by the state agencies that grant recognition to individuals who have met pre-determined qualification [5,6].

Direct clinical practice is the central competency expected from an advanced nurse practitioner [1]. Six additional core competencies that further define advanced practice nursing include expert guidance and coaching, consultation, ethical decision making, collaboration, research skills, and clinical and professional leadership.Further, advanced roles would include autonomous problem-solving and clinical decision-making, advanced assessment, prescriptive authority, and expert nursing care and advanced communication skills, pharmacological and other selected diagnostic and therapeutic procedures [7].

The literatures have examined the impact of certification as it benefits nurses who are certified in their work place. These benefits would include: personal achievement, job satisfaction, validation of knowledge, greater earning potential, commitment to professionalism, and access to a broad range of job opportunities [8], high levels of professionalism, attitude of self-regulation, self-determination, and independence [9]; fewer errors in patient care [6]; Influencing accountability, accomplishment, growth, specialized knowledge, as well as recognition among employers, peers and consumers [10] ; professional fees accepted by the Center for Medicaid and Medicare Services (CMS) [5];and finally reimbursing examination fees, displaying certification credential on nametag and/or business card, and reimbursing for continuing education [11].

In the Philippines, continuous efforts to meet up with the global standards led to the establishment of Advanced Nursing Practice through the adoption of a Nursing Specialty Program and creation of the Nursing Specialty Certification Council (NSCC) [13].This serves as the government's response to the issues faced by the nursing profession such as decreasing quality of nursing graduates, surplus of nurses, increasing unemployment and low compensation [13].

Locally, certification has three (3) levels, namely: Level I- Nurse Clinician I; Level II- Nurse Clinician II; and Level III- Clinical Nurse Specialist. Certifications will be granted to candidates after they have

successfully passed the series of didactic, practical and written examinations and complied with the requirements necessary, such as the following: certified copy of Transcript of Records (TOR) of BSN and graduate M.N. degrees; documents showing completion of the requirement (clinical/academic) for the level applied for; and recommendation of NSCC to Board of Nursing (BON) for the issuance of certification for the level applied for. According to the Philippine Board of Nursing (BON), advanced nursing practice covers the roles of the clinical nurse specialist, who is an expert practitioner within a specialized field of nursing. These nurses participate in a range of sub-roles including direct patient care, research, teaching, consultation and management. Clinical nurse specialists are independent nurse practitioners that could be self-employed and provides professional services to client/patients and their families. These nurses reach out and offer their services rather than expect clients to seek their help.

Although, nurse leaders have exerted efforts to formulate specialty programs for Filipino nurses. The researcher felt that there is a strong need to look into the present conditions of the clinical nurse specialists. What have happened to them after certification? Are they receiving the same recognition and benefits as other international nurse specialists receive? How are they being accepted and utilized in the Philippine health care setting?

Method

Design

Phenomenology seeks knowledge on the basis of the genuine, human experience and aims to describe the phenomena "going to the things themselves" and in the natural experience of the "life-world" [14]. This approach will involve direct exploration, analysis, and description of the acceptance and utilization of Filipino advanced clinical nurse specialists as free as possible from unexamined presuppositions aiming at maximum intuitive presentation and a capacity to stimulate our perception of their lived experiences while giving emphasis on the richness, breadth, and depth of this phenomenon [15].

Selection

Five Filipino advanced clinical nurse specialists, certified by the Philippine Board of Nursing, working in tertiary hospitals in Metro Manila were chosen using Snowball sampling technique. With regard to the recommendation for sampling size [16], in qualitative studies, it is noted that this study had few participants for the reason that qualitative methodology values the understanding of complex human issues rather than generalizability of results.

Procedure

A two-part instrument was developed by the researcher to gather data and information for this qualitative study. It comprises of the participant's demographic profile and a semi-structured in depth interviews comprising of open-ended questions [17] as data gathering tool. The interviewing technique ensured that the study participants spoke on issues pertinent to advanced clinical nursing practice and helped achieve data saturation point. Their sharing revolved around the central question "What describes the acceptance and utilization of advanced clinical nurse specialist in the health care settings?

After securing informed consent, interviews were scheduled based on the participants' availability and convenience. Interviews were taped recorded for the purpose of capturing everything that transpired in the process including the non-verbal cue and clues. Code names were assigned to each recorded audio tape to maintain their anonymity. Interview lasted for an average of one hour. After transcription of the data, the researcher went back to the participants to validate the responses gathered.

Mode of analysis

Tape recorded interviews were personally transcribed by the researcher individually to minimize transcription errors and followed the steps of a descriptive phenomenology method of inquiry as outlined by Swanson-Kauffman and Schonwald [18]. The researcher made every effort to set aside all personal biases and prejudices of the phenomenon [19]. After listening to individual interviews and transcribed the collected data, the researcher analysed all data based on the field texts and processed it with the use of repertory grid. The process involved sorting, categorization (cool analysis) and thematization (warm analysis). Inductive and deductive methods were used to ensure appropriate placement of appropriate themes and finally uncover the central meaning of the phenomenon. Also, the researcher adopted Colaizzi's Seven Steps of Phenomenological analysis [20].

The exhaustive description and the fundamental structure were then validated by qualitative research experts not involved in the study. Member checking procedures were done to ensure truthfulness and trustworthiness of the data [21].

Findings

From the fullness and vividness of the verbalizations of the clinical nurse specialists (CNS), the researcher deduced the phenomenon of "Professional Ambivalence" that described their experiences in the acceptance and utilization of advanced practice nursing in the Philippines. As the study aimed to described and understand the acceptance and utilization of CNS, the phenomenon of Professional Ambivalence Syndrome emerged as shown in Figure 1. Four Clusters of themes delineated their collective experiences and are described as follows: Inspired to perform a new role, Blinded acceptance of the embodied role, Narrowed opportunities to practice area of specialization and Uncertainty to one's own achievements.

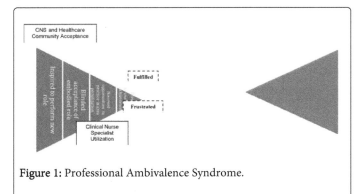

Figure 1: Professional Ambivalence Syndrome.

Professional Ambivalence Syndrome greatly characterized the divergent recognition of the healthcare professionals to the clinical nurse specialists' enthusiasm to commit to practice professional

advancement and maximize their services in the country. Notably, there is an evidence of incongruity in the views of the clinical nurse specialists' and the response of the community of healthcare professionals which was graphically represented by the use of a green laterally inverted triangle. From the enormous commitment of unremittingly improving nursing services, an ambiguous, narrowed response in the community of healthcare professionals was received by the clinical nurse specialist. The shape of a laterally inverted triangle was used to depict the wider perception of the CNS that gradually narrows as the healthcare professionals give limited regard to the value of ANP. Also, the green colour was used to signify the nursing profession.

As the CNSs progress to compete globally, a narrowing regard and acceptance of their specialization was experienced by the clinical nurse specialists' leading to feelings of ambivalence to one's own achievements, from being proud to frustrated, dissatisfied and uncertain to practice confidently and independently as represented by another grey triangular shape in opposing position which highlighted the CNS divided, clouded emotions.

Acceptance

In this study, acceptance is defined as to how the clinical nurse specialists and the healthcare professionals embraced the advance nursing practice in the country. It is clearly highlighted from the two contrasting descriptions of the clinical nurse specialists' positive view to practice independently and the concealing responses of their colleagues and nursing administrators. Contrary to the optimistic views of the nurse to pursue clinical nurse specialization, the healthcare community responded indifferently to the presence of clinical nurse specialists in the healthcare team. Acceptance is further described in the study through the two cluster themes that emerged,(1) Inspired to perform a new role and (2) Blinded Acceptance of Embodied Role.

Inspired to perform a new role

This cluster of theme was characterized by the clinical nurse specialists' positive view to challenge self with the need for professional advancement. For most of participants, Advanced Nursing Practice is a form of specialization that would give them a higher level of advantage in terms of autonomy and authority in their profession, economic stability and degree of worth in the healthcare field. These ideas were clearly depicted by all of the participants' statements as one the participant Nightingale narrated "Through this specialization, I will be able to advance myself both professionally and economically." Moreover, Benner and Orem affirmed that the prestige of being called as a specialist inspired them to become certified.

Additionally, Orem and Roy confirmed their optimistic perception that being a clinical nurse specialists would change their future, be globally recognized and uplift their morale and the nobility of the nursing profession. As Orem stated, "When I heard about the specialization, I was delighted because this could give a new image to Filipino nurses. I was so interested because I felt that this is now the chance to prove to the world that we can be trained and we can excel in our field. This could pave a better future ahead of us. This could open new doors to opportunities and recognition."

Blinded acceptance of embodied role

In this study, blinded acceptance was described by the clinical nurse specialists (CNS) indistinct performance of their perceived role in the healthcare setting and how the patients, administrators and other healthcare professionals appreciated their presence in the area. When Nightingale was asked to describe how her patients, administrators and other healthcare professionals accepted her roles and responsibilities as a Cardiovascular Clinician she strongly responded "Acceptance of the CNS is a big question mark!!There is no well-defined law as to what the scope of the roles and responsibilities of the CNS are. There are even no well-defined competencies that each CNS should be acquired. I am definitely accepted as ICU Nurse but as a specialist in terms of profession I am not. People and even doctors are not even aware that such specialization among nurses exists."

Subsequently all respondents know for a fact that acceptance of their profession is still in question because there is no well-defined laws that explains their scope of practice. "It is so difficult to act especially if you are not guided by the law"; "I really don't know how far I could render care to my patients. It is like practicing the profession without guidelines."

Abdellah distressingly said "Actually, I, myself, am not quite sure of my roles and responsibilities. There are no clear descriptions on what a clinical nurse specialist can do and not do. There are no set of competencies set by the Board of Nursing. I just simply met all the requirements and become certified, that's it! Even as a specialist, I was treated the same way before my certification. There was no big difference at all." Further, Roy added "Even if you are qualified, if your role is not accepted based by law it is nothing."

Utilization

Utilization is defined in the study as to how the services of the clinical nurse specialists are maximized and valued by their patients/public, co-workers and administrators. Two cluster themes described how the CNS was regarded in their area of specialization. First, Narrowed opportunities to perform in area of specialization, second, divided to one's own achievements.

Narrowed opportunities to perform in area of specialization

This cluster of theme outlined the limited regard of the healthcare team to the clinical nurse specialists. As most of the participants validated this experience "Our expertise is only being availed inside the hospital and I think people would still prefer to see a doctor rather than consulting us." But positively some of the respondents shared how public utilization may be made more possible "For the public to utilize our profession the ANP should pass a licensure exam given by the PRC and results must be known to the public"; "People would only believe in us if we have the license as a nurse specialist."

Consequently, this study revealed that utilization of the expertise of these clinical nurse specialists in their workplace depends on how much their colleagues trust them. As Benner shared "You really need to show them that you can because for one doctors would still question and doubt you of our expertise."; "Though advanced nursing practitioners abroad is an autonomous profession, doctors here still claim that they have longer educational preparation than ANPs here and so you always need to prove yourself."; "Some of the doctors allow me to do stoma care especially if they knew that I've undergone

trainings and seminars and am certified as a nurse specialist, but some still don't. It's really a case to case basis."

Lastly, administrators have a great impact as to the utilization of the CNS. These nurse specialists noted that "We are deployed in the clinical area just like other staff nurses."; "It doesn't mean even though you are a new-born screener you'll be automatically assigned in a pediatric or nursery unit as still the hospital administration will decide."In the end such administrative decisions would dictate the path of utilizing the expertise of a clinical nurse specialist because "No special privilege is given to us even after all certifications and trainings we went through to be the expert that we know we are now," a respondent emphatically expressed.

Aggravating to the situation would be the fact that the public is unaware of the existence of such practice as Nightingale and Benner viewed the public and the healthcare professionals' limited regard of their specialization were related to their lack of awareness of such specialization. As Roy affirmed this experience "It is really hard to say that I am truly recognized as a nurse specialist…People will remain seeing us an ordinary staff nurses that happened to have the extra skill,""; "And I don't think people will come to my house for nursing care" Orem skeptically added.

This legal issue that long plagued their profession led to disappointment as experienced by most of the participants as they openly averred "You are just treated the same way as the other nursing staff, even if you went through trainings and certifications. Every day you feel that there's this constant need to prove yourself to your colleagues."; "Yes, you are eventually recognized as skilful but definitely not as a specialist."; "People would usually perceive nurses as secretary of the doctors or assistants"; "What's more disappointing is that you know you are very much capable of doing the tasks and yet you cannot work independently."

Divided to one's own achievements

This emerging pattern surfaced the participants' experience of conflicting emotions in the practice of advanced practice nursing. Being fulfilled of their achievements is coupled with the negative feelings of frustrations based from how they were regarded as members of the healthcare team. As one of the participants verbalized "You are hesitant and most often doubtful of what you can and cannot do because of the lack of a clear scope of practice still plagues the CNS profession," one reflected on the intrapersonal factors that chain the proliferative utilization of such profession in the country today. Moreover lack of confidence and a great feeling of being lost are some of the shared reasons of these respondents as to why they don't assert their profession as much. The following are their verbalizations:

"Being a certified clinical nurse specialist is not an assurance of a promotion" as Nightingale verbalized about its professional gains in their field of practice. Others support his statement by verbalizing that "No special privileges and benefits are given to CNS.; "Definitely I cannot ask for any professional fees, like doctors do, for the special service I've rendered."; "In the hospital that I'm working at, nurse specialists like me are not only overloaded but also can be pulled out anytime of their units to render special care but without any additional compensation." Additionally one responded sums it all why professional gains of these CNS are masked by noting "As what I've observed and experienced myself a CNS obtains promotions not solely based on his/her status as a clinical nurse specialist but mainly because of the skills and the number of years he/she might have rendered in the institution he/she is working at. Sometimes, it's just hard not to compare how well clinical nurse specialists (CNS) are accepted and privileged abroad", one respondent verbalized as he shook his head comparing how Filipino and foreign CNS are accepted in their respective locales.

Discussion

The introduction of advance nursing practice (ANP) has already generated many debates regarding issues such as educational preparation, scope of practice and even the consistency in which these professional roles should be called [22,23]. In the Philippines, ANP became one of the nation's healthcare strategies in improving its global competence [13].However, the same problems arose when regulatory boards failed to address aforementioned concerns surrounding its inconsistencies. Hence this study opted to explore qualitatively the acceptance and utilization of clinical nurse specialists in the Philippine health care settings.

In the study by Niebuhr and Biel [11] both the authors averred that several studies correlated the impact of certification as it benefits to nurses who are certified and how the employment of certified nurse's benefits the workplace. The clinical nurse specialists' positive perceptions of acquiring a specialization in the country were related to the potential advantages of authority, independence and financial stability that accompany it. These optimistic views of Filipino CNS proved the findings of Wynd [9] who emphasized that the value of nursing certification has also been associated with high levels of professionalism, characterized by attitudes of self-regulation, self-determination, and independence. Certified nurses have been shown to possess increased sense of empowerment [11]. Most of the participants in the study initially regard advance practice nursing as giving them the autonomy to achieve their highest level of potential, personal fulfilment and a deeper sense of accomplishment.

Contrary to the Filipino ANPs positive views about the value of certification, this does not directly correlate to an automatic salary increase; promotions are not solely based on their status but mainly because of their skills and most often due to the number of years they have served a hospital or an institution. This variability is parallel to the American Board of Nursing Specialties' Value of Certification Survey4 when only one (1) statement- "Certification increases salary"- did not receive overall agreement from the respondents.

Interviews with the ANP suggest that they collectively view professional gains as being recognized to be skilful and competent at the same time. Competency has been defined as the degree to which individuals can apply the skills and knowledge associated with a profession to the full range of situations that fall within the domain of that particular profession [24]. But without the clear-cut distinction of what an ANP could do and not do, they remain unparalleled to the regular registered nurses (RN). Therefore they will just be recognized as skilful in a particular field but not necessarily a specialist.

Findings of the study also proved how the community of healthcare professionals and their stakeholders can greatly influence the acceptance and utilization of ANP locally. As the study of Niebuhr and Biel [11] identified that lack of institutional support would keep nurses from valuing their specialization. The lack of institutional support was clearly described by most of the study participants in the following situations: First, they felt that they were treated ordinarily by their colleagues and administrators despite their earned specialization. Second, most of the CNSs were assigned to area outside their expertise

prohibiting them from practicing their skills and knowledge, gaining confidence and practicing independently. Third, there were no clear boundaries set by the Board of Nursing in all healthcare institutions to establish their nursing roles and responsibilities as clinical nurse specialists. A need for clarity regarding the core competencies of APN is essential to be able to understand their distinctive role in practice [1].

Narrowed opportunities revealed to be the essence of ANP's utilization in the country. This is due to the lack of public trust to the new found profession. Without public awareness, professional gains for these professionals will remain uninviting. To date the country still experiences paucity when it comes to investigating issues, barriers and efficacy of these professional roles; thereby, contributing to the lack of awareness of the nation with the services that the CNS can offer. Moreover lack of formality when it comes to the scope of practice serves as confusion for both physicians and clinical nurse specialists especially that they utilize the same body of knowledge. Some asserted that when measures of quality and cost are used, the primary care provided by nurse practitioners is equivalent or superior to that provided by physicians [25]. In summary, if the issues about the utilization and acceptance of the Advancednursing practice felt by CNS still remain unheard and not addressed, the evolution of ANP in the Philippines will languish.

Conclusion and Recommendation

Collective analysis of the verbalizations, the Filipino CNS successfully unraveled the eidetic meaning of acceptance and utilization of clinical nurse specialists in the country. An extensive amount of literatures have been published regarding advanced nursing practice, its development, acceptance, barriers and mishaps. Despite those efforts there still exists a paucity of research that digs deep on how advanced nursing practice (ANP) in the Philippines is utilized and accepted. Thus this phenomenological inquiry sought after finding the true essence of both the acceptance and utilization of the aforementioned professional locally.

Philippines continuously geared to move toward global competence; finding ways in improving its resources, practices and services, developing its health care system through the more advanced breed of nurses more known to be called as advanced nurse practitioners (ANP). Driven by their confidence to practice the acquired advanced skills and knowledge, the Filipino clinical nurse specialists (CNS) are initially motivated to improve one's practice and the nation's health. Filipino CNS sparingly enjoys the eminence and appreciation as foreign nurse specialists do. To be able to empower more Filipino nurses to struggle for professional growth and for advanced nursing practice in the Philippines to continue to evolve, it is imperative that Filipino nursing leaders must begin to organize a unified vision of advanced practice nursing to establish the value of advance nurse practice in the Philippines by amending the existing law, delineating the scope of their practice, reviewing the existing requirements for certification and making the healthcare community mindful of the existence and value of such professionals.

As Hanson and Hamric1 noted that the title of advanced practice will have meaning only if it is used consistently to refer to advanced clinical practice rather than being inclusive of other advanced roles in the profession, such as in research, education and administration. All roles whether specialty or advanced practice, are valuable and vital to the profession's continued development [4].

Acknowledgement

The author wishes to express her sincere gratitude to her family for their love, unremitting encouragement and support. To her second home, the UST College of Nursing headed by Dean Susan N. Maravilla, RN, MAN for her appreciation, confidence and trust in her. To her dear friends for sharing their wisdom and expertise in research namely: Iris Chua So, RN, MAN, La. Arnie Lazalita, RN, MAN and Eleanor Lourdes Chua, Tan, RN. Lastly, financial support from the University of Santo Tomas Research and Endowment Foundation Inc. and Commission on Higher Education (CHED) is greatly acknowledged.

References

1. Hanson C, Hamric A (2003) Reflections on the continuing education of advanced nursing practice. Nursing outlook 5:203-211.

2. Savrin C (2009) Growth and development of the nurse practitioner role around the globe. J Pediatr Health Care 23: 310-314.

3. Beitz JM (2000) Specialty practice, advanced practice, and WOC nursing: current professional issues and future opportunities. J Wound Ostomy Continence Nurs 27: 55-64.

4. American Board of Nursing Specialties (2006) Promoting Excellence in Nursing Certification. Aurora, OH:

5. Goudreau KA, Smolenski M (2008) Credentialing and certification: issues for clinical nurse specialists. Clin Nurse Spec 22: 240-244.

6. American Nurses Credentialing Center (2006) Magnet recognition programs.Available at:www.nursingworld.org/ancc/magnet.

7. Bonsall K, Cheater FM (2008) What is the impact of advanced primary care nursing roles on patients, nurses and their colleagues? A literature review. Int J Nurs Stud 45: 1090-1102.

8. Piazza IM, Donahue M, Dykes PC, Griffin MQ, Fitzpatrick JJ (2006) Differences in perceptions of empowerment among nationally certified and noncertified nurses. J NursAdm 36: 277-283.

9. Wynd CA (2003) Current factors contributing to professionalism in nursing. J Prof Nurs 19: 251-261.

10. Byrne M, Valentine W, Carter S (2004) The value of certification--a research journey. AORN J 79: 825-828, 831-5.

11. Niebuhr B, Biel M (2007) The value of specialty nursing certification. Nurs Outlook 55: 176-181.

12. MacDonald JA, Herbert R, Thibeault C (2006) Advanced practice nursing: unification through a common identity. J Prof Nurs 22: 172-179.

13. Philippine Regulatory Commission-Board of Nursing (2011) PRC- BON Resolution No.118. s.2002. BON Newsletter: Philippines 20.

14. Pusa S, Persson C, Sundin K (2012) Significant others' lived experiences following a lung cancer trajectory: from diagnosis through and after the death of a family member. Eur J OncolNurs 16: 34-41.

15. Streubert H, Carpenter D (2011) Qualitative Research in Nursing: Advancing the Humanistic Imperative (5th Edn). Philadephia, USA: Lippincott Williams & Wilkins.

16. Reid K, Flowers P, Larkin M (2005) Exploring lived experience. The Psychologist 18: 1.

17. Patton MQ (1990) Qualitative evaluation and research methods (2nd edn) New York Park,C. Sage Publication, Inc.

18. Wojnar DM, Swanson KM (2007) Phenomenology: an exploration. J Holist Nurs 25: 172-180.

19. Creswell JW (2003) Research design: Qualitative, quantitative, and mixed method approaches. Thousand Oaks, CA: Sage Publication.

20. Collaizi PR (1978) Psychological research as the phenomenologisy views it. In: Vall RS, King M (eds.) Existential Phenomenological Alternatives for Psychology, New York Oxford University Press.

21. De Guzman AB, Tan EB (2007) Understanding the essence of scholarship from the lived experiences of a select group of outstanding Filipino researchers. Educational Research Journal 22: 49-68.

22. Rasch RF, Frauman AC (1996) Advanced practice in nursing: conceptual issues. J Prof Nurs 12: 141-146.

23. Jack B, Hendry C, Topping A (2004)Third year student nurses perception of the role and impact of clinical nurse specialists: a multi-centered descriptive study. Clinical Effectiveness in Nursing. 8: 39-46.

24. Lysaght R, Altschuld J (1999) Beyond initial certification: the assessment and maintenance of competency in professions. Evaluation and Program Planning, 23, 95- 104.

25. Hemani A, Rastegar DA, Hill C, al-Ibrahim MS (1999) A comparison of resource utilization in nurse practitioners and physicians. EffClinPract 2: 258-265.

23

Specific Nursing Care Rendered in Hepatic Encephalopathy: Contemporary Review and New Clinical Insights

Zeljko Vlaisavljević * and Ivan Rankovic

University of Mississippi Clinical Centre of Serbia, Clinic for Gastroenterolgy and Hepatology, Street of Dr Koste Todorovica 2, 11 000 Belgrade, Serbia

*Corresponding author: Zeljko Vlaisavljević, Clinical Centre of Serbia, Clinic for Gastroenterolgy and Hepatology, Street of Dr Koste Todorovica 2, 11 000 Belgrade, Serbia, E-mail: kcszeljko@gmail.com

Abstract

Introduction: Hepatic Encephalopathy (HE) is neuropsychiatric deterioration syndrome due to hepatic insufficiency. HE symptoms appear gradually ranging from altered mental status to deep coma and manifest as disorders of orientation, memory, perception, reasoning, focusing, rigor, and generalized convulsions. Four levels of HE exist with different symptoms.

Aim of the paper: To observe Specific Nursing Care rendered to hepatic encephalopathy patients and determining the significance of nurse education and employment length in HE patient healthcare.

Methodology: This is a cross-sectional study of 70 nurses in (Clinical Center of Serbia, Clinic for Gastroenterology and Hepatology) Between May1 to December15, 2011. The questionnaire was divided into two parts with 18 questions in total. The first part consisted of general questions (sex, professional education, working experience, working hours), while the second part had 13 questions assessing knowledge of nurses about the specificities of HE healthcare

Results: The most common cause of hepatic encephalopathy is ethylic cirrhosis with 69.2%, while 30.8% of patients with cirrhosis and HE died in period from 1.5.-15.12.2011. Nurses (N=70) declared that 91.4% of them had no adequate conditions to provide necessary HE patient healthcare. Out of N=70, 78.6% knew how to recognize first symptoms of HE while 64.3% nurses made no difference between HE and other diseases.

Conclusion: Specificity of HE patient healthcare encompassess nursing interventions and diagnosis. Through continuous education, respecting previous knowledge, it is necessary to focus on specific diseases such as hepatic encephalopathy with the aim of providing healthcare excellence.

Keywords: Healthcare; Hepatic encephalopathy; Nurse

Abbreviation

HE: Hepatic Encephalopathy; CVC: Central Venous Catheter; HCC: Hepatocellular Carcinoma; SDD: Selective Digestive Decontamination; HRS: Hepatorenal Syndrome; DALY: The Disability-Adjusted Life Year; C: College; U: Univeryitet

Introduction

Hepatic encephalopathy (HE) [1] represents potentially reversible reduction of neuropsychiatric functions due to acute and/or chronic liver disease. It occurs most often inpatients with portal hypertension. The beginning is usually insidious, and is characterized by subtle and sometimes periodical changes in memory, cognition, associative higher intellectual functions, as well as altered personality. The liver plays a central role in the regulation of other organ systems through the spectrum of its functions related to energetic metabolism, hormonal and electrolyte balance, immunologic and immunomodulatory status. As a consequence, chronic liver disease causes a number of systemic manifestations that can dominate the clinical course. Some of these complications stem from the reduction in number of functional hepatocytes and the resulting loss of synthetic and metabolic functional capacity. Others consequences are from portal pressure, leading to portal vascular collaterals opening and shunting with bypassing the liver lobules. These manifestations of cirrhosis –reduced synthetic reserve and disrupted perfusion are functionally connected and can change over time depending on various pathophysiological demands. Subtle signs of hepatic encephalopathy can be observed in almost 70% of patients with liver cirrhosis and they are called the subclinical form of hepatic encephalopathy [2]. Hepatic encephalopathy can be provoked by dehydration, excessive protein intake through food and certain beverages, constipation, hypo and hyperkalemia, digestive tract haemorrhages, infections, renal failure, hypoxia, use of barbiturates and benzodiazepine, as well as changes in physical factors(climate and atmospheric disturbances). Hepatic encephalopathy is progressive in terms of its clinical prognostic character. A nurse needs to know well the symptoms of encephalopathy thus being able to react promptly and adequately in taking care of such a patient. Hepatic encephalopathy can manifest itself acutely with a rapid deterioration of mental functions leading to coma, with no previous symptomatology [3]. Being chronic reversible in patients with pronounced portal hypertension, it is caused by certain precipitating factors (constipation, bleeding, and diuretics) which can be identified and removed in most cases. The development of hepatic encephalopathy is a poor prognostic sign and is related to less than 32% of survival rate during first year. The most significant cause of this disease in the developed countries is alcohol abuse [4,5]. In Asia and Africa the most common cause of liver cirrhosis is hepatitis B virus (with or without delta antigens) [6]. The cause of cirrhosis of the liver can also be hepatitis C virus, hepatocellular carcinoma with intraparenchymatous dissemination(the so-called HCC satellite induced HE), various intoxications with heavy metals and poisonous gases, Wilson's disease (hepatolenticular degeneration), metabolic diseases (alpha-1 antitrypsin deficiency, as well as so-called storage diseases, such as hemochromatosis),while other half comprises autoimmune liver disease such as autoimmune hepatitis and primary biliary cirrhosis. HE has four grades of classification, on the basis of West-Haven Classification System [7] (Table1). HE diagnosis is established on the basis of physical clinical examination and biochemical panel. As far as biochemical markers are concerned, blood is taken for a complete blood workup which can indicate the presence of hyperammonemia usually with levels above 50mmol/l, elevated serum transaminases and bilirubin, hypokalemia, hyponatremia and azotemia. Analyses such as metabolic tests of glycaemia, serum osmolality, liver function enzymes, can point out to disorders in metabolism which are indicative for liver cirrhosis. Also urea, creatinine, eGFR, and cystatin C give away the functional capacity of kidneys whose function is also specifically altered in liver cirrhosis. If positive, hemoculture indicates the presence of pathogenic organisms, and administration of adequate antibiotics is mandatory. Coagulation status points to the presence of coagulopathy and low levels of coagulation factors predominantly factor V (with plasma half-life of 3-6h) and factor VII(also referred to as proaccelerin or labile factor) [8]. The biochemical examination of abdominal fluid, ascites (Rivalta test), bacteriological and cytomorphological examination (presence of malignant hyperchromatic cells) can also help determine the etiologic factor of liver lesion. Chest X-ray, ECG, ultrasound with portal system doppler examination and EEG are all basic diagnostic procedures that can be supplemented according to the state of the patient. The assessment of psychological status is conducted using a standardized algorithm preferably number connection test as well as using Glasgow Coma Scale when having severe HE form. Also, we must underline West-Haven criterias which are diagnostic hallmarks. Treatment is conducted through reduction of serum ammonia levels (restriction of animal proteins), administration of oral lactulose, oral or IV antibiotics, giving parenteral solutions with branched-chain amino acids, enemas, transfusions of blood and it's components, and general healthcare [9]. The final and ultimately complete treatment for liver cirrhosis with hepatic encephalopathy is liver transplantation. Transplantation is an incremental factor incuring patients with liver cirrhosis [10,11]. To accurately establish the diagnosis of hepatic encephalopathy it is necessary to determine the severity of liver disease, exclude cerebraltrauma, intracranial vascular and expansive lesions, metabolic disorders, as well as systemic hemodynamic distortions (checking continuously if cardiovascular and renal function is intact) [12]. As stated above, the approach to care differs depending on the level of encephalopathy in patients. It is necessary to establish adequate nursing diagnosis, upon which the planning goals for patient healthcare are defined. How does a patient with second (II) or third (III) grade hepatic encephalopathy clinically present? They speak incomprehensibly, they are often two or three dimensionally disoriented, with clinically pronounced abdomen due to ascites, their skin is sticky, colored from yellow too range. Their odor is sweet, as well as breath, obstipation to diarrhoea is present usually with bimodal incontinence and oliguria. Nutrition in comatose patients is parenteral:

using infusions, with nasogastric or nasojejunal tubes, or with PEG tube in most severe cases with coexisting disorders. Due to altered state of consciousness patients can be aggressive, agitated, and they can try to get out of bed and hurt themselves, therefore, they have to be placed in intensive care units under a 24-hour observation in beds with side rails.

Grade 0 HE	**HE represents the minimal hepatic encephalopathy, known as subclinical, with minimal changes in personality and concentration.**
Grade I HE	Is characterized by trivial lack of consciousness, shortened attention span, insomnia, sleep inversion, euphoria or depression, irritability, decreased intellectual function with altered short term memory which rarely manifests
Grade II HE	clinically features the occurrence of lethargy, apathy, temporal disorientation, incomprehensible speech, inappropriate behavior and somnolence.
Grade III HE	Is characterized by somnolence, disorientation both in time and space, confusion or amnesia.
Grade IV	Represents coma.

Table 1: West-Haven Classification System

Research Material and Methods

Survey data was collected using the self-administration method to ensure the confidentiality and anonymity with a previous oral approval of nurses being questioned. The analysis of medical documentation and official protocols in the Clinic of Gastroenterology and Hepatology of the Clinical Centre of Serbia was also conducted for the time during the study period May 1. to December 15., 2011. Sample size is selected based on criteria that are nurses employed at the Clinic for Gastroenterology and Hepatology - Clinical Center of Serbia, as well as nurses who are working with patients of HE. Employed nurses that are included in the study - 70 of 98. Data processing The SPSS program for Windows, version 17.0, was used for data processing. The comparison of numerical markers between two groups (working experience and level of education) was made using the chi-square (X2) test. Values p<0.05 were taken as statistically significant. Ethical considerations This study was approved by the chief nursing educator, head-chief nurse, and department chief nurses of our clinic where the research was carried out, as well as by the head of the Department of Scientific and Research Work, Education Activity and Human Resources of the Clinic of Gastroenterology, the Director of the Clinic of Gastroenterology, and the Director of the Centre for Scientific Research Work, Education and Teaching Activities and Human Resources of the Clinical Centre of Serbia.

General sample characteristics

Out of the total number of nurses (N=70), 62 of them (88.6%) had only secondary medical school completed, while 8 had college or university degrees (11.4%). According to the length of working experience, 30 respondents had less than 20 years of experience (42.9%), while 40 respondents had over 20 years of working experience (57.1%). The average working experience was 17.3 years. There were 6 male nurses (8.6%) and 64 female nurses (91.4%). 37 respondents worked in shifts (52.9%), while 33 of them worked only in the morning. In the hepatology ward within the Clinic of Gastroenterohepatology, there were 30 grade I and II HE patients and

13 grade III and IV HE patients in the period between May 1 and December 15, 2011. The causes for grade III and IV patients were, results: The findings of this study revealed that the most common cause of hepatic encephalopathy is ethylic cirrhosis with 69.2%, toxic liver disease induced HE with 15.4%, autoimmune liver disease HE with 7.7%, and hepatitis C virus (HCV) HE with 7.7%. Four patients died, or 30.8% of the total number of patients with Grade III and IV HE. 38.5% suffered from portal vein thrombosis, while 66.7% had esophageal varices. Sex distribution consisted of 73.3% of male patients and 13.3% of female patients. Each one of the patients was diagnosed with hepatic encephalopathy (100%) using West-Haven criteria and adjunctive number connection test.

years of professional experience gave correct answer in 62,5%, (p=, 001), and there wasn't any statistical significance relating to the educational level between two groups. On question if they would know to recognise symptoms of HE, first group (one up to 20 years of employment) said that they would recognise (90%), and those over 20 years of experience gave positive answer in 70% (p=,044), while interpreting the educational status, there wasn't any significant statistical difference. Participants up to 20 years would know how to read blood tests (83%) and those over 20 years of employment status answered positively in 50% (p=,004).

Research results (Table 2)

Participants with 20 years of employment status knew that HE is disturbance of consciousness (96,7%), while those with more than 20

Question	N	C%	W%	According to working experience					According to education				
				Less than 20 y. C%	More than 20 y. C%	Less than 20 y. W%	More than 20 y. W%	P	SS C%	C & U C %	SS W%	C & U W %	P
Hepatic encephalopathy is a disorder of consciousness	70	77.1	22.9	96.7	62.5	3.3	37.5	0.001	74.2	100	25.8	0	NS
I know how to recognize first signs and symptoms of HE	70	78.6	21.4	90	70	10	30	0.044	75.8	100	24	0	NS
Can you interpret blood results# of patients with HE	70	64.3	35.7	83.3	50	16.7	50	0.004	61.3	87.5	38.7	12.5	NS
HE is a chronic disease	70	31.4	68.6	26.7	35	73.3	65	NS	27.4	62.5	72.6	37.5	0.044
Do you work in adequate conditions for HE patients care	70	8.6	91.4	10	7.5	90	92.5	NS	4.8	37.5	95.2	62.5	0.002
Are there procedural standards for providing health care to HE patients	70	5.7	94.3	3.3	7.5	96.7	92.5	NS	3.2	25	96.8	75	0.013

Table 2: Knowledge and attitude of nurses toward hepatic encephalopathy Knowledge and attitude of nurses toward hepatic encephalopathy, N – total, C – correct answer, W – wrong answer, SS – Secondary medical school, C – College, U – University, NS-not significant, #Blood results: urea, creatinine, hepatic transaminases

The fact that HE is chronical disease nurses with higher education (C* i U*) knew in 62, 5%, while nurses that just graduated from high school didn't know that (72,6%) (p=,044). Up to 91, 4% of nurses said that they don't have adequate conditions for taking care of HE patients i.e. nurses with high school (95,2%) and those with higher education (62,5%) (p=,044). On question are there standards in healthcare procedures, 94,3% of all replied negatively, and influence of education for this question gave statistically significant result in those with high school in 96,8%, and in those with higher education in 75% (p=,013).

Discussion

Liver cirrhosis represents around 1% of overall global disease burden expressed in DALY (The disability-adjusted life year). The share of cirrhosis in global structure of dying is 1.4% [13]. In line with

this non-negligible percentage, the prevention of this disease is of great importance. And if disease does appear, high-quality healthcare is crucial in the clinical management process. Liver diseases comprised 1.0% of the total mortality rate in central Serbia and Vojvodina in 2000 [14]. Accessing the medical documentation, one can observe that share of cirrhosis in the structure of dying is correlating with prevailing alcohol intake as the primary etiological factor. Regardless of etiology, patients with hepatic encephalopathy have multiple specificities of health care. This paper aims to present the specificities of health care through nursing interventions in the purpose of providing better excellence in healthcare. Adequate care is of utmost importance in all phases of HE [12]. The specificity of health care for such patients would reflect in: Low-protein diet (meat and meat products), mushy and/or liquid food (due to accompanying esophagogastric varices).

Diet regulates protein catabolism and allows the ammonia levels nivelating in blood, simultaneously leading to adequate passage through intestines which prevents the occurrence of constipation. The limited intake of proteins is an important part of therapy, since it enables the correction of nitrogenous substances balance in the organism [12]. The intake of probiotics regulates the gut flora and bowel movement, on the one hand, while it reduces the risk of bacterial translocation and subsequent septicemia as a common secondary complication in HE patients, on the other. The reduction in the possibility of sepsis development improves the prognosis of patients with hepatic dysfunction, thus the intake of yoghurt with added probiotics is recommended as an adjuvant nutritional therapy [15].

The intake of lactulose, a non-absorbable disaccharide which reduces the level of serum ammonia concentration, as well as its absorption, is the cornerstone therapy in the overall strategy of HE treatment [4,16,17]. A patient should not be administered any oral therapy two hours before and after the intake of lactulose to achieve full therapeutic effect of administered drug. The optimal intake of liquid is of great importance due to ascites, with special attention on avoiding the over diuresis syndrome. The effective diuresis larger than 600-800/24h must not be provoked because it leads to prerenal azotemia, which further deteriorates cerebral perfusion, increasing the severity of HE. Every infection can lead to or deteriorate the condition of patients into encephalopathy, thus, for the purpose of monitoring the transaminases in blood, bilirubin, proteins and other biochemical factors, a nurse has to perform venepuncture almost daily. Therefore, placing a CVC is recommended, naturally, only if the coagulation status of the patient allows such an intervention. Infections increase the mortality of HE cirrhotic patients, especially pneumonia, sometimes with the main cause of death in such patients [18]. Special attention should be focused on decubital ulcers which may appear due to prolonged bed lying. The risk of cellulitis also increases because of poor skin integrity and development of peripheral edema [8]. Inadequately treated cellulitis can lead to fasciitis and a potentially lethal phlegmon – Vibrio vulnificus cellulitis. Urinary catheter insertion. Everyday care of catheter should be overall clinical strategy hallmark. Continuous diuresis monitoring with the measurement of urine outputshould be an important parameter which pinpoints the beginning of hepatorenal syndrome (HRS). Time span development of low urine output is the differentiation stigmata between type I and type II of HRS. Type I HRS is the prognostic omen sign of the primary liver disease [19].Rinsing the bladder and clearing or other undesirable contents is beneficial thus preventing post renal insufficiency or azotaemia [20].Treatment of mouth cavity, where candida may appear due to overzealous antibiotic administration should also be considered as the mainstay of therapy. These patients have ascites and large abdominal girth, their skin should be treated with hydrating creams, especially in abdominal region, since there skin is stretched and the feeling of pain and tension is highly pronounced. Positive reciprocal correlation and associated with both hepatic encephalopathy and асцитес as a risk factor for these complications and for death [21]. Abdominal therapeutic and diagnostic puncture and centhesis should be performed rationally and moderately. The use of diuretics and abdominal centhesis leads to positive response in 90% of patients, with the decrease in total body weight being the best indicator of diuretic, nutritional-dietetic and interventional therapy. However, the decrease in total bodyweight must not exceed 10% during a weekly period [22]. The hepatorenal syndrome (HRS) may insidiously overcome compensatory mechanisms and administered therapy and is characterized by acute renal failure with decrease in total urine output.

It occurs in approximately 10% of patients with disease progression [23]. Using diuretics, nutrition and interventional techniques should be cautious respecting hemodynamically over-sensed nephrons. In some patients, progressive oliguria appears with rapid increase in serum concentration of creatinine, and this is type I of hepatorenal syndrome. Type II HRS appears more frequently and it is characterized by increase in serum concentration of creatinine and urea with chronic to moderate progression which usually takes place in the time period of six or over six weeks from the disease starting point (pathological black point).Care of IV cannulas. Every intravenous route is a potential place of infection entry [8]. Bacterial infections are present in about 15% -47% of patients with cirrhosis of the liver, especially in relation to gram-negative bacteria. The most common spontaneous bacterial peritonitis (SBP), urinary tract infection, pneumonia, pleural empyema and sepsis[24].The patient receives infusions through one or preferably more IV routes, most often glucose or 0.9% NaCl with added potassium, magnesium sulfate or concentrated 3%NaCl [25]. Here the nurses role is pivotal giving the therapy strategy cornerstones of not only maintaining IV routes but also recognizing complications early e.g. thrombophlebitis, deep vein thrombosis or apparent hemorrhagic cutaneous or mucosal syndrome. Patients with acute liver failure, with grade III or more importantly grade IV HE, need to be intubated and put on mechanical ventilation following gas analyses every8 hours. This should be standard of nursing monitoring care surveilling respiratory insufficiency (most frequently etiological factor is hepatopulmonary syndrome).Mechanical ventilation should be with sedating agents like fentanyl aiming the protection of respiratory system and/or phenobarbital which is a neurocerebral modulatory agent for early treatment of cerebral edema by decreasing intracranial pressure as well as maintaining sedation [3]. Central nursing fields of intensive treatment should encompass knowing all the principal pharmacodynamics and pharmacokinetics of neuromodulatory agents which have effect on respiratory function. Nurses should be able to recognize overdosing of these agents since they are pulmonary function depressants when used in higher doses. Bleeding in the digestive tract complicates further HE patients treatment since proteins from blood contribute to high levels of serum ammonia. Therefore, intestines should be decontaminated and cleared of its content. This maneuver is called selective digestive decontamination (SDD). Also bleeding induced infections can occur, so proper use of antibiotic prophylaxis should be given respecting pharmacokinetic profiles of given antibiotics. One old and good technique which is in use for decadesis SDD through deep enemas with or without lactulose. Therefore, nurses need to independently perform an intervention of giving deep enemas as an overall therapeutic modality. In the case of hematemesis doctor inserts the Sengstaken-Blakemoor tube with the necessity to provide drainage and skin care around the nostrils. A nurse has to prepare both the adequate material and the patient, and she or he has to assist actively in passing the tube. Blood vomiting usually occurs due to the varicosity in the upper portions of the digestive tract. Esophageal varices are present in 30% of patients with liver cirrhosis and 60% of patients with decompensated liver cirrhosis. Every episode of repeated bleeding carries 20%mortality rate [8,26].The oxygen therapy is necessary in patients with altered consciousness. Oxygen should be administered through a nasal catheter, best using a mask. The continuous assessment of the respiratory status, including the respiratory rate, and oxygen saturation, should be performed through constant gas analyses. Passing an arterial cannula in Gr IV HE patients with acute liver failure should be particularly emphasized, since it allows for a continuous monitoring not only of blood oxygen saturation, but also of lactate and bicarbonate blood levels. The arterial cannulation gives as a clear-cut, always accessible arterial blood pH, without repeated punctures of arteries [22]. When noticing that pH curve is shifting it should alarm the nursing staff that with it hemoglobin oxygen saturation curve shifts as well prompting doctors evaluation and therapeutic intervention. Regular monitoring of total body weight and abdominal girth. Receiving therapy and abdomen ascites centhesis leads to change in abdominal girth and total body weight. Patient should loose from 0.3 to 0.5kg per day, however, if weight loss is greater it can lead to renal failure, since kidneys become more hypo perfused and sensitive to hemodynamic alterations [22]. Multimodality monitoring is tracking of multiple parameters of brain activity (monitoring intracranial pressure, EEG waves). This modern monitoring system has been used worldwide for over 20 years in neurointensive care units [27], facilitating the work of nurses and doctors, and influencing timely and accurately interventions with the improvement in patient's condition through its parameters and clinical status. Patient communication is hampered, i.e. they pronounce words with difficulty and speak incoherently, therefore it is necessary to spend enough time with them to show empathy and understanding. Communication with the patient's family is of utmost importance. Adequate communication with family members in relation to changes in the clinical status and condition offers the family an insight into the actual situation concerning prognosis and course of the disease [8,28]. In a healthcare institution, it is preferable to have a written document stating what kind of information concerning the patient's condition a nurse can convey to patient's family members. From the available medical literature, but above all from the experience of doctors with whom nurses work with, it is a well-known fact that a well educated and problem solving oriented nurse is crucial for the success of intensive care interventional procedures performed by doctors. A nurse offers psychological stability to the entire team led by a doctor, and helps the creation of positive atmosphere when highly complex procedures are performed such as insertion of a hemodialysis two lumen catheter through jugular venous system especially if low access point in the internal jugular vein is chosen or subclavian vein access point. Through their calmness and positive attitude, nurses often make the difference between success and failure of interventions performed by doctors in the intensive care units. This study examines the specificities of healthcare in patients, as well as the influence of knowledge and attitudes of nurses in providing best healthcare to patients with hepatic encephalopathy. Since knowledge is an socio-epidemiological determinant which is also related to informational level of the individual it can be concluded that respondents did not possess a substantial knowledge level of HE. Obtained research results show that correlation between the work quality factors (elaborated in more detail in the conclusion of this study) and ill-informed nurses, i.e. their lack of knowledge (44.3% stated that they did not receive any information at all), is statistically important and it carries a significant statistical relativerisk. Furthermore, the use of the Internet as an universal electronic tool for continuous medical education and self-evaluation is at a very low level, and it speaks of poor motivation of the staff for self-improvement and self-education, which is increasingly present both in contemporary literature and modern medical trends (personalized medical self-education –medline or medline plus networks and medscape internet community). Aspect of interpersonal relationships should also be mentioned, where the flow of information between doctors and head nurses, on the one hand, and ward nurses, on the other, is below the level necessary for further development and improvement of work quality (just 25.7% and 22.9%of staff personnel with secondary education received information from doctors and head

nurses). Speaking of interpersonal relationships, it should be emphasized that they can have a beneficial or adverse influence on all three factors of work quality, defined and explained in more detail in the conclusion chapter of this study. Therefore, interpersonal relationships should be highlighted due to their prospective and universal importance, which makes the man inevitable part of any future epidemiological study dealing with the same or similar medical topic. It is precisely because of the fact that an integrated approach to HE patients is needed, statistically significant percent of nurses need (72.9% of respondents) continuous medical education. Moreover, it is believed that a better organization of continuous medical education would contribute at first hand to the increase in staff interest for further tertiary education, as well as the higher quality of secondary education. Secondly, the choice of topics of continuous medical education should be closely related to the specificities of HE patient care so as to have not only scientific and theoretical, but also practical significance. Thirdly, nurses need to participate actively in education, best in the format of panel discussion which needs to be implemented into continuous medical education, which will allow interactive approach making education clearer and more efficient. Therefore, it is not only sufficient to maintain continuous medical education, but to be modified as well. Since the staff personnel awareness is at respectable level (54.3% of nurses realized the importance of adequate and specific care of HE patients), it is also necessary to introduce the regulated improved official guidelines to nursing care, which would raise the existing awareness of the staff in the HE patient care. Healthcare is part of curative, restorative-healing, invigorating and rehabilitating process. The provided nursing care is of great importance in the treatment of HE patients [29]. Recognition and treatment of encephalopathy is critical for improving survival outcome with less complications in critically ill patients [29]. Managing complications in patients with cirrhosis in intensive care settings requires knowledge of various fields of medicine for doctors [10], which should also apply to nurses. Clinical guidelines already exist for doctors in this institution, but having in mind that the majority of staff recognizes their pivotal role in the complete medical therapy, it is necessary for such guidelines to exist for the nursing staff as well making the roles of doctors and nurses mutually complementary. Furthermore, this would ensure better interpersonal relationships, since it would define the position or place of every nurse in the medical team. Nursing guidelines would contribute to the standardization, as well as uniformity, of educational and interventional factors of work quality. Guidelines could also be modified on the basis of recognizing the importance of adequate and specific care of HE patients thus preparing nurses for addressing adequately any clinical problem and/or complication in HE patients. Clinical nursing guidelines would also allow better medical economics, i.e. pharmacoeconomics, since they would avoid the problems of nursing polypragmasia or economic dispersion in interventional procedures. In addition, such guidelines would define when and which signs, symptoms, i.e. complications, in HE patients call for an alarming situation and establish the list of priorities that would eventually lead to great cost savings. In severe liver diseases, where there is no possibility of curative treatment, it is necessary to provide palliative care. Nurses and doctors are best aware of the symptoms which cause significant quality of patient's life impairment. Their task should be that as a team ensure a general sense of well-being of the patient and a dignified passing if it occurs. It is of great importance to alleviate the final moments of life when it is needed [8], which implies comprehensive engagement of health staff with the provision of organized palliative care. Based on the conducted research in our center, we believe that there are three principal factors that would improve the work of the medical staff with HE patients: economical, educational, and interventional. Hospitals are not only institutions where medical help is provided, but also institutions of social and economic character.

Economical factor

The lack of equipment and working conditions which hinder adequate treatment of HE patients, but also impair further education of the staff with secondary education.

Educational factor

A statistically relevant number of questioned staff with secondary education knows how to recognize the manifestations of HE in patients with liver cirrhosis thus accurately establishing appropriate nursing diagnosis, leading to temporal optimization of therapy commencement. The continuous education and improvement of nurses is of significance when it comes to new medical apprehension and technologies being implemented into practice. Educational factor would ensure that quality of provided care is both effective and efficient. In our research, nurses expressed a good will for continuous education, which should be made possible for them.

Interventional factor

The results show that majority of respondents don't know the difference between the nursing treatment of HE patients and other patients, which results in a poor interventional skills and therapeutic procedures during the course of the treatment.

Conclusion

The specificity of health care in patients with hepatic encephalopathy is of multilevel nature clinically speaking and of great importance in the overall treatment process. Nurses should have the necessary work conditions and continuous education thus enabling effective and efficient care through nursing interventions. The above mentioned three principal factors (economic, educational, and interventional) lead to work improvement of the secondary staff education and better therapeutic modality of HE patient's treatment. These three factors are universal and can be applied as parameters of quality in every health care institution, i.e. at every intensive care unit regardless of the specific clinical pathology. Therefore, this paper has a universal meaning that should help the secondary staff education no matter in which medical institution or ward they are currently employed. The mentioned factors are in a direct correlation with each other and they can be only observed as a whole, where the failure to meet one of the factors is sufficient to make the algorithm of HE patient healthcare unsuccessful. It can be concluded that, apart from the substantial level of staff education, further education process has to improve the other two factors of quality of work, which are: the interventional - therapeutic skills of nursing staff and the upgrade of equipment and improvement of general working conditions.

References

1. Salgado M, Cortes Y (2013) Hepatic encephalopathy: diagnosis and treatment. Compend Contin Educ Vet. 35: E1-E10.

2. Ferenci P (2003) Hepatic encephalopathy. In: Bockus Gastroenterology, Haubrich WS, Schaffner F, Berk JE (eds.,), WB Saunders, Philadelphia, Pa.

3. Kappus MR, Bajaj JS (2012) Covert hepatic encephalopathy: not as minimal as you might think. Clin Gastroenterol Hepatol 10: 1208-1219.

4. Findlay JY, Fix OK, Paugam-Burtz C, Liu L, Sood P, et al. (2011) Critical care of the end-stage liver disease patient awaiting liver transplantation. Liver Transpl 17: 496-510.

5. Singh GK, Hoyert D (2000) Social epidemiology of chronic liver disease end cirrhosis mortality in the United States, 1935-1997: trends end differentials by ethnicity, socioeconomic status end alcohol consumption, Hum Biol. 72: 801-20.

6. Dusheiko G. Hoofnagle JH (1991) Viral hepatitis In: Oxford textbook of clinical hepatology, N. Maclntyre, JP Benhamou, J Bircher, M. Rizzetto, J. Rodes (ed.,) Oxford University Press. 1: 371-92.

7. Kalaitzakis E, Josefsson A, Björnsson E (2008) Type and etiology of liver cirrhosis are not related to the presence of hepatic encephalopathy or health-related quality of life: a cross-sectional study. BMC Gastroenterol 8: 46.

8. Perumalswami PV, Schiano TD (2011) The management of hospitalized patients with cirrhosis: the Mount Sinai experience and a guide for hospitalists. Dig Dis Sci 56: 1266-1281.

9. Mohammad RA, Regal RE, Alaniz C (2012) Combination therapy for the treatment and prevention of hepatic encephalopathy. Ann Pharmacother 46: 1559-1563.

10. Bajaj JS1 (2010) Review article: the modern management of hepatic encephalopathy. Aliment Pharmacol Ther 31: 537-547.

11. Al-Khafaji A, Huang DT (2011) Critical care management of patients with end-stage liver disease. Crit Care Med 39: 1157-1166.

12. Blei AT1, Córdoba J; Practice Parameters Committee of the American College of Gastroenterology (2001) Hepatic Encephalopathy. Am J Gastroenterol 96: 1968-1976.

13. WHO: (2002) World Health Report, Geneva, World Health Organisation.

14. Federal Statistical Office: (2002) Demographic statistics 2000, the Federal Bureau of Statistics. Belgrade. 8-48.

15. Chadalavada R, Sappati Biyyani RS, Maxwell J, Mullen K (2010) Nutrition in hepatic encephalopathy. Nutr Clin Pract 25: 257-264.

16. Jia JD (2012) Lactulose in the treatment of hepatic encephalopathy: new evidence for an old modality. J Gastroenterol Hepatol 27: 1262-1263.

17. Prakash R, Mullen KD (2010) Mechanisms, diagnosis and management of hepatic encephalopathy. Nat Rev Gastroenterol Hepatol 7: 515-525.

18. Hung TH, Lay CJ, Chang CM, Tsai JJ, Tsai CC, et al. (2013) The effect of infections on the mortality of cirrhotic patients with hepatic encephalopathy. Epidemiol Infect 141: 2671-2678.

19. Bruner end Suddarths (2009) Textbook of medical Surgical Nursing. Smeltzer C.S.Bare B.G.Hinkle JL. Cheever KH (ed.,).

20. Martinesen TE (2004) Procedure, Guidance for nurses. Association of Nurses of Serbia. Beograd. 331-333.

21. Almeida JR, Araújo RC1, Castilho GV1, Stahelin L1, Pandolfi Ldos R1, et al. (2015) Usefulness of a new prognostic index for alcoholic hepatitis. Arq Gastroenterol 52: 22-26.

22. Sargent S (2006) Management of patients with advanced liver cirrhosis. Nurs Stand 21: 48-56.

23. Ginès P, Cárdenas A, Arroyo V, Rodés J (2004) Management of cirrhosis and ascites. N Engl J Med 350: 1646-1654.

24. Garcovich M, Zocco MA, Roccarina D, Ponziani FR, Gasbarrini A (2012) Prevention and treatment of hepatic encephalopathy: focusing on gut microbiota. World J Gastroenterol 18: 6693-6700.

25. McCormick PA, O'Keefe C (2001) Improving prognosis following a first variceal haemorrhage over four decades. Gut 49: 682-685.

26. Rankovic I. Stojkovic MLj, Mijac D, Culafic D, Vlaisavljevic Z, Jovicic I.et al. (2012) New therapeutic aspects of acute hepatic insufficiency: early correction of hyponatremia and its consequences.Medicinskicasopis sup. 46: 25-26

27. Wijman CA, Smirnakis SM, Vespa P, Szigeti K, Ziai WC, et al. (2012) Research and technology in neurocritical care. Neurocrit Care 16: 42-54.

28. Olson JC, Wendon JA, Kramer DJ, Arroyo V, Jalan R, et al. (2011) Intensive care of the patient with cirrhosis. Hepatology 54: 1864-1872.

29. Li – Hung Tsai (2008) Nursing Care for Patients with Hepatic Encephalopathy. TzuChi Nursing Journal. 7: 73-79.

24

Professional Nurses' Knowledge level on Type II Diabetes Mellitus at Selected teaching and Training Hospitals in the Central Region of Ghana

Anita Afua Davies[1*] and Christiana Buxton[2]

[1]*Lecturer, School of Nursing, University of Cape coast, Cape Coast, Ghana*

[2]*Lecturer, Department of Mathematics and Science Education, University of Cape Coast, Ghana*

*****Corresponding author:** Anita Afua Davies, Lecturer, MSc Nursing, RN, School of Nursing, University of Cape coast, Cape Coast, Ghana, E-mail: adavies@ucc.edu.gh

Abstract

Background: Diabetes Mellitus is a global public health concern for many nations in the 21st Century with approximately 246 million people worldwide living with diabetes. A large number of research studies have it that nurses' knowledge on diabetes mellitus is poor and that there is the need to increase their knowledge level for effective management of patients with diabetes mellitus. In some cases, nurses' knowledge was adequate but they lacked knowledge in certain aspects of diabetes mellitus care especially, diabetic complications and insulin advancements. Also, there was a general notion in Sub-Saharan Africa that health care workers were insufficiently trained in chronic disease management.

Methods: With this in mind, there was the need to find out the knowledge level of nurses in the Central Region of Ghana, particularly the Central Regional Hospital, the District Hospital and the University Hospital. To arrive at that a modified version of The Michigan Diabetes Research and Training Centre's Brief Diabetic Knowledge Test was administered.

Results: Fourty- four 44 (32.4%) of the respondents' knowledge was good. However, knowledge level in the area of diabetic complications was generally poor among majority (68.4%) of the respondents.

Conclusions: It is recommended that nurses continue to upgrade their knowledge in the area of diabetes mellitus, particularly in the area of diabetes complications and insulin advancements.

Keywords: Nurses; Knowledge; Michigan diabetes knowledge test; Type II diabetes mellitus; Professionals; Selected; Teaching and training hospitals

Introduction

Diabetes Mellitus is a global public health concern for many nations in the 21st Century and approximately 246 million people worldwide have diabetes. Almost 6% the world's adult population have it. About 80% of these clients live in the developing countries, of which 40% are in the 40-59 year group [1]. It is one of the most common chronic diseases in the Western world since 2007 [2]. According to [3] the number of people with diabetes has reached 366 million contributing to approximately 4.6 million of deaths. King et al (1998) cited in [4] predicted that by the year 2025, the number of patients with diabetes mellitus would increase to 300 million [2].

It is becoming an increasing worldwide health problem [5]. The 23 million people represent 8% of the population. Of this 11.5 million are women and 12 million are men, representing 10.2% and 11.2% of the population respectively. It is the seventh leading cause of death and is likely to be underreported as a cause of death [6]. China has the second largest number of people suffering from diabetes in the world. According to WHO, rapid changes in lifestyle and socio-economic developments in Asia will cause major increases in the prevalence of diabetes mellitus in mainland China and India.In 2003, the number of people with diabetes mellitus exceeded 30 million [7].

Apart from the limited number of professional health staff in most developing countries, it has been indicated that health workers are insufficiently trained in chronic disease management [8,9]. It has also been reported that the effort of healthcare professionals has traditionally been spent on developing methods for ensuring compliance with prescribed therapeutic regimens rather than understanding the complexity and reality of managing diabetes on a daily basis [10]. As such it has been suggested that, nurses need to enhance their practical knowledge further by attending courses [4].

The Eastern and the Middle East are the regions with the highest diabetes prevalence rates. In 2007, India had the world's largest diabetes population, followed by China, the USA, Russia, Germany, Japan, Pakistan, Brazil, Mexico and Egypt [1]. The highest prediabetes prevalence is in the European region, with 9% of the adult population being at significant risk of developing type II diabetes mellitus. This escalating diabetes prevalence is underpinned by factors such as an aging population, unhealthy diet, overweight, and obesity, as well as lack of physical activity [1].

Diabetes prevalence is increasing globally and Sub-Saharan Africa is no exception which, according to [9] has the highest growth rates and is among the highest worldwide. Health workers are insufficiently trained in chronic disease management resulting in severe complications and a reduced life expectancy. The health system does not reach a considerable portion of the population, has a focus on emergencies and infectious diseases, and is frequently limited in staff and infrastructure [9]. With diverse challenges, health authorities in Sub-Saharan Africa and international donors need robust data on epidemiology and impact of diabetes [11]. Studies on Diabetes Mellitus in Sub-Saharan Africa are remarkably scarce. Understanding manifestations and associated factors however is essential to guide diagnosis, management and prevention of diabetes mellitus type II [9].

In 2010, 12.1 million people were estimated to be living with diabetes in Africa and this is projected to increase to 23.9 million by 2030. In Sub-Saharan Africa, this trend is emerging in a region grappling with high rates of communicable diseases including the highest global prevalence of HIV, Tuberculosis and Malaria. Impaired glucose tolerance and impaired fasting glucose are predictors of the incidence of type II diabetes mellitus. Prevalence of these suggests that the type II diabetes mellitus is likely to increase further in several countries in the region, including Cameroun, Ghana and Guinea [11]. Non communicable diseases are taking an equally severe, if not more toll on the health of Nigerians than communicable diseases. The mortality and morbidity of acute metabolic complications of diabetes mellitus, particularly diabetic ketoacidosis and hyperosmolar hyperglycemic syndrome are unacceptably high in Nigeria [12].

At an urban site in Ghana, with a sample size of 4735 and a participation rate of 75% the prevalence rate of type II diabetes mellitus was 6.4% with 69.9% undiagnosed. The prevalence of increased glucose tolerance was 10.7% and the prevalence of increased fasting glucose was 6% [11]. In 2003 the prevalence of type II diabetes mellitus rose to 17.9% [11]. There has been scattered report of successful attempts to improve diabetes care delivery and outcome. A team based restructuring of care in Ghana, including in particular nurse-led patient education, resulted in reduced diabetes-related admission rates even that it was funded by a foreign Non-governmental organization, Tropical Health and Education Trust [13].

Ghana Health Service Report [14,15] suggest that health promotion is being seriously embarked on and these are seen to be indicators of the prevention of non-communicable diseases such as diabetes mellitus. Ghana is said to have reached an epidemic where diabetes mellitus is concerned [16] and with researches indicating that knowledge of diabetes mellitus is inadequate among health care workers, it will be necessary to evaluate the knowledge level of Ghanaian nurses on diabetes mellitus.

Ghana's health system is ill-equipped to tackle the country's double burden of infectious and chronic diseases [17]. Statistics, gathered at a regional hospital in Ghana, shows a steady rise in the number of patients who visit the diabetic clinic for review each year. In 2011 the number of patients who visited the clinic for review was 7134. In 2012 the number rose to 8630. As at May, 2013 about 4444 clients had already visited the clinic for review [18,19].The question is how prepared are the professional nurses to handle these patients?

Literature Review

Diabetes Mellitus locally termed "esikyere yeriba", an Akan word in Ghana which literally means "sugar disease", is a disease defined as a chronic illness [7] in which the Islets of Langerhans of the endocrine pancreas, fail to secrete insulin, a hormone necessary to convert excess glucose into glycogen. This is stored in the liver and when the body needs it, it is converted to glucose for the body's need [2,5]. There are

four types of diabetes mellitus which are type I diabetes, type II diabetes, gestational diabetes and diabetes associated with other conditions or Syndrome [4,5].

Diabetes is a chronic disease requiring lifelong medical and nursing intervention and lifestyleadjustment [20]. The importance of regular follow-up of patients with the health care provider is of great significance in averting any long term complications [21]. With the alarming soaring statistics of diabetes mellitus, the role of nurses in helping patients to control associated morbidity and mortality is becoming increasingly important. Nurses, on the front line, can screen patients for early diabetes identification, recognize and initiate corrective measures for inadequate treatment regimens, help patients set and achieve therapeutic goals, and assess diabetes-related complications as they arise.

Diabetic foot disease and its related morbidity and mortality, although preventable has become a serious global burden. It has been reported that the lifetime risk of a patient with diabetes mellitus developing a foot ulcer could be as high as 25% and that every 30 seconds a lower limb is lost as a consequence of diabetes mellitus [22].

Diabetes is largely preventable especially type II diabetes and this is where health education and public awareness becomes critical. Health Care Workers especially nurses constitute important stake holders for the effective delivery of diabetic care and diabetic education [23].Studies have shown that ward nurses are the patient's most frequent contact when it comes to the management of diabetes mellitus [13]. Diabetes self-management is a challenge for both clients and health-care professionals. Healthcare professionals need to understand and address modifiable behaviour-specific variables [1].

Diabetes mellitus in the African continent is hugely affected by epidemiological factors [23] and issues of health care economics [13] and accurate epidemiological studies are often logistically and financially difficult. There continues to be an increasing number of people moving into urban areas from rural environments and this migration is inevitably associated with a shift in lifestyle from a relatively healthy traditional pattern to the urban scenario of increased food quantity, reduced quality, low levels of exercise, smoking and increased alcohol availability [13].

Studies have been carried out to determine the knowledge of nurses in diverse settings among many specialties of nursing. Knowledge of diabetes among student nurses [24] and health personnel is poor. This demands the initiation of educational programmes [3,23,25,26].

Ahmed et al. [3], suggest more hours of training in diabetes especially in the area of insulin and its new advancement. The content of education should be dynamic and needs to reflect current evidence and practice guidelines and expert consensus supports the need for specialized diabetic nurses and educational training beyond academic preparation for the primary instructors on the diabetes team. The one educating has to be evaluated in terms of the person's ability and qualities which should be clinical, pedagogical and personal more than the actual content and quality of the intervention.

Incidence of diabetes is on the increase [26]. It is a growing public health problem in the world [26]. Diabetes is largely preventable [26]. It is important to step up the knowledge levels of health personnel especially nurses since they are the first point of call when it comes to diabetes management, so that effective education as well as care of the diabetic is well taken care of. Knowledge level of health workers on diabetes especially nurses is not adequate to address the health needs of the population [23,27].

Nurses play an important role in diabetes education as they constitute the largest group of health care professionals who have a lengthy contact with patients. Nurses combine science and art to provide health services and seek to eliminate physical, emotional, mental, social-cultural and spiritual patient needs. Since patient care is the first duty of nurses, they play an important role in the care of diabetes mellitus. In developed countries diabetes nursing is divided into several categories, including nurse practitioner, clinical nurse specialist, diabetes nurse, generalist nurse and each of them has clear duties. For example, nurse practitioner focuses on health promotion and disease prevention activities including patient education and consulting [28,29]. It is obvious that with the increasing prevalence of diabetes and its complications, there is undeniable need to train nurse specialist with the requisite skills and knowledge in this field.

The need for nurses to play an active role in diabetes education has been discussed though evidence indicates that this role is not undertaken appropriately [23,24]. One way to reduce the morbidity and mortality from diabetes mellitus is to educate people with diabetes in self-care practices [26]. Lack of knowledge among health care providers has been found to be one of the major obstacles in the management of hyperglycemia in diabetic conditions. Ahmed, Jabber, Zuberi, Islam, Shamim [3], recognized a serious problem with regard to the inadequate knowledge of registered nurses regarding the management of diabetes mellitus.

Other studies have been carried out to determine the knowledge of nurses in diverse settings among many specialties of nursing. In some cases, medical nurses' knowledge was compared with that of surgical nurses. Though statistical significant in their knowledge levels, that of surgical nurses was lower. In some cases, the knowledge was adequate but they lacked knowledge in certain aspects of care of the patient [23]. Yet another study on nurses' understanding of diabetes is not of a desirable level to provide adequate care [3,23].

The cutoff point acceptable for glycosulated haemoglobin is < 7.0%. In their study, the average percentage for glycosulated haemoglobin was 7.54 ± 1.03. Exercise, medication, balancing diets is essential in diabetes mellitus. Glycemic control affects women's visual and memory learning [30]. Also health education and public awareness by health care workers is a key factor in the prevention of this chronic disease [26]. As the incidence, prevalence and diagnosis of diabetes mellitus increases, more people will require care from health professionals [26].

A study by [4] on nurses' perceived and actual level of diabetes mellitus revealedthat overall perceived knowledge was statistically significant and correlated with actual knowledge with a Pearson's co-officient of correlation being 0.32, (p < 0.005). Lack of nurses' knowledge led to patients receiving inadequate health care instruction [4]. The higher the educational level of the nurse the better knowledge level of the nurse on diabetes mellitus [25]. Diabetes self-management education is a cornerstone of diabetes care. However, many diabetic patients in the United Arab Emirates (UAE) lack sufficient knowledge about their disease due to illiteracy[31].

Little information on the knowledge of nurses and indeed other health care professionals who care for patients with diabetes in Ghana is known. This study was to evaluate the knowledge level of nurses in the Cape Coast Metropolis.

Methodology

The study was a quantitative study, cross-sectional and descriptive in nature.The population and sample of professional nurses in a Teaching Hospital and two training centres for health personnel was 220. One hundred and thirty-six professional nurses consented to answer the questionnaire giving a response rate of 61.8%.

The study instrument was a modified version of the Michigan Diabetes Research and Training Centre's Brief Diabetic Knowledge Test. It consists of 23 questions with options. Four questions on diet, five questions on tests, seven questions on diabetic complications and seven questions on diabetes medication. The questionnaire was examined by nurse managers of the three health facilities and also by the nurse in charge of the diabetic clinic in the regional hospital, examiner of the professional nurses' examination of Ghana.

Data analysis

Data was analyzed using the Statistical Package for the Social Sciences (SPSS) program, (version 20). Further analyses that were conducted included the cross tabulation and one way Analysis of Variance (ANOVA). A statistical significant level (p-value) of 0.05 was used in the study.

Results

The results centred on background information percentages of respondents' correct answers to the questions and knowledge level of the respondents in terms of adequacy. The demographics included length of time of training in the area of diabetes (Table 1).

Variable/Statement	n	Percenta ge (%)
Gender		
Female	95	69.9
Male	41	30.1
Age Groups (years)		
20 – 30	90	66.2
31 – 40	25	18.4
41 – 50	12	8.8
51 – 60	9	6.6
Highest level in Nursing Training		
SRN	24	17.6
Diploma (RN)	69	50.7
Degree	31	22.8
Variable/Statement n Percentage (%)		
Post graduate	9	6.6
Missing value	3	2.2
Time spent on Diabetes Mellitus in Nursing School		
< 1 month	87	64

1 month	23	16.9
1 Semester	8	5.9
2 Semesters	14	10.3
3 Semesters	3	2.2
Missing value	1	0.7
Work Experience as Nurse (years)		
1 – 5	91	66.9
6 – 10	3	2.2
11 – 15	8	5.9
16 – 20	4	2.9
>20	10	7.4
Current Job Position/Grade		
Staff Nurse	60	44.1
Senior Staff Nurse	36	26.5
Nursing Officer	23	16.9
Senior Nursing Officer	9	6.6
Principal Nursing Officer	7	5.1
Deputy Director of Nursing Services	1	0.7

Table 1: Background information about Nurses.

Table 1 shows 95 (69.9%) of female and 41 (30.1%) of male participated in the study. More females participated in the study than males. This clearly shows the lack of male interest in the nursing profession. Also among 136 nurses selected for the study, 90 (66.2%) nurses were aged 20-30 years whiles 25 (18.4%) nurses were aged 31-40 years. Twelve (8.8%) nurses were aged 41-50 years. Only 9 (6.6%) nurses were aged 51-60 years. From the data above it could be seen that all nurses were adults and within the working population of Ghana.

On the issue of highest level in nursing training, majority 69 (50.7%) nurses had attained diploma (RN). Also, 24 (17.6%) nurses indicated that they had attained SRN certificate in nursing. The highest level qualification indicated by nurses was Post graduate. This was indicated by 9 (6.6%). Also 31 (22.8%) nurses indicated degree in nursing as their highest level in nursing training. All nurses selected for the study had attained the standard level of qualification to qualify as a nurse in Ghana.

Furthermore, when nurses were asked to indicate time spent on diabetes mellitus during their nursing training, 110 (80.9%) nurses indicated that they did spend less than or equal to a month on teaching and learning of diabetes mellitus. However, 14 (10.3%) nurses indicated that they did spend two semesters in studying diabetes mellitus in nursing school. In all, table two revealed that nurses have had some lessons on diabetes mellitus during their nursing school.

When nurses were asked on their working experience, majority 91 (66.9%) nurses indicated that they had worked as a nurse for about 1-5 years. It was also revealed that 10 (7.4%) nurses had also worked for more than 20 years. Also, 8 (5.9%) nurses indicated that they had

worked as a nurse for 11-15 years whiles 4 (2.9%) nurses indicated to have worked for 16-20 years. Only, 3 (2.2%) nurses indicated to have worked for 6-10 years. Nurses sampled for the study all have had some level of experience to give professional view on the issue.

Majority, 60 (44.1%) nurses indicated that they were staff nurses in their various departments. Also, 36 (26.5%) nurses indicated that they had attained senior staff grade whiles 23 (16.9%) nurses indicated to be nursing officers in their various departments. Furthermore there were 9 (6.6%) nurses who were senior nursing officers and 7 (5.1%) indicating to be principal nursing officers. Only, 1 (0.7%) nurse indicated to be deputy director of nursing services as patriated in the study. Table 2 showing the number and percentages of correct responses to the questions.

Item	n (%)
The diabetes diet is	72(52.9)
Which of the following is highest in carbohydrate?	119 (87.5)
Which of the following is highest in fat?	103 (75.7)
Which of the following is free food?	56 (41.2)
Hemoglobin A1 test measures average glucose level in	35 (25.7)
Which is the best method for testing blood glucose?	104 (76.5)
Effect of unsweetened fruit juice on blood glucose	41 (30.1)
Which should not be used to treat low glucose?	23 (16.9)
Effect of exercise on blood glucose for a person good control	118 (86.8)
Infection is likely to cause?	106(77.9)
The best way to take care of your feet is to	99(72.8)
Eating food lower in fat decreases your risk for	132 (97.1)
Numbness and tingling may be symptoms of	122 (89.7)
Which is usually not associated with Diabetes?	125(91.9)
Signs of ketoacidosis include	43 (31.6)
Changes to make when you have flu?	72 (52.9)
If you have taken NPH or Lente, you may have an insulin reaction in?	58 (42.6)
What do you do if you missed your insulin before breakfast but remember just before lunch?	91 (66.9)
If you are beginning to have an insulin reaction, you should?	65 (47.8)
Low blood glucose may be caused by	105(77.2)
Morning insulin without taking breakfast will	107 (78.7)
High blood glucose may be caused by	110(80.9)

Insulin reaction is most likely to be caused by	50(36.8)

Table 2: Frequency (%) distribution of answers to questionnaire items (N=136).

The mean mark for correctly answered questions was 14.38 (62.5%) for all the study participants. As shown in Table two, 14 out of the 23 questions were answered correctly by at least half of the total respondents. Some of these questions assessed respondents' knowledge on the causes of insulin reaction, low and high blood glucose, effects of unsweetened fruit juice on blood glucose and exercise on blood glucose for a person good control, what should not be used to treat low glucose among others (Table 2). The question that had the least number of respondents answering correctly 43 (31.6%) assessed their knowledge on signs of Ketoacidosis. Majority of the respondents 132 (97.1%) answered correctly the question that assessed their knowledge on the essence of eating food low in fat. Two questions were answered correctly by 52.9% of the respondents. These two questions assessed respondents' knowledge on what a diabetic diet is and changes to make when you have flu.

There is no significant difference between the age groups (Sig. vale = 0.24 > p value = 0.05), current Job position/grade (Sig. value = 0.44 > p value = 0.05) and Highest training in Nursing (Sig. value = 0.77 > p value = 0.05). Hence no significant difference exist between the groups even though there is a difference in the mean scores.

Discussion

The mean for correctly answered question was 14.38 (62.5%) for all the study participants as shown in table i. The question that had the least number of respondents answering correctly 33 (31.6%) assessed their knowledge on signs of Ketoacidosis. This is in line with [8] and Danquah, et al. [9],that health care workers in Sub-Saharan Africa lack knowledge in complicated conditions and that understanding manifestations and associated factors however, is essential to guide diagnosis, management and prevention of Diabetes Mellitus.Majority of the respondents 132 (97.1%) answered correctly the question that assessed their knowledge on the essence of eating food low in fat.

It was observed that all respondents in the following groups: age group 41 to 50 years, Senior Nursing Officers, one month and three semesters training on Diabetes Mellitus at school had at least adequate knowledge on diabetes mellitus. Only respondents who had one month training on diabetes mellitus in school had at least good knowledge in diabetes mellitus. The one and only Deputy Director of Nursing Services had inadequate knowledge on diabetes mellitus. Generally the highest mean scores were obtained in the following groups: females, age group of 20 to 30 years, diploma (RN) holders in nursing, respondents who had training on Diabetes Mellitus for one semester at school, respondents who were Staff Nurses and respondents who had not received any formal training on Diabetes Mellitus apart from Nursing School Training.

Although the level of adequacy of knowledge on Diabetes Mellitus was not in line with researches by [3,4,23,25-27,31] in which nurses had poor knowledge of diabetes mellitus, but supports that of Odili Eke [23] the nurses had adequate knowledge on Diabetes Mellitus but lack knowledge in certain aspects of care.

Further analysis was performed to investigate whether a significant difference existed between the groups with respect to their knowledge level in diabetes mellitus using one way Analysis of Variance (ANOVA). Some of the groups like gender, time spent on diabetes mellitus training in school and had any diabetes mellitus training apart from training school could not meet all the necessary assumptions to enable the use of one way Analysis of variance (ANOVA). There is no significant difference between the age groups (Sig. vale = 0.24 > p value = 0.05), current Job position/grade (Sig. value = 0.44 > p value = 0.05) and Highest training in Nursing (Sig. value = 0.77 > p value = 0.05). Hence no significant difference exist between the groups even though there is a difference in mean scores. This is probably due to the fact that there were a lot of groups which is how Ghana finds itself and also that the group sizes was not large enough to show any significant difference.

Conclusion

This study sought to evaluate nurses' knowledge on Diabetes Mellitus in the Cape Coast Metropolis, particularly, the three health facilities where health personnel have practical training: the Central regional Hospital, the District Hospital and the University Hospital. Nurses in these hospitals who took part in the study were found to have the greater number 66 (48.5%), having adequate knowledge level on diabetes mellitus. They however lacked knowledge in certain aspects of care. This was in the area of diabetic complications.

Recommendations

The nurses' knowledge were found to have a greater percentage being adequate. This is probably so because the questionnaires were left with the nurses and collected at the convenience of the researchers. They probably did not do independent work. Also unknown to the researchers, a more modern instrument existed which could have been used. Future research should use onethat focuses on diabetic complications and insulin advancements.

References

1. Ho AY, Berggren I, Dahlborg-Lyckhage E (2010) Diabetes empowerment related to Pender's Health Promotion Model: a meta-synthesis. Nurs Health Sci 12: 259-267.

2. Kosti M and Kanakari M (2012) Education and Diabetes Review. Health Science Journal (4).

3. Ahmed A, Jabbar A, Zuberi L, Islam M, Shamim K (2012) Diabetes related knowledge among residents and nurses: a multicenter study in Karachi, Pakistan. BMC Endocr Disord 12: 18.

4. Chan MF, Zang YL (2007) Nurses' perceived and actual level of diabetes mellitus knowledge: results of a cluster analysis. J Clin Nurs 16: 234-242.

5. Bare BG, Cheever KH, Hinkle JL and Smelter SC (2010) Brunner & Suddarth's textbook of Medical – Surgical Nursing (12 ed). Philadelphia: Lippincott Williams & Wilkins.

6. Eaton-Spiva L, Day A (2011) Effectiveness of a computerized educational module on nurses' knowledge and confidence level related to diabetes. J Nurses Staff Dev 27: 285-289.

7. Shi Q, Ostwald SK, Wang S (2010) Improving glycaemic control self-efficacy and glycaemic control behaviour in Chinese patients with type 2 diabetes mellitus: randomised controlled trial. J Clin Nurs 19: 398-404.

8. Mbanya JC, Kengne AP, Assah F (2006) Diabetes care in Africa. Lancet 368: 1628-1629.

9. Danquah I, Bedu-Addo G, Terpe KJ, Micah F, Amoako YA, et al. (2012) Diabetes mellitus type 2 in urban Ghana: characteristics and associated factors. BMC Public Health 12: 210.

10. Ruston A, Smith A, Fernando B (2013) Diabetes in the workplace - diabetic's perceptions and experiences of managing their disease at work: a qualitative study. BMC Public Health 13: 386.

11. Hall V, Thomsen RW, Henriksen O, Lohse N (2011) Diabetes in Sub Saharan Africa 1999-2011: epidemiology and public health implications. A systematic review. BMC Public Health 11: 564.

12. Balogun W, Adeleye J (2008) Strategies for prevention of hyperglycaemic emergencies in Nigeria. Ann Ib Postgrad Med 6: 27-30.

13. Gill GV, Mbanya JC, Ramaiya KL, Tesfaye S (2009) A sub-Saharan African perspective of diabetes. Diabetologia 52: 8-16.

14. Okertchiri JA (2011) Ghana has 4m Diabetics.

15. de Graft Aikins A, Anum A, Agyemang C, Addo J, Ogedegbe O (2012) Lay representations of chronic diseases in Ghana: implications for primary prevention. Ghana Med J 46: 59-68.

16. Annual Report: Central Regional Hospital, Ghana 2011

17. Annual Report: Central Regional Hospital, Ghana2012

18. Zolfaghari M, Mousavifar SA, Haghani H (2012) Mobile phone text messaging and Telephone follow-up in type 2 diabetic patients for 3 months: a comparative study. J Diabetes Metab Disord 11: 7.

19. Shrivastava SR, Shrivastava PS, Ramasamy J (2013) Role of self-care in management of diabetes mellitus. J Diabetes Metab Disord 12: 14.

20. Desalu OO, Salawu FK, Jimah AO, Adekoya OA, Busari OA, et al. (2011) Diabetic Foot Care: self Reported Knowledge and practice among Patients Attending Three Tertiary Hospitals in Nigeria. Ghana medical Journal 45: 60-65.

21. Odili VU and Eke I (2010) Knowledge of Diabetes Mellitus among Registered Nurses in

22. Benin City. International Journal of Health Research3 : 145-151.

23. Unadike BC (2010) Awareness and Knowledge about Diabetes Mellitus Amongst Nursing

24. Students in the Niger Delta of Nigeria. Middle East Journal of Nursing, 4.

25. el-Deirawi KM, Zuraikat N (2001) Registered nurses' actual and perceived knowledge of diabetes mellitus. J Nurses Staff Dev 17: 5-11.

26. UnadikeBC and Etukumana EA (2010) Nurses Understanding about Diabetes in a Nigerian Hospital. Pak J Med Sci, 26 : 217-222.

27. Naheed T, Akbar N and Akbar N (2003) Is there Need of Specialized Diabetic Nurses in Pakistan? Pak J Med Sci 19 :75-79.

28. Peimani M, Tabatabaei-Malazy O, Pajouhi M (2010). Nurses' Role in Diabetes Care; A review. Iranian Journal of Diabetes and Lipid Disorders, 9:1–9.

29. Aalaa M, Malazy OT, Sanjari M, Peimani M, Mohajeri-Tehrani M (2012) Nurses' role in diabetic foot prevention and care; a review. J Diabetes Metab Disord 11: 24.

30. Compeán-Ortiz LG, Gallegos EC, Gonzalez-Gonzalez JG, Gomez-Meza MV, Therrien B, et al. (2010) Cognitive performance associated with self-care activities in Mexican adults with type 2 diabetes. Diabetes Educ 36: 268-275.

31. Al-Maskari F, El-Sadig M, Al-Kaabi JM, Afandi B, Nagelkerke N, et al. (2013) Knowledge, attitude and practices of diabetic patients in the United Arab Emirates. PLoS One 8: e52857.

25

Spiritual Needs and Care of Patients from Nurses' Perspectives on ICU

Ya-Lie Ku*

Fooyin University, Kaohsiung, Taiwan

*Corresponding author:** Ya-Lie Ku, Assistant Professor, Fooyin University, Nursing, 151 Chin-Hsueh Rd., Ta-Liao District, Kaohsiung, 831, Taiwan, E-mail: ns126@fy.edu.tw

Abstract

Background: Current studies mainly emphasized the spiritual needs and care of cancer and hospice patients; few deal with the other critically ill patients.

Aim: This study aimed to describe the spiritual needs and care of ICU patients from nurses' perspectives.

Design: This is a qualitative study.

Method: The semi-structured guided interviewing on ICU nurses in a medical center of southern Taiwan was approved by the IRB at the research department of the hospital and data collection was carried out from January to June 2012. The investigator repeatedly read the transcribed text, and found statements relevant to the themes in the transcriptions to form significant statements as the basis of data analysis. To ensure the rigor of this study, the investigator adopted the approach of trustworthiness of qualitative research proposed by Lincoln and Guba.

Results: For the assessment of patients' spiritual needs, the patients were divided into two groups: conscious and unconscious groups. The spiritual needs of the former were assessed by the clinical observation and judgment, while the latter were assessed through family interpretation. In addition, there are six themes in general spiritual care: care skills, interaction promotion, religious belief, cultural care, wish fulfilment, alleviation of grief and terminal care. Spiritual care of the conscious and unconscious patients were also included.

Conclusion: Spiritual needs and care from ICU nurses' perspective were different from the patients; however, both of views were focused on the general spiritual care, while ICU nurses divided spiritual care into the conscious and unconscious patients.

Relevance to clinical practice: The authors suggested that a complete guideline of spiritual care for critically ill patients integrating with the cultural care and interdisciplinary cooperation could be developed on the basis of the results of this study in the future, which could provide more empirical data as the nursing reference.

Keywords: Spirituality; Patients; Intensive care nursing

Introduction

The Intensive Care Unit (ICU) is a medical-labor-intensive critical care department equipped with specialized instruments, where most of these patients undergo endo-tracheal intubation and, in addition, may be restrained physically or given sedatives or hypnotics; meanwhile, all these practices may impair patients' senses such as vision, hearing, or touch which caused difficulty in their verbal expression so that nurses were unable to understand their inner needs [1]. Although many critically ill patients cannot express their inner needs due to the diseases or treatment, it does not mean that they have no spiritual needs. However, such needs are either not recognized, or often are simply neglected. The health care team in the ICU traditionally emphasized on stabilizing patients' vital signs and relieving their physiological symptoms, but rarely paying attention on the patients' psychological and spiritual needs [1].

Meanwhile, [2] conducted a content analysis of 15 adult ICU from United States and Canada to identify the forms of documentation and results shown spiritual support as not well-prepared. Continuously, most of studies on spiritual care needs were focused on the general, cancer, and hospice patients and the studies on the spiritual needs of patients with critical illnesses were greatly scarce. Again, Rodriguez et al. [3] reported that only 16% of 31 ICU nurses would provide the end of life spiritual care commonly. Simiarly, Turan and Karamanog lu [4] survey 123 ICU nurses from four Turkey hospitals about their perceptions and practice levels of spiritual care and identified that inappropriate spiritual care practices were found.

Purpose of the Study

The study aimed to describe the spiritual needs and care of ICU patients from nurses' perspectives.

Literature Review

In terms of spiritual needs, Timmins and Kelly [5] overviewed the spiritual assessment for ICU/CCU nurses and suggested that nurses in such units better selected the assessment tools as fit into the definition of spirituality as well as the mission statement and philosophy of care based on the patients' point of view. Chao et al. [6] used hermeneutic study to explore the essence of spirituality among terminally ill patients by in-depth interviews with six terminal cancer patients in the hospice ward of a teaching hospital. The results comprised four patterns as communion with self, others, nature, and a higher being. Additionally, Papathanassoglou et al. [7] explored the experiences of 8 critical patients who have lived in the ICU by using phenomenology and identified three themes as transformation, transcendence, and rebirth as well as critical illness being conceptualized as a cocooning phase to transform self, promote spirituality, and personal growth. Continuously, Murray et al. [8] explored the spiritual needs of dying patients by in-depth qualitative interviews with 20 patients with lung cancer and 20 patients with terminal heart failure. Whether or not the patients held religious beliefs, they expressed the need for love, meaning, purpose and transcendence.

In terms of spiritual care, Hsu [9] divided the intervention strategies for satisfying the spiritual needs of terminal patients into two categories: general spiritual care and special spiritual care. The general spiritual care included palliative care, group psychotherapy, supportive treatment, depth psychotherapy, practice guided therapy, and treatment for demoralization. The special spiritual care included alternative therapy, such as therapeutic touch, acupuncture, biofeedback, relaxation techniques and aromatherapy, psychotherapy with deity, logo-therapy and dignity therapy. Furthermore, Lin et al. [10] proposed spiritual nursing interventions in the aspect of "communion with self", therapies such as life review or reminiscence, supported by logo-therapy, in particular when the patients felt that life had lost its meaning and value under the threat of death. In addition, the patients could be assisted to accomplish their wishes. In the aspect of "communion with others", nurses could play the role of a bridge to help the patients to maintain and reconstruct relationships with others. In the aspect of "communion with nature", nurses could teach the patients to achieve spiritual relaxation through aromatherapy, music therapy or imagery therapy, or to understand their inner feelings through painting or writing. When the patients felt frightened or anxious, playing the patient's favorite soft music could help to ease their perturbed emotions. In the aspect of "communion with a higher being", nurses could introduce religious beliefs to the patient as own needed, and arrange for priests or religious leaders to hold special religious rituals such as praying, chanting, worshiping, etc., with the aim of establishing communication between the patients and the higher being of their beliefs.

Currently, Lundberg and Kerdonfag [11] interviewed 30 Thai nurses from 6 different ICUs with the aim of exploring how they provided spiritual care to the patients in the qualitative study. The study found five themes related to the provision of spiritual care by nurses: giving mental support, facilitating religious rituals and cultural beliefs, communicating with patients and their families, assessing the spiritual needs of patients, and showing respect and facilitating family participation in spiritual care. Continuously, Zeilani and Seymour [12] used narrative approach to explore the 16 Muslim women's experiences of suffering in ICU and they interpreted suffering with physical, social, spiritual, and technological themes, including pain, unfamiliar environment, feeling uncertainty. However, religious beliefs and cultural norms as well as social supports were identified as the essential variables for them to adjust the suffering.

Method

This study used a qualitative approach to describe the nature, meaning and values of phenomena in specific life experiences [13]. Samples were ICU nurses in a medical center of southern Taiwan selecting by purposive sampling with the criteria as follows: (1) had worked in a medical ICU for at least two years, (2) were interested in spiritual care or had such care experiences and (3) had taken at least two hours of courses on spiritual care. The numbers of interview samples for this study were closed when the data approaching saturation during analysis. The proposal of this study was approved by the Institutional Review Board (No.100- 3745C) at the research department of the hospital before data collection. Data collection of this study was conducted for 6 months from January to June 2012. An interview guide was developed based on the study objective, literature validation, and personal clinical experiences of the principal investigator, and was revised once after the first pilot test. The place to conduct the interview was decided by the participants either at their homes or workplaces with one-to-one face in the natural surroundings without disturbance. Each interview took about 40 to 60 min. After each interview, all data were transcribed into an original, true and complete verbatim context, and conducted data analysis one case following the other until data saturation.

As for ethical consideration, the principal investigator followed the principles of interests, dignity and justice [14] for the benefit of participating ICU nurses. Conforming to the principle of interests, this study had assured no physical harm to any nurses, no criticism of their thoughts and conduct, and no overstimulation of their emotions. To express the appreciation for sharing their precious experiences, the principal investigator gave a small present when the nurses agreed to participate in this study. Conforming to the principle of dignity, the principal investigator did not threaten, bribe, or coerce the nurses to participate in this study with the superior authority in the hospital. The participants were fully informed about the objective of the study, the procedure, and were required to agree to audio record their interview with a written consent prior to the study. However, samples who wished to stop the recorded interview or terminate their participation could do so at any time. Conforming to the principle of justice, confidentiality and anonymity would be maintained, nurses' names would not appear in the documents, but replace them with the numbers, so that the individual identities would not be revealed or implied, and finally an integral presentation would be given in the study results.

The investigator was the main instrument of this study, which owned an RN license with working in an ICU at a medical center for 15 years, and had, took a two-credit course on qualitative research for 36 h during studying in the graduate school of nursing in an university. In this study, data analysis and collection were simultaneously conducted. First, the principal investigator cast aside previous views on ICU nurses, adopted an open attitude, and repeatedly read the transcribed text, tried to understand the context and the integral concept, and then found statements relevant to the research themes in interview transcriptions to form significant statements as the basis of data analysis. Moreover, the investigator sought to deepen the understanding of ICU nurses' experiences and employed descriptive analysis to extract meaning from significant statements, grouped common features of significant statements into themes, gave an exhaustive description of grouped themes and expounded on the essential structure of the phenomena. During the interviews, the statements of informants were reviewed once again by each informant to ensure that the contents reflected their empirical experiences.

To ensure the rigor of this study, the principal investigator adopted the approach of trustworthiness of qualitative research proposed by Lincoln and Guba [15] which involves establishing credibility, confirmability, dependability and transferability. First, to maintain the credibility of data, the principal investigator held neutral, open, and impartial attitudes to the feelings and thoughts of informants while interpreting their experiences. Second, for the confirmability, the principal investigator asked typical participants to read, review and discuss analyzed themes and transcriptions during the whole process of analysis to ensure that the results reflected the real experiences of participants. For dependability, the principal investigator cooperated with an expert, who had taught the spiritual nursing course and engaged in qualitative and quantitative research on spirituality for more than 10 years with publishing many relevant articles, reports and case studies about spiritual care in Taiwan and abroad, to review and ensure the consistency of data analysis. For transferability, the principal investigator used purposive sampling referred as much as possible to informants' rich clinical experiences of spiritual care in the data analysis of interviews, which could be transferred to the clinical practices of other ICU nurses.

Results

These 11 participants are all single, female, university graduates, with an average age of 35 years old, and mostly Taoists. Their average nursing experience and ICU experience were 15 and 12 years, respectively. Following are the axis and perspectives for the nurses' assessment of patients' spiritual needs and nurses' providing of patients' spiritual care for conscious and unconscious patients.

Nurses' assessment of patients' spiritual needs

The axis of assessment of patients' spiritual needs contained two perspectives: Conscious patients and unconscious patients.

Conscious patients

The perspective of conscious patients was clinical observation and judgment.

Clinical observation and jugement

In clinical situations, while nurses could directly ask conscious patients about their spiritual needs, the responses might come as verbal and non-verbal behaviors. For example:

"With conscious patients, we could understand their thoughts. Some patients may know they are going to leave the world. They seem to be able to foretell the end is near (crooking the index finger, which means to die). Generally, we would tell him/her not to dwell upon unnecessary issues. We would observe what they need and immediately provide help. If they could write, we will let them write. If not, they could let us know the needs by gestures. If the patient used to pray or listen to something at home, we would let him continue to do so." (Case 1)

Unconscious patients

The perspective of unconscious patients was family interpretation.

Family interpretation

As many ICU patients were unconscious, nurses should have greater sensitivity and pay more attention on the family. For example:

"The family decided all. When the patient needed some support, what he/she needed is to be accompanied by the family. Some families might think everything was unnecessary, like pictures were unnecessary, etc. No! No! Nothing is necessary! (In Taiwanese) Some families might decide everything for the patient because the intubation patients could not speak, express, and showed no reactions. The family was the big influencing the mind of the patient. Success or failure depended on the family. For the patients, the most important connection was from the family, not us. But when the family dismissed patients' feelings, their spirituality would be shut off with a closed door and simply ignored. (Case 8)

Nurses' providing of patients' spiritual care

The axis of spiritual care by nurses contains three perspectives: General spiritual care, spiritual care for conscious and unconscious patients.

General spiritual care

The perspective of general spiritual care includes six themes: care skills, interaction promotion, religious belief, cultural care, wish fulfilment, alleviation of grief and terminal care.

Care skills

In clinical spiritual care, nurses should patiently take time to understand patients' needs, establish good relationships with patients, and provide as the bridge of communication between the patients and their families. For example:

"We tell jokes to patients to divert their attention. It depends on patients; some like to be Sometimes we may chat or tell jokes while the nurse is treating the patient. In such a way, the patient may divert his/her attention and the time may appear to pass faster. The patient may feel different and better if we sometimes tell jokes or talk about our families. In that way, we treat the patient as a family member and he/she wouldn't feel like a patient." (Case 3)

Interaction promotion

When critically ill patients are admitted into the ICU, nurses can timely provide patients with companionship and concern of familiar persons, allow them to keep habitual, familiar or meaningful articles at bedside or somewhere they can see, ask the family to tape record words of encouragement, play the tapes of the patient, his/her family or some familiar people's voices or singing, and guide the family to interact and communicate with patients. For example:

"We guide the family to interact more with the patient. How to guide depends on the condition. When the family sees so many tubes in the patient, they may get scared, not knowing which part of the patient they can or cannot touch. Usually we would instruct the family to give the patient a massage and help exercise the muscles and joints of the patient's limbs. Above all, patients desire their families. They need their families. When they are nervous and scared, they require the company of a familiar person, a family member. Yes! They hope to be accompanied by their family. We guide the family to talk with the patient, to bring family photos or tapes for the patient and sometimes ask the family to record tapes with words of encouragement. The family does it, too. We let the family accompany the patient as much as possible, when it's necessary. It is very meaningful and helpful to a patient's spirit when many people come to see and care for him/her. When you are sick, you feel particularly vulnerable and you wish for more attention and care. In that way, you won't feel abandoned." (Case 3)

Religious belief

Nurses can provide spiritual care in the following ways: allowing patients to listen to Buddhist sutras, Amitabha, religious music or hymns via a player and to recite along, allowing patients to wear Buddhist prayer beads or Buddha figure pendants and placing Buddhist sutras, the Bible or crosses on their clothes, below the pillow, at the bedside or somewhere that the patient can see, which should be noted down on the shift checklist; placing god figures or pictures; providing worship halls, asking Protestant ministers or Catholic priests to lead the worship in the ward, pray or sing hymns with the patient; asking the religious workers to accompany and talk to the patient. For example:

"Patients may say they want to recite Amitabha with a Buddhist sutra player or to read something. We offer it accordingly and assist as much as we can, but only if their conditions permit. It would be better if the religion can give patients support. They may need articles such as Buddhist sutras, prayer beads, Buddha figures, etc. Some may wear Buddha figure pendants, pictures of Jesus, Bodhisattva or Mazu, or place them at their bedside. These are not expensive articles, such as Buddhist prayer beads that the patient used to pray with, or a god figure or a picture of Guanyin put on the patient or posted on the ward bed." (Case 1)

"For Protestants or Catholics, a crowd may come to the ward for worshipping or praying, not simply to visit. It is better for the patient and, I think, the effect is more obvious. The patient sees people praying for him/her. In particular, it makes more difference if the priest also comes for him/her. All people come to pray for him/her, making him/her feel like a god. After the worship, he/she would feel more hopeful about his/her condition. If you just put a god figure and tell the patient "God bless you", his/her feelings may not be as strong! I think, other people's praying would be more powerful. Only placing some charms on the patient's body cannot have such effects. Christians are quite united; they may come to the hospital particularly on Sunday to pray for the patient; even the priest comes quite often. For the patient, seeing the priest is like seeing the light! Wow! he/she becomes hopeful and uplifted. The patient feels honored." (Case 4)

Cultural care

Spiritual care is often influenced by personal beliefs and social culture, and nurses should have insights into different cultural backgrounds and customs of the patients for providing the sensitive cultural care. Clinically, we often find that the family may make the patient wear a necklace, amulet, or incense bag blessed by the temple or a diviner, take the patient's clothes to the temple for passing-over-fire ritual, feed the patient worshiped incense ash, place a round container like an incense burner with turtle eggs or stones inside, set Taoist Wang Ye flags by the bed headboard, make the patient wear divine clothes, Wang Ye's headband or a whole yellow top, i.e., yellow cloth for the dead, spray sacred water on the patient's body and all

around the ward or dab the patient's lips with the water, or place leaves by the pillow of the patient to drive off evil spirits. For examples:

"A necklace! They would wear a necklace sought from the temple! It is frequent that the family goes to seek divine advice. Once the patient is admitted to the ICU, the family would not only look for medical assistance, but also seek folk treatment or divine advice. The family may bring back many incense bags or clothes with red temple stamps, which are believed to remove bad luck. Taking the patient's clothes to the temple for passing-over-fire ritual is also for the same purpose, to remove all the bad luck and to ensure safety. The clothes are put on the patient, cover the patient, or put by the pillow, as the family particularly requests. We would help to put them by the pillow or on the patient. When the family comes, they would change the clothes themselves." (Case 1)

"They may bring some incense bags for ensuring the patient's safety. I have even seen the family put leaves on the patient or by the pillow, saying that it could drive off evil spirits. The family may also spray sacred water on the patient and all around the ward or dab the patient's lips with it." (Case 2)

"They may tell the patient, "The incense bag will bless your safety. Gods are taking care of you (In Taiwanese)." They would say some words to put the patient at ease and the patient might think, "You see! My family also heads to the temple to pray for me." Some families have sought sacred water or incense bags for the patient. We let the family put them on the patient. Some also have wanted to feed the patient incense ash given by gods for blessing their safety. We respect that and do not intervene. I tell them to do it themselves if they have such needs because I respect the patient. When the patient or the family hopes to place the incense bag by the head, on the body or near an organ of the patient, we give them all our respect." (Case 7)

"Some want to place a round container like an incense burner with turtle eggs, stones, charms or divine clothes inside. They may ask if it is allowed to set Taoist Wang Ye flags by the bed headboard, some in small size and some large ones. The divine clothes will cover the patient. It could be a short Wang Ye headband or a yellow top. Moreover, terminal patients may want to be covered with a large piece of yellow cloth for the dead." (Case 10)

Wish fulfillment

Nurses can help the patient to fulfil wishes. For example:

"Some patients knew that they would soon leave the world. They might foretell the end of life. You can ask the patient if he/she wants to see any person, to see a son or daughter who lives at a distant place or abroad and then help him/her to ask his/her family to come back. Or, you can ask if he/she has any wish or wants to do something special and then help him/her to fulfill it. Recently, we took care of a very young patient. He was unconscious when he was admitted into the ICU. His consciousness returned after the treatment, but he became very agitated. It was through his handwriting that we learned he wanted to see his wife, son and daughter." (Case 1)

Alleviation of Grief and Terminal Care

Nurses should help the family to alleviate their grief and pay attention to the mental status of the family. The care should cater not only to the patient, but also to the family. With empathy, nurses can give the family a buffer period. For example:

"No one suggested doing this, but I felt I should do it. All of a sudden, her condition deteriorated and her cancer spread all over her body. I discussed it with her husband. They wanted to follow the patient's wish; it would be better not to insert her trachea tube. At that time, her child was about four, the age of innocence. So we thought to encourage the child not to fear and ask the child to accompany the mother until she took her journey to heaven. Then the patient passed away. But at least, I think, the patient passed away very peacefully and serenely. We helped her to clean up and comb her hair while the child stayed close by. At least, I think, no shadow of fear would be left in the child's mind. This was an impressive case. The family was grateful that we let them hold her hands and accompany her when she passed away, instead of letting her leave the world alone." (Case 4)

Perspective of spiritual care for conscious patients

Nurses' spiritual care for conscious patients should contain the following interventions: listening, comforting, encouraging and accompanying the patient, communicating with the patient face-to-face, talking with the patient about his/her needs, trying to understand what he/she thinks, fulfilling the wishes of the patient, letting the patient listen to religious scriptures, offering newspapers or magazines to the patient, helping the patient to find the physician or nurses that he/she has trusted, letting the patient read or watch TV, letting the family accompany the patient when the patient has the need and satisfying the patient's needs, assisting with the communication between the family and the patient,. For example:

"He might want to look for the doctor whom he/she trusted before, or he/she wants to find some nurse. Or he/she said he/she wanted to listen to Buddhist sutras, or read the Bible. He/she wanted to read a book or watch TV. Normally, those with clear consciousness feel bored in the ICU and their only desire is to leave the hospital soon and go home. We would try to comfort him/her, telling him/her to wait patiently for the meeting hours since the family is not allowed to enter the ICU now. If it's truly necessary, we can still timely help him/her to arrange for the family to visit and keep him/her company, which will make the patient feel safe and at ease. Then we tell the patient that his/her family is waiting in the lounge and won't leave, so they can be found anytime. Or, we tell him/her that it is hard for his/her family to take turns caring for him/her and that it would be better to let the family go home for a rest and come back to visit him/her later. Many patients can accept it!" (Case 7)

Perspective of spiritual care for unconscious patients

As for nurses' spiritual care for unconscious patients, since nurses cannot understand the thoughts of the patient, nursing care puts greater emphasis on the family: Encouraging the family to have physical contact with the patient or to speak with the patient, letting the patient hear the voice of the family, letting the family accompany the patient or prolonging visiting hours if necessary, letting the patient listen to the tapes with the recorded voice of the family, being accompanied by a radio, guiding the family to let the patient go at the end of his/her life. This is the moment when the family usually needs more care and communication than does the patient; nurses should have greater sensitivity and ask for the intervention of a palliative care coordinator or social worker if necessary. For example:

"For patients without clear consciousness, more attention should be paid to the family. Some care very much for the patient and cannot let the patient go at the end of life. We all know that the time is almost over, but the family just cannot accept it. Then we have to tell the family that the patient has suffered for a while and it might be better to let the patient go since he/she is in such a poor state of health. Tell the family to let go and that everyone has done his/her utmost." (Case 1)

"For unconscious patients, we would suggest for the family to give the patient a body massage and to help move and stretch the patient's limbs. The family can continue to speak to the patient, letting the patient hear the voices of the family. We can't do too many things to the patient, because he/she may already be in a coma when we intervene. So the focus would be on the family. After all, ICU patients are mostly in the worst health conditions; they may be unconscious, in a coma or slowly recovering from unconsciousness after a period of treatment." (Case 3)

Discussion

By using a qualitative approach, this study described the experiences of ICU nurses on the spiritual care for critically ill patients, including nurses' assessment of patients' needs and spiritual care by nurses. Based on our data analysis and literature review, the authors offer the following discussion.

Nurses' assessment of patients' spiritual needs

Although Timmins and Kelly [5] suggested ICU nurses choosing the assessment tools of spiritual care based on the patients' point of view, the results showed that two perspectives in the assessment of patients' spiritual needs: conscious and unconscious patients, including two themes: clinical observation and judgment, and family interpretation, were all from the nurses' point of view. However, the current literature explored conscious patients' spiritual needs from both the perspectives of patients and nurses, but appeared to know little about unconscious patients' spiritual needs from the nurses' point of view as the findings in this study. Additionally, four patterns of communion with self, others, nature, and a higher being as well as three themes of transformation, transcendence, and rebirth with the need for love, meaning, purpose were considered as the core essences of spiritual needs for the critical patients [6-8].

Nurses' providing of patients' spiritual care

The results of this study showed that the 11 ICU nurses divided their spiritual care according to general spiritual care, and spiritual care for conscious and unconscious patients, which was different from Hsu [9] divided the spiritual intervention strategies into general and special spiritual care. The previous study was based on the patients' point of view, rather than this study was focused on the nurses' point of view. Specifically, comparing the previous studies on non-ICU units with the present study, the following aspects of spiritual care by non-ICU and ICU nurses were majorly on general six themes, including care skills, interaction promotion, religious belief, cultural care, wish fulfilment, alleviation of grief and terminal care. For instance, the aspects of spiritual care by ICU nurses included psychological, cultural, and religious perspectives of care through assessment and communication with the patients and their family members in the respectful attitudes [10], which were all similar to the themes underlined in the general spiritual care of this study. Additionally, Zeilani and Seymour [12] suggested the religious beliefs, cultural norms, and social supports as the essential components for ICU patients to adjust their suffering, which were also comparable to the themes underlined in the general spiritual care of this study. Nevertheless, the results of this study showed that spiritual care for conscious and unconscious patients were different from Lin et al. [10] proposed spiritual nursing interventions in the aspect of communion with self, others, nature, and a higher being.

Conclusion and Suggestions for Future Studies

Using a qualitative method, this study described the ICU nurses' experiences of spiritual care for critically ill patients. For the assessment of patients' spiritual needs, the patients were divided into two groups: conscious and unconscious groups. The spiritual needs of the former were assessed by means of clinical observation and judgment, while the needs of the latter were assessed through family interpretation. In addition, the spiritual care by nurses includes general spiritual care, as well as spiritual care for conscious and unconscious patients. Six themes in general spiritual care included care skills, interaction promotion, religious belief, cultural care, wish fulfillment, alleviation of grief and terminal care. Furthermore, spiritual care of the conscious and unconscious patients were also included.

In conclusion, spiritual needs and care from ICU nurses' perspective were different from the patients; however, both of views were focused on the general spiritual care, while ICU nurses divided spiritual care into the conscious and unconscious patients. The spiritual needs and care of the former were focused on the patients' point of view, whereas the needs and care of the latter were assisted through family interpretation. Additionally, among the guidelines of spiritual care, none is available for critically ill patients. Since this study found that the spiritual needs and care of critically ill patients who were highly culturally influenced, Penrod et al. [16] conducted an integrated palliative nursing care into ICU as quality improved program and suggested to apply the interdisciplinary training for ICU health professionals as well as Hughes et al. [17] integrated Chaplain to 12 ICU units with the cooperation of critical care and palliative nurses for spiritual care assessments. The cultural bound spiritual care in Taiwan was deeply involved into the Taoist religion, including wearing the divine cloth and a yellow headband, as well as eating of ash that all symbolized the way of protection the critical ill patients from getting evil spirits and could recover soon. Therefore, the authors suggested that a complete guideline of spiritual care for critically ill patients integrating with the cultural care and interdisciplinary cooperation could be developed on the basis of the results of this study in the future, which could provide more empirical data as the significant nursing reference.

References

1. Tsai YS, Lin YL, Huang SJ (2007) End-of-life care in critical illness. Taiwan Journal of Hospice Palliative Care 12: 312-319.
2. Clarke EB, Luce JM, Curtis R, Danis, Levy M, et al. (2004) A content analysis of forms, guidelines and other materials documenting end-of-life care in intensive care units. Journal of Critical Care 19: 108-117.
3. Rodriguez E, Johnson GA, Culbertson T, Grant W (2011) An educational program for spiritual care providers on end of life care in the critical care setting. Journal of Interprofessional Care 25: 375-377.
4. Turan T, Karamanog lu AY (2012) Determining intensive care unit nurses' perceptions and practice levels of spiritual care in Turkey. Nursing in Critical Care 18: 70-78.
5. Timmins F, Kelly J (2008) Spiritual assessment in intensive and cardiac care nursing. Nursing in Critical Care 13: 124-131.
6. Chao CS, Chen CH, Yen MF (2002) The essence of spirituality of terminally ill patients. The Journal of Nursing Research 10: 237-245.
7. Papathanassoglou EDE, Patiraki E (2003) Transformations of self: A phenomenological investigation into the lived experience of survivors of critical illness. Nursing in Critical Care 8: 13-21.
8. Murray SA, Kendall M, Kirsty B, Worth A, Benton TF (2004) Exploring the spiritual needs of people dying of lung cancer or heart failure: A prospective qualitative interview study of patients and their carers. Palliative Medicine 18: 39-45.
9. Hsu CG (2008) Intervening strategies and promoting the satisfaction of spiritual needs for terminal patients. Counseling and Guidance 275: 5-12.
10. Lin YH, Liou SH, Chen CH (2008) Spiritual care in nursing practice. Journal of Nursing 55: 69-74.
11. Lundberg PC, Kerdonfag P (2010) Spiritual care provided by Thai nurses in intensive care units. Journal of Clinical Nursing 19: 1121-1128.
12. Zeilani R, Seymour JE (2010) Muslim women's experiences of suffering in Jordanian intensive care units: A narrative study. Intensive and Critical Care Nursing 26: 175-184.
13. Hu YH (2008) Qualitative research: Theory, methods and indigenous women's studies. Sage Publishing, London.
14. Lee S (2011) Nursing Research and Application, Farseeing Publishing Co., Ltd, Taipei.
15. Lincoln YS, Guba EG (1985) Naturalistic inquiry, Sage, New York.
16. Penrod JD, Luhrs CA, Livote EE, Cortez TB, Kwak J (2011) Implementation and evaluation of a network-based pilot program to improve palliative care in the intensive care unit. Journal of Pain and Symptom Management 42: 668-671.
17. Hughes B, Whitmer M, Hurst S (2007) Innovative solutions: A plurality of vision. Dimensions of Critical Care Nursing 26: 91-95.

26

Tailoring an Evidence-Based Practice Fellowship to Meet Learning Needs of Bedside Nurses

Donna J. Plonczynski[1*] and **Donna Kruse**[2] RN, MS, CCRN-CMC-CSC

[1]*Associate professor, Northern Illinois University, USA*

[2]*Clinical Educator/Magnet Program Director, Advocate Sherman Hospital, USA*

*Corresponding author: Donna J. Plonczynski,** Associate professor, Northern Illinois University, 1240 Normal Rd, DeKalb, IL 60115, USA,
E-mail: djplonz@niu.edu

Abstract

The ability for nurses to practice to the fullest level of their education and expertise in order to optimize patient care is an ideal vision for nursing practice. While healthcare quality has improved over the past decades, delays continue in transferring current information from research to patient care. Many nurses are not experienced in transferring research into practice. This paper describes the process for planning, implementing and evaluating the evidence-based practice (EBP) Fellowship that transferred these critical skills to five bedside nurses. All five Fellows implemented evidence in their area of practice with significant positive changes in patient outcomes. The results from the Fellowship indicate that we met and exceeded the goals of transferring the knowledge, skills and attitudes for EBP to bedside nurses. Unexpected outcomes included the development of leadership and presentation skills as all five of the Fellows disseminated the results of their successful projects regionally and nationally.

Background

In a powerful Lancet article, it was estimated that overall 20-25% of patients receive treatments are that are either unnecessary or potentially harmful and that 30-40% patients do not receive evidence-based practice (EBP) care [1]. The United States Department of Health and Human Services (DHHS) has prioritized "high value, safe and effective health care" for U.S. healthcare systems [2]. The Department has set goals to be met by the end of 2015 toward the decline of preventable injuries in hospitals by 40%, as well as the reduction of readmissions by 20% annually. The realization of these goals could save the lives of 60,000 patients as well as prevent over 1.5 million patients from complications annually. This goal would also reduce Medicare costs by $50 billion dollars over 10 years, in addition to the reduction in other payer's costs.

Literature Review

It is well established that patients are admitted to acute care hospitals because they are in need of nursing care to address their health status or manage an acute health problem. The quality of that nursing care is based on the nurse's education, as well as the state of the environment in which she works [3]. According to the National Sample Survey of Registered Nurses, the average age of registered nurses in the United States is 46 years of age [4]. Most of these nurses have graduated decades earlier in programs that did not have an emphasis on research application or the implementation of EBP. Because of this gap in professional education, many nurses are not adept at interpreting current healthcare research or using the results to change practice in a timely manner.

The environment in which the nurse works is also being evaluated in order to address discrepancies. The Agency for Healthcare Quality and Research Quality publishes a report that compares quality of hospital outcomes over a decade [5]. This recent report has demonstrated improvements, but important disparities remain. In this analysis, no hospitals worsened, and a few showed no improvement at all over the previous decade. However, 77% of hospitals that have demonstrated overall improvement over the past 10 years continue to have safety concerns. A mere 38% of hospitals demonstrated improvement on their safety measures.

The Institute of Medicine (IOM) articulated a vision for nursing care that fosters practice to the fullest level in order to optimize care [6]. While healthcare quality has improved over the past decade, delays in transferring research to the bedside continue. A recent survey indicated that nurses are interested in - and are hopeful of - being active in EBP [7]. Because nurses are interested in providing optimal care, resources are needed in order to address the skills and knowledge needed to positively impact care throughout a hospital and healthcare system. Robert Wood Johnson advocates for partnerships to assist with the advancing of knowledge and education for nurses [8].

The implementation of an EBP nursing Fellowship is an ideal mechanism to deliver evolving healthcare knowledge into practice for the benefit of hospitalized patients. While evidence-based nursing practice is a priority for nursing care, the development of Fellowship mentoring programs are evolving. One Midwestern community hospital conducts a one-year researchship to educate 8 Fellows annually on the generation of research by conducting studies within the hospital [9]. Other hospitals have changed from this type of Fellowship into an EBP model that translates current research into nursing practice [10,11]. One system shortened the timeline of the Fellowship to less than one year in order to implement changes more quickly [12]. Because of the time-intensive nature of the education and mentoring, along with a safety imperative, Fellowships include limited numbers of Fellows. This paper will describe the process by which a tailored Fellowship was developed, maintained, and evaluated in order to address bedside nurse's educational and environmental needs.

Methods

This Fellowship plan began with a vision by nursing administrative leadership. The question posed to the Council of Application of Research and Evidence (CARE) was: "What are the most effective methods to conduct an ideal EBP program in order to address the learning needs of bedside nurses in order to improve patient outcomes?" The draft outline of the Fellowship was determined from published literature and from practices at other hospitals and academic centers [11]. It was tailored to meet the needs of this hospital's nurses. Brainstorming, a draft proposal, and subsequent revisions as a Council were developed as a result of this challenge from nursing leadership.

The purpose of the nursing Fellowship program was to promote quality care for the patients by providing the knowledge, skills and attitudes to bedside nurses for implementation of EBP. This purpose was accomplished by the incorporation of research into practice, which will close the time delay now seen nationwide between knowledge generation and its implementation.

The reality of healthcare practice includes the need for funding. Funding was needed for a research and statistical consultant, the salary of 92 work hours per Fellow, supplies, and the costs of poster generation and conference attendance for subsequent presentations. Disseminating the results of the EBP was critical to the program's success. The hospital sought and obtained funding from a local community foundation and a local benefactor. Similar support from the hospital included technological, logistic, and coordinator support for the duration of the program. In addition, continuing education credits that count toward re-licensure were provided for the Fellows through the hospital.

A foundational consideration was the choice of a model used for the program. The process by which research is initially identified, transferred throughout the nursing staff, and used in patient care follows a nursing practice framework. Multiple clinical and academic settings use the Iowa Model [13,14], which uses an algorhythm that nurses 'find intuitively understandable" [15]. The well-established Iowa model and educational program were used as a template for the Fellowship after evaluating multiple other models [14].

The modifications of the original educational program from a more research-focus are listed below [16]. These modifications were made in keeping with cost accountability and timeline considerations:

- timeline reduced from one-to-two years to three months;
- reduced class meetings from 12 to 4 days;
- placed locating evidence on first day, rather than third;
- removed conference attendance as part of initial Fellowship timeline;
- added discussions each meeting to foster collaboration and problem-solving as a group; and
- included creation and presentation of poster and oral presentation to leaders and mentors as part of the Fellowship timeline.

Once the plan was complete and funding obtained, the application and review process were developed by the CARE council. The application form included suggested topics for an EBP project, but choosing one of the suggested topics was not used as a criterion for selection. The application process was announced via the hospital's newsletter, emails and nursing forums and was available on-line and in paper formats in various locations. Each applicant submitted an interest statement, an outline of previous professional changes he/she had implemented and their outcomes, as well as an EBP project idea. Completed applications were blinded and forward to the CARE council members by the chair for review and scoring. Applicants were then notified via letter of results and comments. Those applicants that were not selected were given feedback on methods to improve their application for the next submission.

Each chosen Fellow obtained a letter of support from his/her leader and signed a contract to ensure clear communication of expectations. Each Fellow agreed to attend and participate at all EBP workshop sessions. In addition, they agreed to meet individually with their identified mentor and nurse leader at least one hour per month. Furthermore, they agreed to complete the EBP project in the three months of the Fellowship and promote the further implementation of their EBP across departments and committees in subsequent months. Finally, the Fellows agreed to develop and deliver a poster and podium presentation and submit their work for a regional or national conference.

The five selected Fellows were mentored for 92 hours over three months. The Fellow was provided with 32 hours of workshop time and used the remaining 60 hours toward mentored implementation and evaluation of the new practice. The Fellowship hours were separate from his/her usual practice responsibilities on the department schedule and did not count toward the departmental productivity goals.

It was determined that the Fellowship was best presented in a workshop format with an application focus with each topic. The consideration of the program as a workshop was critical to its success for bedside nurses. Each presentation, whether on searching literature, evaluating literature, or entering excel data was followed by a mentored practice session on computers with Internet access.

Our topics were modified for bedside nurses. The following were topics covered during the workshops:

Organizational and leadership support of EBP
The Iowa Model
Defining the EBP project's development with PICOT (population, intervention, control or comparison group, outcome, and timing)
Action plan
Feasibility analysis and team building
Literature and web resource searching
Evaluating resources for quality
Obtain evidence (baseline data)
Excel data entry
Role of statistics
Writing a protocol/procedure/guideline
Implementing change
Poster and podium presentation development

Table 1: Topics covered during the workshops.

Application to practice was the rationale for reducing sections on literature reviews and literature synthesis. For example, there was no use of research critique forms. This Fellowship did not include some models such as the research translation model, nor did it include research language such as independent and dependent variables. The focus of the research parts of this Fellowship focused on the use of high-quality evidence, such as from internationally recognized sources. The purpose of the statistical presentation was to enhance understanding of statistics without explaining how to conduct the analyses.

Our modifications also included the use of notebooks to track progress, ideas, and barriers for problem solving by the individual with the mentor or with the Fellowship group. Each workshop concluded with a review of assignments that were to be completed prior to the next meeting.

To ensure that the process was understandable, the planner and major presenter continually linked the EBP process to the nursing process of assesses, diagnose, plan, intervene and evaluate, which was labeled the 'Iowa Model in a nutshell' : (Table 2)

Steps in EBP process	Nursing process
Identify an issue of concern; and Assemble and evaluate evidence in literature and current best practices	Assess
Measure baseline data and determine exact issue that can be addressed	Diagnose
Develop implementation and outcome measurement steps	Plan
Pilot protocol	Implement
Measure process and outcomes	Evaluate

Table 2: Iowa Model in a nutshell.

The goals of this Fellowship were accomplished in three months with meetings held approximately every three weeks. The remaining time was spent on individual mentored development of the project. A recognition event was held at the end of the three months with mentors and leaders. At that time, Fellows presented their posters and a podium presentation to the leadership, followed by several weeks of presentations to various audiences, including the funders, the hospital staff and medical staff.

Results

The projects all were a success in many ways. There were significant improvements in each of the five EBP changes. The projects:

- reduced delirium by using a wake-up protocol for patients who were intubated;
- improved breastfeeding rates and maternal bonding by allowing for daily maternal nap and quiet time;
- provided pain relief for children using distraction techniques on Ipads©;
- improved discharges to home instead of to extended care facilities by developing a comprehensive walking program; and
- reduced the risk of errors by implementing a medication-passing program.

The feedback from the Fellows at each workshop was positive. The total of the feedback forms (n=75) from the Fellows on the evaluation of each of the seven presenter's effectiveness was labeled to a 'great extent' (95%, n=71), 'moderate extent' (4%, n=3), and 'slight extent' (1%, n=1). For the summed feedback (n=30) on the extent course objectives were met each workshop, 90% (n=27) stated 'great extent', while 10% (n=3) stated 'moderate extent'.

At the conclusion of the Fellowship, the Fellows were asked to provide overall evaluations, as well as barriers and facilitators to the program. The comments were as follows: 'Excellent'; 'Met and exceeded goals'; 'Improved confidence as nurse'; 'Improved ability to publically speak'; 'Added leadership role to department'; 'Improved written communication skills'; 'Expanded understanding of research'.

The two barriers identified by the Fellows were difficulties scheduling off department time and the short time to complete the project. The three identified facilitators were 'Excellent feedback'; 'Support systems: Mentors, Leaders, Coordinator'; and 'Resources for getting project done'.

To determine the impact of the Fellowship further out in time, the Fellows, Mentors and Leaders were asked to anonymously critique the program six months after its completion. By that time, all the projects had been expanded or were in the process of being expanded in other departments. Additionally, several Fellows had joined the CARE council and had been active in promoting EBP in units. All of the Fellows had presented their posters and PowerPoint's locally, and all were accepted to present at a national EBP conference. Furthermore, two of the Fellows had enrolled in Advanced Practice Nurse (APN) Master's degree programs.

One leader wrote in 6-month follow-up evaluation that this was a "Great Fellowship, I'm glad to see it's continued. I believe this will shape nursing practice at this Hospital for the better in the future, and will plant the seeds for many great changes." Furthermore, the Chief Nursing Officer (CNO), who had originated this program's vision provided feedback. She stated that the Fellowship "Had a positive impact on patient outcomes; increased the value of EBP in our organization; provided new opportunities for poster and project presentations in the region and nationally; and elevated/advanced the practice of nursing".

Discussion

This Fellowship met the DHHS goals of providing safe, effective patient care that is cost-effective [2]. In hospitals, because the care provided by nurses is instrumental for optimal patient outcomes, the use of EBP by nurses is crucial to meeting the DHHS goals. In each project, the Fellow demonstrated improved patient outcomes with EBP care.

This Fellowship was in keeping with Robert Wood Johnson's [8] encouragement of interdisciplinary partnerships to advance knowledge for nurses, with the use of an informaticist, educator, researcher, case manager, data manager, and coordinator.

These Fellows volunteered for the program and demonstrated great interest in being active in EBP, similar to what is found in the literature [7]. Because nurses are interested in providing optimal care, resources are needed in order to address the skills and knowledge needed to positively impact care throughout a hospital and healthcare system. Financing and health system resources were made available through administrative and community support. This was a critical factor in the program's success.

The Fellowship fostered improvements in patient care at multiple levels by implementing EBP rapidly to the bedside. This result is in keeping with the IOM's vision for nursing to provide practice at an optimal level to ensure safe and effective patient outcomes [6].

In answering the CNO's challenge about her vision for evidence-based nursing practice, the CARE council implemented the Fellowship outline from published literature and from best practices at other hospitals and academic centers [11]. Because most of the Fellows did not have experience in EBP implementation, the Fellowship required a tailored, bedside-focused workshop format.

The results from the Fellowships indicate that the goals of providing the knowledge, skills and attitudes to bedside nurses for implementation of EBP were met and exceeded. The mentored process has further developed these excellent nurses and recognized them for their investment in optimizing patient care. Additionally, the work of the Fellows was at such a high level, that they each have presented their work regionally and nationally. A final, and unexpected result of the Fellowship was the development of leadership skills in these nurses, who have gone on to mentor other nurses, pursue further degrees, and assumed membership in health system committees.

Future implications

The positive transformational impact of mentoring process on nurses has been well recorded in residency programs [17], but not in EBP Fellowships. Therefore, an analysis of the impact on process and outcome measures such as leadership roles and nurse retention has yet to be studied extensively. Research on these issues would help direct future programs.

For this Fellowship, the facilitators and barriers as well as feedback from the Fellows, Mentors, and Leaders were used to further develop the structure of the Fellowship. With Fellows now serving on the CARE council, their feedback will be used in future planning, thereby closing the feedback loop. This process further supports the culture of EBP in the health system.

Acknowledgements

The Fellows who have successfully navigated EBP changes.

Their leaders and mentors

Judy Balcitis, RN, MSN, CNO

Benefactors for the program funding

References

1. Grol R, Grimshaw J (2003) From best evidence to best practice: effective implementation of change in patients' care. Lancet 362: 1225-1230.

2. U.S. Department of Health and Human Services (DHHS, 2010). Strategic plan and priorities: Fiscal years 2010-2015.

3. Aiken, L., Cimiotti, J., Sloan, D., Smith, H., Flynn, L., & Neff, D (2011) Effects of nurse staffing and nurse education on patient deaths in hospitals with different nurse work environments. Medical Care, 49(12): 1047-1053.

4. Federal Division of Nursing (2010) The registered nurse population: Findings from the 2008 national sample survey of Registered Nurses. Department of Health and Human Services, Washington, USA.

5. Rockville MD (2012) Agency for Healthcare Research and Quality. National healthcare quality report.

6. Institute of Medicine (2010) The Future of nursing: Leading change, advancing health. National Academies Press Washington, USA.

7. Soukup M, McCleish J (2008) Advancing evidence-based practice: a program series. J Contin Educ Nurs 39: 402-406.

8. Robert Wood Johnson (2011) The nursing profession: development, challenges, and opportunities. Mason D, Isaacs S and Colby D (Eds.), Wiley, Jossey-Bass: Hoboken, USA.

9. Turkel MC, Ferket K, Reidinger G, Beatty DE (2008) Building a nursing research fellowship in a community hospital. Nurs Econ 26: 26-34.

10. Gattusso, J., Hinds, P., Beaumont, C., Funk, A., Green, J., et al. (2007) Transforming a hospital nursing research fellowship into an evidence-based practice fellowship. Journal of Nursing Administration, 37 : 539-545.

11. Weeks S, Moore P, Allender M (2011) A regional evidence-based practice Fellowship: Collaborating competitors. Journal of Nursing Administration, 41: 10-14.

12. Milne D, Krishnasamy M, Aranda S (2007) Promoting evidence-based care through a clinical research fellowship programe. Journal of Clinical Nursing 16: 1629-1639.

13. Krom Z, Batten J, Bautista C (2010) A Unique Collaborative Nursing Evidence-Based Practice Initiative Using the Iowa Model: A Clinical Nurse Specialist, a Health Science Librarian, and a Staff Nurse's Success Story. Clinical Nurse Specialist 24: 54-59.

14. Titler MG, Kleiber C, Steelman VJ, Rakel BA, Budreau G, et al. (2001) The Iowa Model of Evidence-Based Practice to Promote Quality Care. Crit Care Nurs Clin North Am 13: 497-509.

15. Gawlinski A, Rutledge D (2008) Selecting a model for evidence-based practice changes: a practical approach. AACN Adv Crit Care 19: 291-300.

16. Cullen L, Titler MG (2004) Promoting evidence-based practice: an internship for staff nurses. Worldviews Evid Based Nurs 1: 215-223.

17. Kramer M, Maguire P, Halfer D, Budin WC, Hall DS, et al. (2012) The organizational transformative power of nurse residency programs. Nurs Adm Q 36: 155-168.

27

The Implementation of Nursing Process and Associated Factors among Nurses Working in Debremarkos and Finoteselam Hospitals, Northwest Ethiopia, 2013

Nurilign Abebe[1*], Habtamu Abera[1] and Mulatu Ayana[2]

[1]Nursing Department, Medicine and Health Sciences College, Debre Markos University, Debre Markos, Ethiopia

[2]Public Health Department, Medicine and Health Sciences College, Debre Markos University, Debre Markos, Ethiopia

*Corresponding author: Nurilign Abebe Moges, Nursing Department, Medicine and Health Sciences College, Debre Markos University, Debre Markos, Ethiopia, E-mail: nure113@gmail.com

Abstract

Background: The aim of this study was to describe the level of implementation of nursing process and associated factors among nurses working in DebreMarkos Referral Hospital and Finote Selam District Hospital, northwest Ethiopia, 2013.

Materials and methods: A total of 124 nurses with one year and above working experience in the respective hospitals gave complete response out of 139 total nurses. Self-administered questionnaire from standardized and pre-tested tool were adopted to collect data. The data was entered using Epidata version3.1 and analyzed using SPSS software. In addition to descriptive statistics both bivariate and multivariate logistic regression model fitted to identify possible factors associated with nursing process implementation. Then those variables with P-value of <0.05 at 95% confidence interval (CI) was declared as statistically significant.

Results: Among 124 total respondents 72 (58.2%) were female nurses, the ages of the respondents were between 20 and 62 years with median age of 29 years. They implemented nursing process at various degree of consistency 46 (37.1%) practice it very much, 62 (50%) practiced somewhat and the rest 16 (12.9%) not at all and not really practiced. Low knowledge negatively associate with nursing process implementation, Adjusted odds Ratio (AOR) 0.16, at 95% CI=0.07-0.39) and Presence of patients with uncomplicated case facilitate nursing process implementation (AOR=5.67, at 95% CI=2.52-12.73).

Conclusion: The level of nursing process implementation is low among nurses. Factors associated with implementation of nursing process among nurses working in hospitals were; presence of patients with complicated case and low level of knowledge about nursing process. Nurses' patient care knowledge in general and nursing process in particular should be evaluated and monitored periodically in order to provide on service training.

Keywords: Nurse; Debre Markos; Finote Selam; Hospital; Nursing process; Knowledge; Implementation; Ethiopia

Abbreviations:

SNCPs: Standardized Nursing Care Plans; USA: United State of America; WHO: World Health Organization

Introduction

In the eighties, the nursing process was introduced as a systematic method of planning nursing care internationally [1]. The nursing process has been used for over 25 years as a systematic approach to nursing practice [2]. Yet hospitals confront challenges with regards to nursing involvement, including scarcity of nursing resources; difficulty engaging nurses at all levels from bed side to management; growing demands to participate in more, often duplicative, and quality improvement activates[3].

Nursing process is a systematic method of planning, delivering, and evaluating individualized care for clients in any state of health or illness. Based on the scientific problem-solving method, it constitutes the foundation for nursing practice [4].

Because nurses are the key caregivers in hospitals, they can significantly influence the quality of care provided and, ultimately, treatment and patient outcomes. Consequently, hospitals' pursuit of high-quality of patient care is dependent, at least in part, on their ability to engage and use nursing resources effectively. This will likely become more challenging as these resources become increasingly limited [5]. The scarcity of nurses is a major challenge for hospitals because it impact to not only their ability to provide nursing coverage for patient care, but also to provide adequate nursing resources for other key activities, such as quality improvement [3].

Despite their knowledge of the nursing process, certain factors limited the ability of nurses to implement it in their daily practice, including lack of time, high patient volume, and high patient turnover [6]. Despite these hurdles, the daily application of the nursing process is characterized by the scientific background of the professionals involved since it requires Knowledge and provides individualized human assistance [6]. An investigation of the steps of the nursing process actually implemented in the routine of a university hospital showed that all phases were performed however; problems were identified in the nursing process, involving recording the history and implementing nursing perception. The evaluation of expected results, in particular, was not adequately recorded [7].

Though the government of Ethiopia give due emphasis on quality of health service in general and quality of nursing care in particular [8], there is still huge gap on the implementation of nursing process among nurses working in hospitals [9]. Therefore this study tried to assess the level and factors associated with nursing process implementation among nurses working in the two hospitals.

Factors affecting the implementation of nursing process

Studies have shown that the implementation of the nursing diagnosis is a challenge for nurses [10]. A study conducted in Nigeria on factors influencing the implementation of nursing process indicated that knowledge factor has the highest predictive value of 0.350 in the use of nursing process, followed by institutional factor (B=0.222) and professional factor (B=0.063) the least is the attitude factor (B=0.019). The result concluded that the knowledge factor has the most important influence on the use of nursing process [11].

It is believed that "most nurses are resistant to change, professional development and advancement. Some nurses tend to hold onto previous knowledge and skills without making efforts to improve and maintain new skills. Many nurses are not willing to accept the challenges of staying abreast with education and development of new skills in nursing practice [12].

Study done in Ethiopia shows that the characteristics work place, nurses who were working in a stressful environment were 0.357 times significantly and less likely to implement nursing process than those worked in a disorganized environment (COR: 0357, 95%CI (0.157-0.814), P: 0.014). Neglecting working environment had no significant association with implementation of nursing process. Hence nursing process implementation needs a safe and encouraging working environment [13].

Material and Methods

Study Design

Institutional based cross-sectional study design was conducted.

Study area

The study was conducted in DebreMarkos referral hospital, Amhara Regional State of Ethiopia Debre Markos is the administrative town of East GojjamZone and it is found in the North West part of the country bounded by Gozamenworeda in the North, South, and East, and Anededworeda in the West. Debre Markos is located on the main road of Addis Ababa to Bahir-Dar. It is 300 km away from Addis Ababa and 265 km from Bahir-Dar. It has 01 referral hospital, 03 governmental health center, 07 health post, 16 private pharmacies, 22 private clinics, 02 diagnostic laboratories and 12 traditional healer service provider and Finote Selam is the administrative town of West Gojjam Zone and it is found in the North West part of the country. It is Located on the main road of Addis Ababa-Bahir-Dar and 387 km away from Addis Ababa and 178 km from Bahir-Dar. It has 01 District hospital, 01 governmental health center, 02 health post, 06 private pharmacy, 08 private clinics, and 05 traditional healer service provider.

Study period: The study was conducted from March 2013 to May 2013.

Source population: All nurses who have been working in DebreMarkos Referral Hospital & Finote Selam District Hospital, North West Ethiopia.

Study population: Nurse who fulfill the inclusion criteria.

Inclusive criteria: Nurses who are working at Debre Markos Referral Hospital & Finote Selam District Hospital for at least six months. Both diploma and degree nurse were included

Exclusive criteria: Nurses who will not be available due to sick leave, temporary reassignment, annual leave; Nurse working for free service.

Sampling technique: All nurses in the two hospitals, there are 108 and 31 nurses in DebreMarkos referral Hospital and FinoteSelam District Hospital respectively was included. These Hospitals were purposively selected based on the general service they have been provided and their number of nurses for study area.

Dependent variable: Implementation of nursing process (Yes/No).

Independent variable: Year of experience; Knowledge of nurses; Nurses demographics; Nurses skill; Hospitals organizational structures.

Operational Definition

Skill: Daily nurses practice performed for participant. Those respondents who have scored >26 are highly skill full; 18-25 are moderately skill full, and <17 are low skill full group out of 30 [13].

Knowledgeable nurses: Nurses awareness about nursing process. Highly knowledgeable nurses are those 80% of the questions, moderately knowledgeable nurses are those answered in between 55-79.9%, and low knowledgeable nurses those scored < 55% [13].

Data Collection Tools and Method of Data Collection

Data was collected by using structured self-administered questionnaire. Structured English version questionnaire which is adapted from previous study. It was collected by trained graduating nursing students after one day training is given on the general purpose, data collection methods and data handling techniques.

Data quality assurance

Pretests were done among health center nurse who were not later include in the main study. The principal investigators supervise during data collection time and each night there were a discussion to correct any misunderstanding accordingly.

Data processing and analysis

Data were entered using Epidata software version 3.1 and exported to SPSS version 16 for further analysis. Descriptive statistics was performed on mean, median; range and percentage of dependent and independent variables. Binary logistic regression was run to identify statistically significant independent variables. Both bivariate and multivariate logistic regression model was fitted to select associated factors and to control cofounding respectively. Those variables significantly associated with nursing process implementation at P-value of 25% were included for further analysis in multivariate analysis and final decision was made on p-value 0.05 at 95% CI for the significant association of nursing process implementation.

Ethical consideration

Ethical clearance was obtained from Debre Markos University Medicine and Health Sciences College, Department of nursing. Before the beginning of data collection permission letter was provided to the two hospitals administrative body for data collection. After that participants oriented about the purpose and procedure of data collection, and that confidentiality and privacy is ensured. It was also cleared that participation was fully based on the willingness of participants using written consent.

Result

Socio demographic characteristics of the respondents

In this study 139 nurses were included out of which 124 nurses give complete response from Debre Markos Referral hospital and Finote Selam Disrtict hospital with response rate of 89%. Among the respondents 72 (58.2%) were female nurses, the age of the respondents were between 20 and 62 years with median age of 29 years. Age distribution of study participants was not normally distributed so that we use median to group it. So that 64 (56.6%) of nurse were at age of 29 and bellow. Majority of them were Amhara in ethnic origin 115 (92.7%) fifty nine (46.6%) were married Table 1.

Characteristics	Frequency	Percentage (%)
Sex		
M	52	41.90
F	72	58.10
Age (median)		
<29 years	64	51.60
>29 years	60	48.40
Ethnicity		
Amhara	115	92.70
Others*	9	7.30
Marital status		
Single	38	30.60
Married	59	47.60
Others (divorce, widowed and separate)	27	21.80
*others=Tigray, Oromo		

Table 1: Socio-demographic characteristics of Nurses in Debre Markos and Finote Selam Hospitals, Northwest Ethiopia, 2013 (n=124)

Organizational and nurses related factors

Work experience of nurse varies from one to twenty seven years while majority lies on less than five years (mean 6.64 and median 4 years). Nurses whose clinical service was less than and equal to four years were 72 (58.1%) and the rest 52 (41.9%) nurses had greater than four years. Since it is not normal distribution we took the median. Nurse who respond as they have no enough equipment necessary for

patient care was 71 (57.3%) and with the necessary equipments 43 (42.3%). Working hours, number of patient get care by nurses and other organizational factors are given bellow in Table 2.

Characteristics	Frequency	Percentage (%)
Working experience (median)		
<4 years	72	58.10
>4 years	52	41.90
Daily working hours (Ethiopian civil servant working hrs)		
< 8 hrs	113	91.10
>8 hrs	13	8.90
Number of patients get care per day by a nurse (mean)		
<14 patients	78	62.9
>14 patients	46	37.1
got orientation		
Yes	34	27.4
No	90	72.6
Knowledge		
Knowledgeable	72	58.1
Low knowledge	52	41.9

Table 2: Organizational and nurses related factors for Nursing process implementation in Debre Markos and Finote Selam Hospitals, Northwest Ethiopia, 2013 (n=124)

Study participants respond on the influencing factors for the implementation of nursing process rated according to reason listed here; patients discharge before completing the planned intervention 116 (93.5%), non-cooperative patients 101 (81.5%), inability to collect require data 88 (71%) and present of patients with complicated case 64 (51.6%).

Knowledge and practice of nurses on nursing process

Among the ten questions about knowledge that measure in percentage rated as highly knowledgeable those who answer 80% correctly, moderately knowledgeable those who give correct response for 65% and less than those who give correct answer for less than 65% were grouped as low knowledge. Based on this 72(58.1%) were highly knowledgeable, 38 (30.6%) were moderately knowledgeable and 14 (11.3%) were under the group of low knowledgeable category. But for the purpose of analysis and we believe that there is no as such difference between the moderate and low knowledge we combine them together and have two category only high and low knowledge. Study participants responded for the frequency of implementing nursing process that 46 (37.1%) practice it very much, 62 (50%) practiced somewhat and the rest 16 (12.9%) not at all and not really practiced.

In the bivariate analysis of logistic regression, seven variables were statistically significantly associated with the level of nursing process implementation. Namely working experience of more than 4 years was almost double more likely to implement nursing process than working experience of less than or equal to 4 years, (COR=2.60, 95% CI=1.23-5.50). Availability of necessary equipment's for patient care in the hospital were three times more likely to implement nursing process than inadequate one (COR=3.30, 95% CI=1.54-7.09). Those nurses got orientation during the entrance of the respective hospitals were more likely to implement nursing process (COR=2.96, 95% CI=1.31-6.67). Patients who were cooperative during patient care were three times more likely to get nursing process than those not cooperative (COR=3.35, 95% CI=1.32-8.56). Patients who presented with no complication were about six times more likely to get nursing process (COR=5.67, 95% CI=2.52-12.73) and nurses who were knowledgeable were more likely to implement nursing process Table 3 and 4.

Characteristics	Frequency	COR at 95% CI	p-value
Sex			
M	52	1.95 (0.93-4.09)	0.08
F	72	1	
Age (median)			
<29 years	64	1	
>29 years	60	1.69 (0.81-3.51)	0.17
Marital status			
Single	115	92.70	
Married	9	7.30	
Marital status			
Single	38	1	
Married	39	1.32 (0.57-3.08)	0.52
Others (divorce, widowed and separate)	27	0.96 (0.37-2.37)	0.94

Table 3: Bivariate logistic regression analysis of factors associated for the implementation of nursing process among nurses in Debre Markos and Finote Selam Hospitals, Northwest Ethiopia, 2013 (n=124)

Characteristics	Frequency	COR at 95% CI	p-value
Working experience (median)			
<4 years	72	1	0.000*
>4 years	52	2.6 (1.23-5.50)	
Daily working hours (Ethiopian civil servant working hrs)			
< 8 hrs	113	1	
>8 hrs	13	1.64 (0.41-6.51)	0.48

Number of patients get care per day by a nurse (mean)			
<14 patients	78	1	0.25
>14 patients	46	1.54 (0.74-3.21)	
necessary equipment's for care			
Yes	42	3.30 (1.54-7.05)	0.002*
No	82	1	
got orientation			
Yes	34	2.96 (1.31-6.67)	0.009*
No	90	1	

Table 4: Bivariate logistic regression analysis of factors associated for the implementation of nursing process among nurses in Debre Markos and Finote Selam Hospitals, Northwest Ethiopia, 2013 (n=124)

In multivariate logistic analysis including variables significant at bivariate analysis with other variable considered as significant from other literatures were analyzed and two variables were statistically significant to associate the implementation of nursing process by nurses working in hospitals. These were nurses with low knowledge was 0.16 times less likely to implement nursing process (AOR=0.62, 95% CI=0.07-0.39) and nursing process was not implemented almost six time more likely than patients who present without complication (AOR=4.33, 95% CI, 1.40-13.41) Table 5.

Characteristics	Frequency	COR at 95% CI	P-value
Knowledge			
Knowledgeable	72	1	0.000*
Low knowledge	52	0.16 (0.07-0.39)	
patient discharge before completing the planned			
Yes	116	1	
No	8	1.02 (0.23-4.48)	0.98
Patient are cooperative			
Yes	23	3.35 (1.32-8.56)	
No	101	1	0.011*
Ability to collect the required material for care			
Yes	36	2.98 (1.34-6.64)	0.008*
No	88	1	

Complicated case presentation			
Yes	64	1	0.000*
No	60	5.67 (2.52-12.73)	

Table 5: Bivariate logistic regression analysis of factors associated for the implementation of nursing process among nurses in DebreMarkos and FinoteSelam Hospitals, Northwest Ethiopia, 2013 (n=124)

COR: Crude Odds Ratio; CI: Confidence Interval, *statistically significant at 95% CI with P-value<0.05.

Discussion

This study describes the level of nursing process implementation and associated factors among 124 nurses in Debre Markos Referral Hospital and Finote Selam District Hospital northwest Ethiopia.

About 37.1% of nurses were implementing nursing process very much and the rest 62.9% fall from not all practicing to somewhat practicing. This was measured from skill assessment scores based on 1 not at all, 2 not really, 3 undecided, 4 somewhat and 5 very much. Inline to this there were six skill questions from that respondent who score 26 and above were considered as very much implementing nursing process. Similar study among nurses working in selected government hospitals in Addis Ababa, Ethiopia revealed that 52.1% of nurse implemented nursing process [13]. Regarding their level of skill towards nursing process 37.1% were highly skillful, 50% were moderately skillful and 12.9% were low in skill. Level of skill was similar with findings in Addis Ababa. Another study conducted on factors influencing the implementation of standardized nursing care plan in Sweden show that 98% of the respondents used standardized nursing care plan in their everyday work [14]. This huge discrepancy (37.1Vs 98%) may be because of the difference between the two countries socio demographic factors for nurses, patients and organizational facilities that facilitate nursing process. Additionally, the later study was done in university hospitals in which many of nurses are believed to have better knowledge to practice nursing process.

In the bivariate analysis of logistic regression, seven variables were statistically significantly associated with the level of nursing process implementation. Namely working experience of more than 4 years was almost double more likely to implement nursing process than working experience of less than or equal to 4 years, Availability of necessary equipment's for patient care in the hospital were three times more likely to implement nursing process than inadequate one. Those nurses got orientation during the entrance of the respective hospitals were more likely to implement nursing process Patients who were cooperative during patient care were three times more likely to get nursing process than those not cooperative. Patients who presented with no complication were about six times more likely to get nursing process and nurses who were knowledgeable were more likely to implement nursing process.

This finding is consistent with study done in Nigeria on factors affecting the use of nursing process on health institutions [11]. This study identifies the four basic predictors of nursing process implementation. Our result in work experience, knowledge of nurses and caring for patients with complicated case can be grouped under professional and attitudinal factors that predict nursing process implementation. Availability of necessary nursing care equipment's and orientation while joining the organization can be under institutional factors that inhibit implementation of nursing process.

Therefore the above factors the influence implementation of nursing process can be grouped under knowledge related, institutional issues, professional factors and attitudinal factors as it also indicated in [11].

In multivariate logistic analysis including variables significant at bivariate analysis with other variable considered as significant from other literatures were analyzed and two variables were statistically significant to associate the implementation of nursing process by nurses working in hospitals. The first factor is nurse who were knowledgeable were more likely to implement nursing process. This result is in line with study in Ethiopia [11,13]. However, despite their knowledge of the nursing process, certain factors limited the ability of nurses to implement it in their daily practice, including lack of time, high patient volume, and high patient turnover. Despite these hurdles, the daily application of the nursing process is characterized by the scientific background of the professionals involved since it requires Knowledge and provides individualized human assistance.6 this is true because knowledge is a prerequisite to practice. Therefore, nurses should have adequate training in nursing process implementation. The second statistically significant factor was the present of patients with complicated case. This might be due to the increase of work load on nurse that hider the full practice of nursing process which is vital for such type of patients. Under a heavy work load, nurses may not have sufficient time to perform tasks that can have a direct effect on patient safety [13] Table 6 and 7.

Characteristics	Frequency	COR at 95% CI	AOR at 95% CI	P-value
Sex				
M	52	1.95 (0.93-4.09)	1.42 (0.52-3.86)	0.49
F	72	1	1	
Age (median)				
<29 years	64	1	1	0.90
>29 years	60	1.69 (0.81-3.51)	1.09 (0.30-4.02)	
Working experience (median)				

<4 years	72	1	1	0.28
>4 years	52	2.6 (1.23-5.50)	2.07 (0.55-7.84)	
Daily working hours				
< 8 hrs	113	1	1	0.08
>8 hrs	11	1.64 (0.41-6.51)	0.16 (0.02-1.22)	
Number of patients get care				
<14	78	1	1	0.70
>14	46	1.54 (0.74-3.21)	1.24 (0.42-3.72)	

Table 6: Bivariate and Multivariate logistic regression analysis of factors associated for the implementation of nursing process among nurses in DebreMarkos and FinoteSelam Hospitals, Northwest Ethiopia, 2013 (n=124)

Characteristics	Frequency	COR at 95% CI	AOR at 95% CI	P-value
Knowledge				
Knowledgeable	72	1	1	0.0
Low knowledge	52	0.16 (0.07-0.39)	0.12(0.04-0.39)	01*
Patient are cooperativeness				
Yes	23	3.35 (1.32-8.56)	1.63(0.41-6.52)	0.4
No	101	1	1	9
present of the patient with complication				
Yes	64	1	1	
No	60	5.67(2.52-2.73)	4.33(1.40-13.41)	0.011*

Table 7: Bivariate and Multivariate logistic regression analysis of factors associated for the implementation of nursing process among nurses in DebreMarkos and FinoteSelam Hospitals, Northwest Ethiopia, 2013 (n=124)

AOR: Adjusted Odds Ratio; COR: Crude Odds Ratio; CI: confidence interval; *statistically significant at 95% CI with P-value<0.05.

Conclusion

The study indicated that the level of nursing process implementation was low among nurses working in DebreMarkos Referral Hospital and FinoteSelam District Hospital, northwest Ethiopia during the study period.

Factors associated with implementation of nursing process among nurses working in hospitals were; lack of clinical experience, lack of orientation in the hospital, lack of necessary equipment's for patient care, uncooperative patients with complicated case and low level of knowledge about nursing process identified in this study.

Recommendation

It is identified that the level of nursing process implementation was low so that the following measures should be taken to minimize the burdensome of factors affecting implementation of nursing process.

To Nurses and nurse educators

Nurse and nurse educator should update their knowledge on nursing process theoretical aspect as well as practical aspect especially fresh graduates should be monitored

Additional qualitative research should be conducted in large scale from the nationwide to recommended feasible actions for the concerned stalk holders

Nurse should approach systematically in way to provide full access for nursing care for patients with complicated case.

To health institutions

Health institutions should avail all necessary equipments for patient care since it highly affects the implementation of nursing process for patients

Newly graduated nurses should be also oriented on how to provide nursing care, available resources for nursing care and other work related issues.

Nurses' patient care knowledge in general and nursing process in particular should be evaluated and monitored periodically in order to provide on service training.

Acknowledgments

First we would like to thank Debre Markos University for ethical approval and support for necessary materials while doing this study. Second data collectors, study participants and administrative bodies of the two hospitals.

Author contributions

NA writes the proposal, design the study, and participate in supervision of data collection. HA and MA participate in the data analysis, written up of results, discussion. All of the authors contributed in manuscript preparation, critical evaluation of the study result.

References

1. Müller-Staub M, Needham I, Odenbreit M, Lavin MA, van Achterberg T (2007) Improved quality of nursing documentation: results of a nursing diagnoses, interventions, and outcomes implementation study. Int J Nurs Terminol Classif 18: 5-17.

2. Marilynn E (2003) Application of Nursing Process and Nursing Diagnosis an Interactive Text for Diagnostic Reasoning. (4thedn), New York, United States of America.

3. de Moraes Lopes MH, Higa R, Dos Reis MJ, de Oliveira NR, Christóforo FF (2010) Evaluation of the nursing process used at a Brazilian teaching hospital. Int J Nurs Terminol Classif 21: 116-123.

4. Carpenito-Moyet LJ (2004) Nursing diagnosis: application to clinical practice (10th Ed) Philadelphia.

5. Revisalid A (2002) Applying Nursing Process collaborative care. (5th Ed), New York.

6. Clarke SP, Aiken LH (2003) Failure to rescue. Am J Nurs 103: 42-47.

7. Reppetto MA, de Souza MF (2005) [Evaluation of nursing care systematization through the phases of nursing process performance and registration in a teaching hospital]. Rev Bras Enferm 58: 325-329.

8. FMOH (2011) Nursing care practice standards, Reference manual for nurses and health care managers in Ethiopia. Addis Ababa, Ethiopia.

9. Fisseha Hagos, Fessehaye Alemseged, Fikadu Balcha, Semarya Berhe, Alemseged Aregay (2014) Application of Nursing Process and Its Affecting Factors among Nurses Working in Mekelle Zone Hospitals, Northern Ethiopia," Nurs Res Pract 2014: 9.

10. Lee TT (2005) Nursing diagnoses: factors affecting their use in charting standardized care plans. J Clin Nurs 14: 640-647.

11. Florence O Adeyemo, Adenike A A E Olaogun (2013) Factors Affecting the Use Of Nursing Process In Health Institutions In Ogbomoso Town, Oyo State.

12. OGBUOKIRI, Grace Udochi (2011) Challenges facing nursing in Nigeria award winning essay. School of Nursing, Ahmadu Bello University Teaching Hospital, Zaria, Kaduna State.

13. Asratie M (2011) Assessment on factors affecting implementation of nursing process among nurses in selected governmental hospitals, Addis Ababa, Ethiopia.

14. Jansson I, Bahtsevani C, Pilhammar-Andersson E, Forsberg A (2010) Factors and Conditions that Influence the Implementation of Standardized Nursing Care Plans. Open Nurs J 4: 25-34.

28

The Teaching Method and Problems of Patient Information Handling in the Nursing Education Curriculum in Bachelor Course

Mikiko Natsume[*1] and **Katusmasa OTA**[2]

1Department of Nursing College of Life and Health Sciences, Chubu University, Japan

[2]Nagoya University Graduate School of Medicine Doctor of Medical Sciences, Japan.

[*]**Corresponding author**: Mikiko Natsume, Master of nursing, Department of Nursing College of Life and Health Sciences, Chubu University, 1200 Matsumoto-cho,Kasugai,aichi, 487-8501, Japan, E-mail:nmikiko@isc.chubu.ac.jp

Abstract

Objective: The purpose of this paper is to describe the problems that arise in relation to nursing students' handling of patient information as well as the current status of students' instructions on the matter. The instructions needed to avoid these problems are also presented.

Methods: Research was conducted by giving self-report questionnaires to nursing faculty at Japanese nursing colleges as well as those directly instructing nursing practice.

Results: At present, these problems are not occurring by chance, but instead stem directly from students' low awareness of information privacy issues—suggesting that there is a need for more thorough instruction. Nursing faculty felt that the instruction they were already giving was effective for the most part in preventing most privacy problems. However, even instructions that a great number of nursing faculty members are implementing have been shown to be ineffective in some regards.At the same time, while detailed, time-consuming instruction and instruction that requires coordination with hospitals have been shown to be effective, there are few instructors who have experience carrying these out. In order to determine the appropriate features of instruction that would effectively prevent problems from occurring, a survey was again conducted on "necessary instruction". As a result, a diverse set of eighteen instruction items were identified, among them "emphasis on prohibited actions" and "implementation of review when problems occur".

Conclusion: The type of instruction deemed necessary is critical for the proper handling of patient information and includes basic content that can be applied outside of Japan as well.

Keywords: Patient information; Clinical practicum; Nursing education; Nursing teachers; Information privacy

Introduction

Privacy has been considered the "right to be left alone" however, nowadays the handling of personal information is not limited to the maintenance of confidentiality, but also includes the concept of "information privacy" [1], which includes ethical aspects related to the handling of information based on the Right to control of One's Own information. The HIPPA privacy rule [2] was enforced in the medical field in 1996, and official regulations when the patient information dealt with all medical institutions have been clarified.

The nursing student collects sensitive information of the patient in the clinical practice and records it and performs a nursing care. The literature reveals that in the course of this process, nursing students encounter a host of problems related to the handling of patient information, among them ethical issues related to privacy during information collection [3], problems with information sharing between students in academic settings [4], problems related to access to digital patient records, [5], and a lack of knowledge about patient information privacy. The American Association of Colleges of Nursing states that its baccalaureate program prepares the graduate to "uphold ethical standards related to data security, regulatory requirements, confidentiality, and clients' right to privacy" [6,7], suggesting that there is a need for education on protecting confidentiality when it comes to patient information. Hospitals must also deal with several confidentiality issues when it comes to patient information, including the sharing of that information among hospital staff [8,9] and issues related to the security of patient information given the increasing use of information technology [10]. There is therefore a need for education that fosters the capabilities needed to handle this information appropriately within basic nursing clinical practice programs. In looking specifically at the kinds of students that should be the targets of this instruction, we find that many university websites post cautions and the like related to how patient information is to be treated. Still, although many countries have instructional guidelines designed to prevent the leakage of patient information through social media sites and similar channels [11,12], a search for other types of instruction did not reveal a single specific policy. Given this situation, this indicates that nursing faculty themselves are struggling as they provide students with instruction on patient information privacy and consider the results of that education from the students' point of view [13].

	Included	Not included	Don't know
Caution regarding the location of the acquisition and handling of clients' personal information	58(100.0)	0(0.0)	0(0.0)
Explanation and consent of users related to handling of personal information	53(91.4)	5(8.6)	0(0.0)
Caution regarding accessing clients' personal information (in printed media/electronic media)	53(91.4)	3(5.2)	2(3.4)
Restrictions on copying clients' personal information (prohibition of photocopying, etc.)	56(96.6)	2(3.4)	0(0.0)
Ensuring anonymity of clients' personal information once acquired	58(100.0)	0(0.0)	0(0.0)
Preventing leakage of clients' personal information once acquired	58(100.0)	0(0.0)	0(0.0)
Caution regarding restrictions on transportation of records related to practical nursing practice during nursing studies (paper records, computers, storage media, etc.) (including data transfers), and storage locations	55(94.8)	3(5.2)	0(0.0)
Methods of handling personal information during learning activities within the university, etc. (conferences, creating papers/instructions)	53(91.4)	4(6.9)	1(1.7)
Methods of storage and destruction of records related to practical nursing practice during nursing studies upon the completion of nursing practice	51(87.9)	7(12.1)	0(0.0)

Table 1: References in clinical practice guidelines to university rules in regard to the handling of patient information during clinical nursing practice (n=58)

	Attribute	Number of participants	%
Age	30s	28	21.2
	40s	42	31.8
	over50	60	45.5
	NA	2	1.5
Gender	male	14	10.6
	female	118	89.4
Experience in teaching	under 5years	16	12.1
	5-10years	42	31.8
	over10years	73	55.3
	NA	1	0.8
Position	assistant	3	2.3
	research associate	31	23.5
	lecturer	35	26.5
	Associate professor	17	12.9
	professor	45	34.1
	NA	1	0.8

Table 2: Background of respondents (n=132).

If policies were in place regarding the content of instructions and methods for evaluation regarding the appropriate handling of patient information by student nurses, it is believed that it would be possible to include the requisite content in nursing practice. In order to achieve this, research was done in Japan with the aim of proposing necessary instruction on patient information handling to be given to students undergoing on-site nursing practice -instruction on which consensus could be reached.

Study purpose

Identify the current status of instruction on nursing students' handling of patient information and associated problems. Propose the necessary instruction for preventing these problems from occurring.

Methods

Data collection

This study was comprised of the following two self-report questionnaires .

(1) Regarding the provision or otherwise of regulations within the university related to the handling of patient information by student nurses

The following survey was implemented in order to understand the existence or otherwise of regulations regarding consistent, instructions as a university on the handling of patient information.

Scope of survey:

Heads of nursing departments or nursing faculties at all nursing universities in Japan (217 in total) (hereinafter, referred to as "nursing department heads").

Survey method:

Self-report questionnaires. Surveys were distributed by mail, with responses collected by being directly mailed back.

Contents of survey

Nine categories directly related to the practice of students out of a total of 13 categories requiring consideration when guidelines are produced, according to "Hints for the creation of guidelines regarding the handling of personal information during nursing practice" [14] issued by the Japan Association of Nursing Programs in Universities, were selected and respondents were asked to comment on whether or not references to regulations related to university instructions were included within the clinical practice guidelines.

(2) Problems experienced by individual members of nursing faculty and instructions to ensure that said problems do not occur

In order to clarify the problems experienced by individual nursing faculty members along with what instructions has been experienced to ensure that said problems do not occur, the following survey was carried out among nursing faculty directly responsible for instructions.

1) Subjects

Nursing faculty directly responsible for practice instructions, with three or more years' experience providing clinical practice instructions. These subjects were selected because they are considered to have an understanding of the state of problems and instructions. In the current study, the objective was to extract problems occurring during practice in hospitals, etc., and consequently, nursing faculty working in areas of regional and home-based care were excluded.

2) Survey procedure

Nursing department heads at all nursing universities in Japan (217 in total) were requested to distribute survey documents, with those nursing department heads who cooperated asked to distribute documents to nursing faculty fulfilling the criteria. Responses were mailed back directly by the survey subjects.

3) Survey method

(1) Selection procedure for survey items

The survey items used in this survey were extracted after semi-structured interviews with ten nursing faculty members directly responsible for clinical practice instructions, resulting in 24 problematic cases related to students' handling of patient information, along with 24 necessary instructions in order to prevent these problems from occurring . To these items were added aspects obtained from literary research, with any necessary instructions limited to those implemented by nursing faculty directly responsible for clinical practice. The results were organized into similar itemss by two researchers engaged in nursing practice studies, resulting in a total of 29 problematic cases, comprising "Caution regarding the location of the acquisition and handling of clients' personal information (4 cases)," "Ensuring anonymity of clients' personal information once acquired (5cases)," "Preventing leakage of clients' personal information once acquired (13cases)," "Caution regarding restrictions on transportation of records related to practical nursing practice during nursing studies and storage locations (1 case)," "Methods of handling personal information during learning activities within the university, etc. (conferences, creating papers/instructions) (4cases)," and "Methods of storage and destruction of records related to practical nursing practice during nursing studies upon the completion of nursing practice (2 cases)." Furthermore, in terms of any necessary instructions, a total of 27 survey instructions were extracted, covering "Thorough adherence to prohibitions (4instructions)," "Creating awareness of information privacy (3 instructions)," "Building systems to ensure management methods that do not cause problems (13instructions)," "Creation of management methods that minimize

damage if a problem occurs (4instructions)" and "Reviewing behavior when problems occur (3 instructions)."

(2) Response method

Respondents were asked to select between three responses – "experience frequently," "experience occasionally," "have never experienced" – in regard to their own experience during clinical practice instructions of the problematic cases, when student nurses handle patient information. Furthermore, they were asked whether or not they felt the problematic cases were in fact problems, using the responses "Think it is a problem," "Don't think it is a problem" and "Can't say." Furthermore, respondents were asked to provide details of any other problems they had experienced in their own words, along with whether or not they still consider them problems. In terms of any necessary instructions, they were asked whether they had experience with providing such instructions, using the two responses "Have experience" and "Have no experience," and nursing faculty with experience were further asked whether or not they felt it was effective, using the five responses "The problem stopped occurring," "The problem occurred less frequently," "The problem was made smaller," "There was no particular effect," and "Don't know." Furthermore, respondents were asked whether they considered instructions necessary, using the three responses "Consider it necessary," "Do not consider it necessary" and "Can't say."

4) Survey to confirm the instructions required to ensure that problems do not occur

In this survey, cooperating subjects were asked to comment on their experience with providing instructions, the effectiveness of instructions and the need for instructions in regard to instructions considered necessary, with the results used in order to implement a second survey on the need for instructions. While this paper does not propose specific guidelines, items deemed necessary by 51% or more of respondents were considered "necessary instruction items" in order to pinpoint potentially critical items.

Data analysis

The responses obtained were subjected to frequency analysis using SPSSVer18.0 as well as disparity verification (where $p \leq 0.05$) based on the attributes of subjects (educational experience). The free answer areas were qualitatively compiled.

Survey period

The survey was conducted from November 2015 to February 2016.

Ethical considerations

When requesting permission to conduct the survey, the subjects received a written explanation of privacy protection and ethical considerations. The explanation included the maintenance of confidentiality of data collected, the fact that the data and contacts would not be used outside the purposes of the study, the maintenance of anonymity in terms both university surveys and unidentified surveys, and the fact that the contact details, names and other responses provided in order to facilitate repeat surveys would be separately stored in such a way that respondents could not be identified. Before beginning this research, we received approval from the Nagoya University School of Medicine Ethics Committee regarding the ethical considerations related to this research.

Results

The survey results below address three key points with regards to whether universities issue written clinical practice guidelines or the like in order to regulate the handing of patient information throughout the institution: (1) Whether or not Clinical Nursing Practice Guidelines include reference to rule as university on the handling of patient information, (2) Problems that arise when nursing students handle patient information and the current status of instruction from nursing faculty, and (3) Necessary instruction to prevent problems. Hereinafter categories are marked "___," while cases and instructions are marked '___.'

1. Whether or not Clinical Nursing Practice Guidelines include reference to rule as university on the handling of patient information

A total of 217 subjects were asked to cooperate with the survey, of which responses were received from 58 (response rate 26.7%). The results are shown in Table 1. These indicate that in all categories, 85% or more of universities make reference to university regulations in their clinical practice guidelines. Even in categories with lower numbers of universities making reference to regulations, 87.9% of respondents noted "Methods of storage and destruction of records related to practical nursing practice during nursing studies upon the completion of nursing practice".

2. Problems that arise when nursing students handle patient information and the current status of instruction from nursing faculty

Cooperation was obtained from 49 colleges, with 394 questionnaires distributed and 132 responses obtained (response rate 33.5%). Respondents' attributes are shown in Table 2. The majority of respondents were aged 50 or above (45.5%), female (89.4%), had 10 years or more teaching experience (55.3%), and were professors (34.1%).

1) Problems related to the proper handling of patient information

Table 3 indicates experience with potential problem items.

Nursing faculty reported 14 of the items have been experienced by at least 51%, with 80% or more experiencing (1) the disclosure of information that could identify individuals, including actual names, at conferences with the practicum groups nursing practice (which falls under "methods of handling personal information during learning activities within the university, etc. (conferences, creating papers/ instructions)" and (2) the disclosure of highly sensitive personal information, including life history and lifestyle conditions, at conferences with the practicum group. Of the problematic case given, 25 were seen as problems by at least 51% of nursing faculty.

However, when nursing faculty were asked whether they thought these problematic cases were actually problems, many of them said that they included cases that they had experienced but did not consider problematic.

2) Instructions given to prevent problems

Responses related to experience in implementing instructions, its effectiveness and the necessity for such instructions when asked about instructions implemented to avoid problems are shown in Table 4. In terms of the effectiveness of instructions, "Instructions were effective" is considered indicated by the total number who responded "The problem stopped occurring," "The problem occurred less frequently" and "The problem was made smaller."

At least 51% of nursing faculty reported experience implementing 18 of the instruction items, and the majority felt that 15 of those items were effective. Although at least 51% of nursing faculty reported implementing the other three ('nursing faculty should demonstrate the appropriate handling of students' personal information in order to ensure students gain an awareness of the appropriate way to handle personal information', 'students are instructed to write their own name on all notes and nursing practice sheets', and 'if records of nursing practices or pamphlets for patient education are created using electronic media, students are instructed to take care in regard to the storage of media'), less than 51% felt they were effective.

In addition, there were seven items where less than 51% of nursing faculty reported implementing instruction, yet the majority felt that such instruction was effective. These included 'request that hospital staff demonstrate correct handling of patients' personal information (management of records, etc.) in order to ensure students gain an awareness of the appropriate way to handle personal information' and 'notebooks are coil-bound and covered with a white cover to prevent loss'.

3. Necessary instruction to prevent problems

There were 22 instruction items that least 51% of nursing faculty indicated as necessary to prevent problems.

Second survey was implemented among cooperating subjects to establish appropriateness in regard to instructions considered necessary in order to prevent problems from occurring. In this second survey, 45 questionnaires were distributed and 41 responses obtained (response rate 91.1%). Instruction was deemed necessary for 18 items on the second survey. Table 5 shows the results. At least 51% of nursing faculty reported experience implementing instruction in 17 of the 18 items.

Discussion

Current problems arising with nursing students handling patient information

At least 51% of nursing faculty reported experience with 14 case items. These included not only accidents and situations where students were simply not careful, but a good number of incidents that occurred because students lacked proper awareness about how patient information had to be handled—such as 'records of nursing practice were created in a public place (on a train or in a restaurant, etc.' and 'actual name, profession, age, or other information making it possible to identify individuals was recorded on memos'. It has been said that this is a result of nursing faculty stressing these issues throughout the curriculum—not just during nursing practice, but during various lecturing and teaching opportunities as well [15]. It would seem that students need to be trained to handle patient information not only during nursing practice, but also need to be made aware of it during their academic courses, practice exercises, and the like.

Among the items that at least 51% of nursing faculty had experienced and at least 80% considered problems were 'records of nursing practice were forgotten or dropped (including those in electronic format)' and 'medical records or records of nursing practice were left open on a desk such that patient information was visible'—which fall under the category of "preventing leakage of clients' personal information once acquired". Although issues like these are covered in the clinical practice guidelines and similar codes at all universities, the survey results indicate that there is a need for detailed and thorough instruction from nursing faculty to prevent them from occurring.

Of the items indicating potential issues with handling patient information, there were three that many (though less than 51% of) nursing faculty felt were in fact problems. Two of these were 'information that can identify individuals, including actual names, etc., was disclosed at conferences with the practicum group' and 'highly sensitive personal information, including life history and lifestyle conditions, was disclosed at conferences with the practicum group'—both of which fall under "methods of handling personal information during learning activities within the university, etc. (conferences, creating papers/instructions)". Over 51% of nursing faculty had experienced these three items, indicating that students were sharing the information they had collected from patients as they participated in joint learning activities within their practicum groups. However, there are studies that show that patients themselves want their personal information shared only with the people directly involved in their lives [16], making it entirely possible that they would not agree to students not directly involved in their care having access to it. The National Student Nurses' Association writes, "in discussing client cases in the academic setting, care must be taken to avoid breeching confidentiality and violating HIPAA regulations; this includes appropriate selection of the time and place of discussion, people attending the discussion, and omitting data that is not necessary to the purpose of the discussion or that discloses the client's personal identity [17], which points to a need to creatively address the ways in which information on patients other than one's own is provided to others.

Current instruction aimed at preventing problems

It is clear that instruction being carried out on the university level in Japan today is based in regulations.

In addition, most of the nursing faculty who give this instruction feel that much of it is effective.

At the same time, at least 51% of nursing faculty surveyed said that although they issued instructions to the effect that (1) nursing faculty should demonstrate the appropriate handling of students' personal information in order to ensure students gain an awareness of the appropriate way to handle personal information, (2) students are instructed to write their own name on all notes and nursing practice sheets, and (3) if records of nursing practices or pamphlets for patient education are created using electronic media, students are instructed not to store them on their computers, less than half thought that these approaches were effective. It may be that awareness is low regarding the effectiveness of these instruction items because they are difficult to implement thoroughly and sufficiently communicate to students. However, it is most likely necessary to continue teaching them.

In the opposite category were seven instruction items that less than 51% of nursing faculty reported implementing, though a majority felt they were effective. Four of them (including 'notebooks are coil-bound and covered with a white cover to prevent loss', 'students are instructed to confirm the whereabouts of their records of nursing practice sheets at the beginning and end of each nursing practice session, based on a checklist', and 'nursing faculty check lockers and changing rooms to ensure that no records of nursing practices etc. have been left behind, after students go home') require tremendously detailed and time-consuming instruction, which is probably why this instruction is not being carried out. The other three, which included 'request that hospital staff demonstrate correct handling of patients' personal information (management of records, etc.) in order to ensure students gain an awareness of the appropriate way to handle personal information' and 'request that hospital staff not only provide nursing care, but also give instructions in the handling of patient information', require coordination with hospitals, suggesting that these instruction items are difficult to implement as well. Still, at least 51% of respondents indicated that these forms of instruction were needed (Table 3).

	potentially problematic case	Experience or otherwise regarding the issue		Considered to be a problem or not?		
		Never	Experienced	Dont consider it a problem	Consider it a problem	Cant say either way
Caution regarding the location of the acquisition and handling of clients personal information	Collection from patient or medical records of information not required for nursing purposes	36.4	61.4	5.3	60.6	28
	Viewing of information in medical records related to patients other than the student is treating	69.7	28.8	10.6	65.2	18.9
	The student communicates information to a patient that he/she did not acquire directly from the patient, but rather from his/her medical records	63.3	33.3	12.9	75	7.6
	An ID or password used to browse electronic medical records has been shared between students	75	22.7	9.8	68.2	17.4

Ensuring anonymity of clients personal information once acquired	Name of hospital and ward on which practical nursing practice undertaken was recorded in the records of nursing practice	30.3	67.5	18.9	65.9	10.6
	Name of scheduled transfer hospital or hospital to which transfer occurred was recorded in the records of nursing practice	67.4	30.3	9.8	74.2	7.6
	Actual age, profession or other information making it possible to identify individuals was recorded in the records of nursing practice	28	68.9	11.4	58.3	25
	Actual name, profession, actual age, or other information making it possible to identify individuals was recorded on memos	0.8	74.3	7.6	68.2	16.7
	Patient's initials were recorded in the records of nursing practice	28.8	67.4	15.2	59.1	20.5
Preventing leakage of clients personal information once acquired	File used to store the records of nursing practice was transparent, allowing recorded contents to be seen through the cover	66.7	31	13.6	70.5	9.8
	Records of nursing practice were forgotten or dropped (including those in electronic format)	25	73.5	3.8	92.4	0
	Records were stolen as a result of theft from a parked car, etc	91.7	6.8	8.3	83.3	1.5
	A memo containing patient information was dropped	36.4	62.1	3	91.7	0
	Original records of nursing practice containing patient information were left in the photocopier	38.6	59.8	3.8	90.2	0
	Medical records or records of nursing practice were left open on a desk such that patient information was visible	37.1	60.6	6.1	84.8	5.3
	Conversations regarding nursing practice was held in a public place (on a train, etc.)	50	47.7	3	89.4	3.8
	Records of nursing practice were created in a public place (on a train or in a restaurant, etc.)	68.9	58.8	6.8	86.4	3.8
	Student told his/her own family information that the patient did not wish to be known	81.1	14.4	6.8	87.9	1.5
	Information about nursing practice was uploaded on a blog or social networking service, etc.	64.4	33.3	6.1	89.4	0.8
	The patient's family was told information that the patient him/herself did not wish to be communicated	92.4	5.3	6.8	81.1	5.3
	A patient was told information about another patient	87.1	12.1	6.8	81.1	8.3
	Patient information was communicated to a visitor	90.2	9.1	8.3	75.8	11.4

Table 3: Experience or otherwise regarding the issues (n=132%).

They require that nursing faculty maintain close communication and collaboration with the nurses who carry out nursing practice instruction at hospitals, which in turn suggests that nursing faculty must be the ones to reach out [18]. In short, nursing faculty must take the initiative to ensure that communication with nursing practice hospitals is robust enough to support the implementation of such instruction.

Instructions agreed upon as necessary

The first survey showed 22 items for which instruction was necessary in order to prevent problems from occurring, while consensus was reached about the necessity of all but four (18 items) in the second survey. Of the 18 items identified as necessary instructions, at least 51% of nursing faculty reported having experience with 17 of them. This leads us to determine that high-priority instruction items are also practical in terms of their ability to be taught. There was only one item for which there was consensus regarding their necessity but which were being implemented by less than 51% of nursing faculty, and it was 'Students are instructed that if records of nursing practices are created using electronic media, they should confirm deletion at the end of nursing practice'. Examples were found of American universities posting detailed warnings regarding digital records on their websites, such as "students must encrypt portable devices (e.g. laptops and USB drives, etc.) used to store patient or individual research data, and encrypt data files with Protected Health Information (PHI) if stored on a portable device that is not encrypted [19]. Although many nursing faculty feel that it is necessary for students to delete their digital records once their nursing practice is complete, it seems there is still a need for more specific, detailed instructions to this effect in cases were those digital records are being created.

The 18 necessary instruction items spanned all categories—Thorough adherence to prohibitions, Creating awareness of information privacy, Building systems to ensure management methods that do not cause problems, Creation of management methods that minimize damage if a problem occurs, and Reviewing behavior when problems occur—and indicate the need for diverse instructional approaches that address information privacy both before and after problems arise.

	Details of instructions	Experience (%)			Need for instructions		
		Experience (proportion who said instructions were effective)	No experience		Required	Not required	Can't say
Thorough adherence to prohibitions	Give an explanation, based on completed documents, of prohibited actions in regard to handling patient information	92.4	(57.4)	6.8	98.5	0.0	1.5
	Give instructions, using practical examples, of specific cases of handling patient information in which problems have arisen	91.7	(65.3)	8.3	97.0	0.8	2.3
	Give instructions regarding prohibited actions in regard to handling patient information, ensuring that the reasons can be understood	92.4	(61.4)	6.8	97.7	0.8	1.5
	Give instructions regarding the fact that information regarding nursing practice must not be disclosed on blogs or social networking services	81.8	(54.6)	18.2	97.7	0.0	2.3
Creating awareness of information privacy	Request that hospital staff demonstrate correct handling of patients' personal information (management of records, etc.) in order to ensure students gain an awareness of the appropriate way to handle personal information	24.2	(75.0)	74.2	60.6	7.6	31.1
	Request that hospital staff not only provide nursing care, but also give instructions in the handling of patient information	37.9	(68.0)	61.4	62.1	10.6	27.3
	Nursing faculty should demonstrate the appropriate handling of students' personal information in order to ensure students gain an awareness of the appropriate way to handle personal information	69.7	(46.8)	28.0	81.1	1.5	16.7
Building systems to ensure management methods that do not cause problems	Students are instructed to use notebooks for note-taking that cannot have single pages torn out of them	90.2	(69.8)	8.3	94.7	1.5	3.0
	Notebooks are coil-bound and covered with a white cover to prevent loss	37.9	(80.0)	59.8	43.9	12.1	43.9
	Students are instructed to write their own name on all notes and nursing practice sheets	69.7	(50.0)	28.0	68.9	12.9	18.2
	Students are instructed to confirm the whereabouts of their records of nursing practice sheets at the beginning and end of each nursing practice session, based on a checklist	22.0	(82.7)	76.5	40.9	9.8	47.7

Category	Item					
	Students are instructed to keep all records of nursing practice sheets together in a file and keep the file in a paper bag, etc.	90.2	(71.6)	8.3	96.2	0.0	3.8
	If records of nursing practices or pamphlets for patient education are created using electronic media, students are instructed not to store them on their computers	58.3	(55.9)	40.2	76.5	6.8	15.9
	Notes and conference records are collected at the end of nursing practice by nurse faculty	53.0	(61.3)	45.5	53.8	20.5	25.8
	Students are instructed to record patients using numbers, which cannot be traced to their names	85.6	(69.0)	13.6	88.6	3.0	7.6
	Students are instructed to record "50s" or "60s" rather than the actual age of patients	68.9	(67.0)	31.1	65.9	6.8	27.3
	If records of nursing practices or pamphlets for patient education are created using electronic media, students are instructed to take care in regard to the storage of media	70.5	(49.5)	28.0	78.8	7.6	12.1
	In conferences, etc., patient names are encoded to ensure that identification is not possible before being published	43.9	(65.6)	53.8	41.7	31.8	25.8
	Students are instructed that if records of nursing practices are created using electronic media, they should confirm deletion at the end of nursing practice	47.7	(50.8)	50.0	68.9	12.9	18.2
	Nursing faculty check lockers and changing rooms to ensure that no records of nursing practices etc. have been left behind, after students go home	28.8	(60.5)	70.5	30.3	42.4	26.5
Creation of management methods that minimize damage if a problem occurs	When copying records of nursing practices, students are instructed to use photocopiers available only to hospital staff	48.5	(70.3)	47.0	59.1	15.9	22.7
	When copying records of nursing practices, students are instructed to confirm in pairs that no original documents have been left behind	12.9	(21.2)	82.6	38.6	22.0	35.6
	Students are instructed not to record any information that enables patient identification in notes	90.2	(65.5)	7.6	86.4	0.0	13.6
	Students are instructed not to use clear-covered files to store records	61.4	(70.4)	37.1	81.8	3.0	15.2
Reviewing behaviour when problems occur	If records are left behind, etc., the student is contacted immediately and made to understand the seriousness of his/her actions	72.7	(71.9)	26.5	99.2	0.0	0.8
	If a problem occurs, a member of the nursing faculty works with the student to review the cause, etc., and provide instructions	75.0	(76.8)	25.0	97.7	0.0	2.3
	Every time a problem occurs, students are cautioned and given instructions to ensure that he/she learns the correct behavior	81.8	(68.5)	17.4	98.5	0.8	0.8

Table 4: Experience in regard to instructions, its effectiveness n=132%.

*In terms of the effectiveness of instructions, "Instructions were effective" is the total number who responded "The problem stopped occurring," "The problem occurred less frequently" and "The problem was made smaller."

		need for instruction (n=41)%		
	Details of instructions	Required	Not required	Can't say
Thorough adherence to prohibitions	Give an explanation, based on completed documents, of prohibited actions in regard to handling patient information	100	0	0

Give instructions, using practical examples, of specific cases of handling patient information in which problems have arisen	100	0	0
Give instructions regarding prohibited actions in regard to handling patient information, ensuring that the reasons can be understood	100	0	0
Give instructions regarding the fact that information regarding nursing practice must not be disclosed on	100	0	0

	blogs or social networking services			
Creating awareness of information privacy	Request that hospital staff demonstrate correct handling of patients' personal information (management of records, etc.) in order to ensure students gain an awareness of the appropriate way to handle personal information	46.3	19.5	34.1
	Request that hospital staff not only provide nursing care, but also give instructions in the handling of patient information	48.8	29.3	22
	Nursing faculty should demonstrate the appropriate handling of students' personal information in order to ensure students gain an awareness of the appropriate way to handle personal information	75.6	17.1	7.3
Building systems to ensure management methods that do not cause problems	Students are instructed to use notebooks for note-taking that cannot have single pages torn out of them	92.7	0	7.3
	Notebooks are coil-bound and covered with a white cover to prevent loss	24.4	24.4	51.2
	Students are instructed to write their own name on all notes and nursing practice sheets	68.3	9.8	22
	Students are instructed to confirm the whereabouts of their records of nursing practice sheets at the beginning and end of each nursing practice session, based on a checklist	14.6	34.1	48.8
	Students are instructed to keep all records of nursing practice sheets together in a file and keep the file in a paper bag, etc.	100	0	0
	If records of nursing practices or pamphlets for patient education are created using electronic media, students are instructed not to store them on their computers	73.2	4.9	22
	Notes and conference records are collected at the end of nursing practice by nurse faculty	34.1	26.8	39
	Students are instructed to record patients using numbers, which cannot be traced to their names	95.1	0	4.9

	Students are instructed to record "50s" or "60s" rather than the actual age of patients	65.9	12.2	22
	If records of nursing practices or pamphlets for patient education are created using electronic media, students are instructed to take care in regard to the storage of media	85.4	2.4	12.2
	In conferences, etc., patient names are encoded to ensure that identification is not possible before being published	22	41.5	36.6
	Students are instructed that if records of nursing practices are created using electronic media, they should confirm deletion at the end of nursing practice	78	2.4	19.5
	Nursing faculty check lockers and changing rooms to ensure that no records of nursing practices etc. have been left behind, after students go home	14.6	48.8	36.6
Creation of management methods that minimize damage if a problem occurs	When copying records of nursing practices, students are instructed to use photocopiers available only to hospital staff	31.7	17.1	43.9
	When copying records of nursing practices, students are instructed to confirm in pairs that no original documents have been left behind	17.1	19.5	56.1
	Students are instructed not to record any information that enables patient identification in notes	97.6	0	2.4
	Students are instructed not to use clear-covered files to store records	82.9	4.9	12.2
Reviewing behaviour when problems occur	If records are left behind, etc., the student is contacted immediately and made to understand the seriousness of his/her actions	97.6	0	2.4
	If a problem occurs, a member of the nursing faculty works with the student to review the cause, etc., and provide instructions	92.7	0	7.3
	Every time a problem occurs, students are cautioned and given instructions to ensure that	95.1	2.4	2.4

	he/she learns the correct behavior			

Table 5: Need for instructions (second survey)%.

Conclusion

As a result of this survey, it has become clear that when student nurses handle patient information during clinical practice, a range of problems occur in areas including "Preventing leakage of clients' personal information once acquired" and "Ensuring anonymity of clients' personal information once acquired" Moreover, in order to prevent these problems, a total of 18 instructions of required instructions were extracted, ranging from "Thorough adherence to prohibitions" through to "Reviewing behavior when problems occur."

Limitation

As a result of this study, problems occurring when student nurses handle information, along with the instructions required to prevent them from happening, were comprehensively studied. As the scope of the study was limited, however, it is not possible to state that its results cover all the required instructions. Furthermore, multiple factors contribute to the effectiveness of instructions, making it difficult to focus on a single factor when discussing effectiveness.

Nursing practice at nursing colleges takes many forms in different countries, and cannot be treated as a general category. At the same time, information privacy concepts are specified in the eight OECD Privacy Principles [20], which surely include content that can be incorporated into instructions given in any country.

Acknowledgement

The authors would like to thank all the department heads and nursing faculty at the nursing universities cooperating with this survey.

References

1. Bélanger F, Crossler R.E (2011)Privacy in the digital age: a review of information privacy researchin information systems, MIS Quarterly 35: 1017-1041.

2. U.S. Department of Health & Human Services (1996) Health Information Privacy

3. Reis Pessalacia, Juliana Dias, Tavares et al (2013) Perception of nursing students about behaviors and ethical aspects involved in patient data collectionInvestigation and Education 31:210-217.

4. MatlakalaMC,MokoenaJD (2011) Student nurse's views regarding disclosure of patient's confidential information, South Africa family Practice 53:481-487.

5. Luke Davis, Jennifer. A. Domm , Michel.R Konikoff (1999) Attitudes of First-year Medical Students toward the Confidentiality of Computerized Patient Records, Journal of American informatics Association 6:55-60.

6. Kapborg ID, Berterö CM (2009)Swedish student nurses' knowledge of health statutes: a descriptive survey, International nursing review 56 : 222-229.

7. American association of college of nursing (2008)The Essentials of Baccalaureate Education for Professional Nursing Practice:19

8. Claire McGowan(2012)Patient's Confidentiality, Clinical care nurse32:61-65

9. Nahid Dehghan Nayeri, Mohammad Aghajani(2010) Patients' privacy and satisfaction in the emergency department: A descriptive analytical study. Nursing ethics 17:167-177

10. Elizabeth J (2008) Ethical Issues and electronic health records. The Health Care Manager 2:165-176.

11. National Student Nurses Association. (n.d.) Recommendations for: Social media usage and maintaining privacy, confidentiality and professionalism.

12. Royal College of Nursing (2009) Legal advice for RCN members using the internet.

13. Mikiko NATSUME, KatsumasaOTA (2013)Problems in nursing students' handling of patient information in clinical practicums, and instruction methods to prevent them, Japanese Journal of Nursing and Health Sciences11:1-9. (in Japanese)

14. Japan Association of Nursing Programs in Universities (2005) For the purpose of creating guidelines regarding the handling of personal information during practical clinical practice in nursing. in Japanese

15. Paige W, Isakson J, Walden D (2005) HIPPA and Nursing Education-How to Teach in a paranoid Health Care Environment, Journal of Nursing Education 44:489-492.

16. Katsumasa OTA (2007) Study on Information Sharing of Patient's Information in Nursing considering Information Privacy 2003-2005. Grant-in-Aid for Scientific Research(C) Results of research report.

17. National students nurse association (2009) Code of Ethics: Part IICode of Academic and Clinical Conductand Interpretive Statements (in Japanese).

18. Satoko YAMADA, Katsumasa OTA(2012) Essentialroles of clinical nurse instructors in Japan: A Delphi study. Nursing and HealthSciences14:229-237

19. Columbia university, Confidentiality, Electronic Media,& Protected Patient Information

20. OECD (2013) Flows of Personal Data Guidelines on the Protection of Privacy and Transborder Flows of Personal Data.

29

Unveiling the Meanings of Coronary Artery Disease for Menopausal Women: A Descriptive Study

Líscia Divana Carvalho Silva[1*] and Marli Villela Mamede[2]

Universidade Federal do Maranhão. São Luís, MA, Brazil

*Corresponding author: Rua Parnaíba, 1 Apt. 700 - Casa do Morro, Torre Marcos Regadas, CEP: 65075-839. São Luís, MA, Brazil, E-mail: liscia@elointernet.com.br

Abstract

Objective: To understand the meaning attributed by menopausal women to coronary artery disease.

Method: A descriptive and exploratory study of qualitative - quantitative approach, carried out between June and August 2013 in the cardiology service in north eastern Maranhão - Brazil. It was used the symbolic interactionism and the method of content analysis. In the quantitative phase, the data collection instrument was the Menopause Rating Scale with forty (40) women; from these 40 women, twenty five (25) took part in the qualitative phase.

Results: The coronary artery disease is described as a serious and incurable manifestation of multifactorial nature, with intense symptoms, feelings and emotions (rapid heartbeat, palpitations, fatigue, pain, disability, dependence).

Discussion: A change is revealed in their daily lives, what turns them into fragile, insecure women. A conflict between the desirable world and the real world, endowed with meaning and significance.

Conclusion: Heart disease is responsible for the biggest changes in their lives, a threat to their physical and emotional integrity, placing them in the sick role.

Keywords: Climacteric; Menopause; Coronary disease

Introduction

In the Brazilian population, women are more numerous and have higher life expectancy. From a total of 195.2 million people, 100.5 million (51.5%) are women, a higher number than the 94.7 million men (48.5%). The female gender is not only more expressive; there are 5.8 million more women; they are also in older age groups. Women predominate among the population above 30 years old, unlike men, who stand out in the younger segments of the population [1].

Cardiovascular disease remain the main cause of women's morbidity and mortality in many countries, especially among those above 50 years of age and, with an increasing elderly population, it is conceivable that it will continue to remain as the main cause of morbidity and mortality [2]. In this age group there are more deaths of women from cardiovascular disease (41.3%) than the next seven causes of death together, a risk six times greater of dying from the disease than from breast cancer. Recent data from the American Heart Association (AHA) show that only 46% of women are aware of this fact. Studies suggest that, when receiving therapy with estrogen and progestogen, post-menopause women has an increased risk of coronary artery disease (CAD), while others warn that the risk is no longer present when women start hormone replacement right after the menopause [3].

The increased risk of CAD in women over the age of 50 appears to be related to menopause because of the consequent estrogen deprivation, since the advantages related to cardioprotection offered by estrogens gradually cease in the climacteric [4]. However, the relationship between menopause and risk factor for CAD is still unclear. The high prevalence of hypertension, hyperglycemia and endothelial dysfunction in postmenopausal women may be related to obesity and not only to menopause [5].

The hospital mortality rate of the DAC is higher in women; they have twice the chance of death, have narrower lumens of the coronary artery and less collateral circulation when compared to men, which can lead to an increase in ischemia, especially during actions that require effort or stress [6]. Such evidence has caused a great worldwide interest in understanding how heart disease is present in the female population. Increasingly, studies are echoing this reality and trying to approach the way men and women experience and feel their illness as a means to improve the efficiency in the fight against diseases and especially against the CAD [7].

The answer to the question: "What meaning climacteric women attribute to coronary artery disease?" was the challenge of this research, with the assumption that not always the CAD-related symptoms are perceived by women as a sign of the disease, but it is often confused with the climacteric, so the symptoms is often undervalued by women themselves. The aim of the study was to understand the meaning assigned by menopausal women with coronary artery disease by analyzing the relationship they establish when experiencing these episodes: climacteric and CAD.

Method

A study conducted at the University Hospital of the Federal University of Maranhão (HUUFMA), an agency of the federal government, from the city of São Luís - Maranhão, Brazil, which operates in the areas of care, teaching, research and extension in the area of health and the like; it is a state reference for highly complex procedures in the cardiovascular area. Study participants were women seen in HUUFMA Cardiology Clinic between June and August 2013, aged between 45 and 65 years, referencing climacteric symptoms, with CAD confirmed by examination of coronary arteriography. Confirmation of climacteric symptoms was made by applying the instrument Menopause Rating Scale – MRS [8]. The participants were also investigated about their menopausal status and history of depression.

Forty women were identified with climacteric symptoms according to MRS; three of which (03) were excluded from the study because they had been previously submitted to oophorectomy, and five (05) because they have undergone hysterectomy. It was also considered as an exclusion criterion women with speech difficulties, mental disorders, those submitted to oophorectomy and hysterectomy; hormone replacement therapy users (HRT) in the last five years; and those who have not identified any climacteric symptoms in MRS scale.

The study was conducted in two phases. In the first one, a quantitative and recruitment phase, forty women (40) participated, when it was investigated the menopausal status and history of depression. The second one, a qualitative phase, which was conducted through focus groups, there were twenty five (25) participants of the first phase. It was used as an eligibility criterion for the second phase the following: the women who had participated in the first phase were randomly contacted by phone and invited to participate in focus groups to continue the research. The determination of this quantity was given by the data saturation criterion and the satisfactory service to the proposed objectives. Focus groups took place in the same sector of the hospital at a time and date previously scheduled. Six (06) sessions of the focus group were performed and the central theme for them was directed to understand what women know about perimenopause/menopause and CAD, seeking the meanings that they construct in relation to heart disease and his own life.

For the analysis and interpretation of the qualitative data, it was used the symbolic interactionism [9] supported by the Bardin [10] content analysis method. The use of interactional perspective aimed to apprehend behaviors, feelings and expectations in the perception of the dynamic interactive processes among women experiencing CAD; how the environment, other people and the social context, endowed with value and meaning, revealing the meanings women attach to the situation they experience. The project was submitted for the consideration of the Ethics in Research Committee of the Ribeirão Preto Nursing School of the University of São Paulo, having received an opinion under number 293900.

Results

Summarizing the sociodemographic characteristics of the participants, they were women with a mean age of 58 years, with a stable union, low education, housekeepers, Catholics, the average age of menarche was 13 years and the menopause age was 45 years old; they had no more than three abortions and ten children, and only one used HRT for more than five years.

The climacteric symptoms most often reported were, according to the MRS scale, anxiety, heart complaints, irritability, muscle and joint problems, shortness of breath, sweating, hot flashes, physical and mental exhaustion, sleep problems, depressed mood, sexual and bladder problems, as well as vaginal dryness. Analyzing the answers to the MRS and the intensity of the symptoms, it is observed that in descending order there were the muscle and joint problems, followed by anxiety, uneasiness of the heart, physical and mental exhaustion, irritability and shortness of breath, sweating, hot flashes, depressed mood, sleep problems, sexual problems, bladder problems, and, the less intense, vaginal dryness. It was verified that despite that the muscle and joint problems were not the most frequent symptom when analyzed by the intensity (score), they were considered as the most intense by most participants (Table 1).

Symptoms	Frequency n=40	Percentage	Score	Average score
1. Shortness of breath, sweating, hot flashes	35	87	22.8	0. 57
2. Malaise heart	38	95	25.6	0.64
3. Sleep problems	34	85	19.7	0.49
4. Depressive mood	32	80	21.9	0.55
5.Irritability	38	95	23.1	0.58
6. Anxiety	39	97	26.2	0.65
7. Physical and mental exhaustion	35	87	24.1	0.6
8. Sexual problems	30	75	18.5	0.46
9. Bladder problems	20	50	11.6	0.29
10. Vaginal dryness	15	37	6.7	0.17

| 11 Muscle and joint problems | 36 | 90 | 26.4 | 0.66 |

Table 1: Frequency, percentage, score and average score of climacteric symptoms in women in the Cardiology Clinic of the University Hospital of UFMA. Sao Luis - MA, 2013, Menopause Rating Scale (MRS).

With regard to qualitative data, in order to understand the significance of CAD for climacteric women, four categories were identified: The first category was "serious and incurable problem"; the second category "the trigger process of CAD", with the following subcategories: "heredity and emotional changes" and "diet, hypertension, diabetes, smoking and physical inactivity"; the third category was "significant changes in coping with the disease", which have as a subcategory "lifestyle changes"; the fourth category was "fragility".

a) A serious, incurable problem

Finding the seriousness of the problem and the high value added to the chronicity and severity of CAD has proven to be, in many cases, one of the most difficult times of their lives. It meant therefore a serious and incurable problem that shook their physical and emotional conditions, as reported:

- It is very bad. It is an incurable disease. I say so because it has no cure, it is very bad. It is not easy, if you do not have a medicine to cure it, heal it, then we depend on it all the time. All my time I depend on the medicine. I am still depending on the medicine for blood pressure, cholesterol, diabetes and heart - the four, all the time (P25).

b) The DAC triggering process

- Heredity and emotional changes

Women identify within their subjective reality signs of the origin of their CAD episode, among which they highlight heredity and emotional stress, classifying them as important components that triggers this disease, as reported:

- In my family this heart problem is hereditary. My father died of heart problem, as well as my grandmother, my aunt and my sister. I have an 11 year old nephew who makes treatment; my sister has died one year ago from heart problem, two months after she had a baby. In my family it is hereditary (P21).
- I worried a lot about my son. He went to the street; I did not know what time he would come, I stayed awake till one, two hours in the morning. My mother always said, 'You should want to be a child, but should not want to be a mother' ...I think that all this stirred my heart, which gave this heart problem. I think it's when you have a very large family problem (P3).

In the speaking of some women, it is evident the multifactorial nature involved, such as genetics, lifestyle and environmental conditions. It was perceived that while identifying changes in their emotional condition as responsible for the ACD episode, women announced different positions for this marker, connecting and taking sometimes a position that this was the cause of the ACD and in another as the very symptom of the disease, as suggested by the following depositions:

- My sister, my problem is nervous. I cannot be nervous because I get accelerated; I feel a burning sensation in the chest, feel that thing tighten me here (in the chest); I have to cry out for it to get out. If someone gives me bad news, I get stressed. I have to cry out for it to get out (P13).
- I'm nervous, but I find it is caused by my heart. I did two catheterization and one angioplasty. It is a very serious problem, we live in a bad expectation all the time, we are never quiet (P24).

Besides heredity and emotional stress, women reported the existence of other causative factors of CAD such as diet, hypertension, diabetes, smoking and physical inactivity, which shows that, for them, the disease brings with it a multifactorial nature and that developing CAD can be seen as part of a process:

- For me I think that the main cause of heart problems is cholesterol and also some family problems that we have. (P2).
- For me, heart trouble is because of high blood pressure and these foods of today, which have too much fat, many things that formerly we did not have; now we have so much trouble that it helped a lot in these diseases, and also a very thick blood...I think a clot is formed in the arteries, in the passages, the thick blood. (P3)

However, in a tireless attempt to reconcile the performance of their roles and the social responsibilities, the experience has shown the recurrence of the symptoms of CAD even when following appropriate treatment, as described as follows:

- I felt a pain here (in the back). I think it was no back problem; it was already a heart problem (P7).
- I feel very tired. When I walk a lot, climb a hill, I have to stop in the middle of the slope to rest to be able to go ahead. That strong palpitation, a strong beat, so quickly, I feel it from time to time, not so much (P19).

Tachycardia, palpitations, fatigue and especially chest pain and back pain were the most reported symptoms besides other less common symptoms reported such as dizziness and pain in the left arm.

c) Significant changes in coping with the disease

- Change in lifestyle

- The changes happen from beliefs and values, which are built and resized. The change of some habits precedes a process of awareness that can transform not only the person, in a narrower sense, but the family, the community, the society, thus helping to promote a healthier life, as the psychological meanings are also social meanings. The findings showed that for women, living healthily inevitably refers to the past, which is expressed through the memories of a way of life that they had before the disease. A normal life without restrictions, limitations and care is confronted with a conscious and permanent reality of the seriousness of being a carrier of CAD. The women's report indicates changes in lifestyle, especially those related to diet:
- Another thing I liked was fried food. I stopped eating fried food; I had to eliminate this frying stuff. The flour, frying, I quit for my own well; drinking too (P21).

d) Fragility

What comes to anchor the meaning of CAD in these women's life seems to be a deep sense of helplessness and vulnerability due to the disease process, which is represented as something that limits life itself, as described:

At that stage now, things are getting more complicated, because we will become increasingly more fragile even physically, psychologically. Now the trend is gradually to get worse and worse (P8).

Discussion

In view of the prospect that the symbols can be considered as images or signs of psychological realities of many species, these women perceive the situation that they experienced as a serious and unsolvable problem. People do not have a collection of random, confused thoughts about themselves, rather they organize their view of the "I" that each one is in consistent schemes that influence the way that they interpret new things that happen to them [11]. In the speaking of some women, it is made evident the multifactorial nature involved in the coronary artery disease, such as genetics, lifestyle and environmental conditions.

The similarity of depression, anxiety and ACD symptoms can further complicate the diagnosing process of heart disease in women [12]. The diagnosis of depression in the presence of heart disease is complicated by the similarity of symptoms, because lack of energy, sadness, appetite and fatigue, insomnia and difficulty concentrating are related to both conditions, and often also to menopause [13]. Stress becomes a negative factor to the body when a person feels she cannot face the environment, and therefore, the stress is related to the way the person understand the objective world [14].

The changes that arise from the knowing the causes of the illness may influence the performance of roles, providing an atmosphere conducive to awareness of health. It is understood that the experiences are unique, that is, each person perceives the sensations that cause them malaise and name them according to their understanding and interpretation of the differences of their health status, giving meaning to their own experience with the illness. The women's attitude towards their health condition reveals the level of assessment that they make on the significance of CAD in their lives. Man is not a neutral observer of the world, but a constant evaluator of what he sees and the social experience of each one plays an important role in shaping attitudes.

There is a need to pay attention to the symptom time interval related to CAD, particularly when symptoms are prodromal or acute, since little has been described when patients are women [12]. The presence of pain in the dorsal region is twice as big in women than in men; in addition, women are more prone to certain types of symptoms when they are under emotional stress, as well as to disregard for themselves the possibility of health problems and are more likely to incorporate the symptoms of coronary disease as inherent to the stage of life that they are experiencing, as in the case of climacteric [15,16]. "Back" pain can be understood as lower back pain and not evoke an understanding or discomfort description in the upper back rear shoulder, whose description is relevant in the definition of cardiac disease suspicion.

Changes happen from beliefs and values, which are built and resized. The change of some habits precedes a process of awareness that can transform not only the person, in a narrower sense, but the family, the community, the society, thus helping to promote a healthier life, since psychological meanings are also social meanings. The discovery of heart disease caused a significant change in these women's behavior, influencing decisively in it. The ACD presents itself as an incurable disease that triggers intense feelings and emotions that interfere with daily life.

All human life is a result of the conflict between the world of desires and the real world that does not bend to these desires. In this conflict there is also a precarious balance. The conflict between the desire for independence and the reality of dependence, lived deeply, is distressing [17]. Suffering of any kind is a singular space of search for meaning. Faced with suffering, the human being prove for himself his ability to resist, to face the toughest and adverse situations, to assign a meaning to the reality that he lives and that surrounds him; it is an essential school for the discovery of meanings and senses [18]. Hope reflects the desire for a better future, whose expectation is needed to help people not to give up on their goals and to move forward toward fulfilling their dreams and be happy, despite their health condition. The ability to give great value to what one have or want is a virtue that cannot be missed and professionals should encourage it.

Frailty is a present feeling when women perceive themselves as limited to perform daily activities with the same quality they used to perform before, and so they feel sick, sad and unhappy, changing the image of their role in the professional, social and family contexts [19]. This can lead to internal conflicts. Studies reveal that the frailty is not necessarily related to aging or to a specific disease condition, but may be worse in people with diseases [20,21]. The meaning of fragility as expressed by these women is present probably because of the imminent fear of a threat, specifically the proximity of aging or, in fact, its very existence, of complications of the disease and the appearance of others or even death. Coronary artery disease reveals the close contact with finitude, because of the constant threat of death that it provides, reflecting in a rather negative way at that stage of life.

The concept of malaise does not refer to disease perception models, but to the sociocultural process of interaction and negotiation throughout the episode. It can then be understood that, for women, the experience of menopause/perimenopause through the malaise manifestations, predicted the presence of the CAD episode, but without the clarity and awareness about the possibility of getting the disease. So the episode of the disease is not a diagnosis or a category or a perceptual model, but a process that emerges through the interactions of the actors involved throughout its duration [22].

When talking about the CAD, the participants configured their roles in the social space as "sick" persons, since they described clearly the sick role that they represent in the social context, that is, they enjoy the rights associated with "being sick". Thus, being excluded from the obligations of the activities related to their social roles and having the obligation as a sick person to seek professionally competent assistance are required to assume the sick role, since spontaneous recovery cannot be expected quickly [23].

Conclusion

Menopause was defined for women as a difficult phase, steeped in physical and emotional symptoms - locomotor, vasomotor, cardiac, emotional symptoms, etc. - revealing that this is a major health status change marker, i.e. a period in which they are very prone to consider themselves as ill (disease). The symptoms related to the climacteric and menopause seem to be confused with the problems of age and perceived more strongly in the presence of musculoskeletal diseases, hypertension, diabetes or coronary artery disease itself.

The experience of menopause/perimenopause through the manifestation of malaise predicted the presence of the ACD episode, but without the clarity and awareness about the possibility of getting the disease. So even though these women may identify a number of complaints when speaking about their menopause experience, only from the diagnosis of ACD they assume the sick role. When talking about the CAD, the participants set themselves in the social space as "sick" persons, since they described clearly the sick role that they represent in their social context, that is, they enjoy the rights associated with "being sick".

The discovery of the CAD proved to be one of the most critical and difficult moments of their lives, translated as a serious and incurable problem, which brings restrictions, limitations and requires care, so being a condition that defined them as being sick. They recognize the multifactorial nature of ACD and emphasize transformations after the discovery of the disease such as the change in their diet and role. The experience of this situation goes beyond the physical suffering, but also involves psychological, emotional and social suffering; they show themselves physically debilitated and psychologically vulnerable.

This sense of instability and imbalance imposes limits, restrictions, anguish and frustration, which turns them into fragile, insecure women. It proves to be a conflict between the desirable world and the real world, a concrete reality of limitations, a threat to their lives and physical and emotional integrity. It results in a reworking of their identity process and consolidation of the self, placing them in the sick role. Suffering drives them to reach the limits of the perception of the disease severity and the importance of changing their behavioral habits.

As a limitation in this study, it is emphasized the peculiarities of a qualitative research as the knowledge of a reality of a specific group, the fragment cut and specific and pre-defined moments, the geographic region and the data collection where the study was conducted. Therefore, the generalization of the findings of this study shows limitations, but it is suggested that this research proposal be expanded to other realities, services and other social markers such as family members or health professionals.

References

1. Brazilian Institute of Geography and Statistics, Brazil: Complete mortality: 2010, 2011.

2. Fernandes EF, Pine NJSL, Gebara OCE (2008) Brazilian guidelines on cardiovascular disease prevention in climacteric women and influence of hormone replacement therapy (HRT) of the Brazilian Society of Cardiology (SBC) and the Brazilian Association of Climacteric (Sobrac). Brazilian Archives of Cardiology, Rio de Janeiro.

3. Toh S, D Henández Logan R, Rossouw JE, Hermán MA (2010) Coronary heart disease in postmenopausal recipients of estrogen plus progestin therapy: Does the Increased risk ever disappear? Ann Intern Med 152: 211-217.

4. Achutti A (2012) Prevention of cardiovascular diseases and health promotion. Chemist Public Health 17: 18-22.

5. Antonicelli R, F Olivieri, Morichi V, Urbani, More V (2008) Prevention of cardiovascular events in early menopause: a possible role for hormone replacement therapy. Int J Cardiol 130: 140-146.

6. Lion AP, Eikevicius CP, DD Ferreira, Boschin HBC, Vieira LG, et al. (2011) Causes of myocardial infarction: the understanding of patient woman. Rev Soc Cardiol 21: 28-32.

7. Cantus DS, Ruix MCS (2013) Ischemic heart disease in women. Latin American Journal of Nursing 19: 19-26.

8. Heinemann K, Ruebig A Potthof P, HPG Schneider, Strelow F (2004) The menopause rating scale (MRS): The methodological review. Health What Life Outcomes 2:45.

9. Cancian R (2009) Symbolic Interactionism: Applicability.

10. Bardin L (2011) Content analysis.

11. Assagioli R (2006) The basis of modern and transpersonal psychology, São Paulo: Cultrix.

12. Norris, CM, KM Hegadoren, Patterson L, Pilote L (2008) Sex differences in prodromal symptoms of patients with acute coronary syndrome: A pilot study. Prog Cardiovasc Nurs 23: 27-31.

13. Serrano JCV (2011) Depression, emotional state and coronary artery disease. Rev Soc Cardiol.

14. Aronson, Wilson TD, Akert RM (2013) A social psychology, Rio de Janeiro: LTC.

15. Sjostrom-Strand, Fridlund B (2008) Women's descriptions of symptoms and reasons delay in seeking medical care at the time of the first myocardial infraction: A qualitative study. Int J Nurs Stud 45: 1003-1010.

16. Potsch AA (2003) A Bassan care and pre-hospital treatment of acute myocardial infarction. In:. Timmerman A Feitosa GS (Eds.). Acute coronary syndromes. Rio de Janeiro: Atheneu 231-242.

17. Mazzetti L (2010) The seasons of life. São Paulo: Editora Educacional.

18. Selli L (2007) Pain and suffering in tessitude life. The World Health, São Paulo 297-300

19. Galter C, Rodrigues GC, Galvão ECF. The perception of cardiac patients to active life after recovery from heart surgery. Journal of the Health Sciences Institute, São Paulo 28: 255-258.

20. SCC Fabricio Rodrigues RA P (2013) Literature review of fragility and its relationship to aging. RENE Magazine 9: 113-19.

21. Flag I C (2010) Fragility in the elderly: an integrative review. In: Work Completion of course (Diploma in Nursing) - Nursing School, Federal University of Rio Grande do Sul, Porto Alegre.

22. Langdon EJ (2012) Reviews for "disease versus Illness in General practice", by Cecil Helman G Fields. Antropol Rev Soc 10: 113-7.

23. Richardson W (1971) Ambulatory use of physicians' services in response to illness episodes in a low-income neighborhood. Chicago: Center for Health Administration Studies, University of Chicago.

30

Beyond the Language Barrier 'Speak', 'See', 'Help Me'

Shirin Badruddin* and **Shazia Arif**

King Faisal Specialist Hospital and Research Center, Surgical Intensive Care Unit, Riyadh, Saudi Arabia

*Corresponding author: Shirin Badruddin, King Faisal Specialist Hospital and Research Center, Surgical Intensive Care Unit, Riyadh, Saudi Arabia, E-mail: shirin_badruddin@msn.com

Abstract

Introduction: King Faisal Specialist Hospital and Research Center (KFSHRC) workforce is composed of close to 67 different nationalities. Diversity in the nursing workforce is unique in the hospital reason being the expatriates outnumber the Saudi nationals. Staff from different backgrounds provides a different perspective to the clinical care ensuring the hospital standards and policies are adhered to. In the Intensive Care Unit (ICU), when these new nurses arrive, their grasp of Arabic is limited. It is essential that nurses understand the language of their patients. In intensive care setting, patient's condition is critical and highly specialized nursing care is paramount to the safety of the patient. It poses a challenge for non-Arabic speaking nurses to overcome the language barriers, to ensure high quality care is provided to the patient, maintain patient satisfaction and confidentiality. Therefore, communication tool kit is developed to overcome the language barrier. The tool kit is an educational instrument for non-Arabic speakers by expediting learning most frequent terms and words in Arabic.

Aim: The purpose of this study is to focus on the importance of implementing a communication toolkit to enhance the communication between the nurse and the patient. Moreover, this study attempted to evaluate the efficacy of this communication tool prepared for non-Arabic health care providers.

Method: Descriptive Quantitative pre and post-test study design was used. This study included all adult intensive care units and non-Arabic speaking nurses from KFSHRC in Riyadh. The pre and post questionnaire was developed by a panel of experts working in the ICU. The communication toolkit was created by direct care staff nurses working alongside the multidisciplinary team to address communication barriers. Baseline assessment was conducted which highlighted the common words and culturally appropriate images used by the Arabic patients.

After the approval of the ethics and research board the study was conducted. Recruitment of the participants was performed on a voluntarily basis. On the basis of the sample size, 95 percent level of confidence, 73 participants were recruited. The communication toolkit was distributed for the duration of three months. Follow up was performed by the investigators after three a months' time frame.

Results: The results of the study showed that 90 percent of the nurses did not study Arabic prior to their arrival in the hospital. 72 nurses completed the pre and post questionnaires. Majority of the nurses were from Asian countries and few were from Western countries. Most of the nurses were using interpreters to overcome the language barrier. With regards to the questionnaire 94 percent of the nurses viewed that this toolkit will overcome their language difficulties.

19 percent used the toolkit daily, 55 percent used it twice per week and 16 percent used once per month. In regards to the efficacy 83 percent stated that this toolkit is a good mode of communication with the patients. 50 percent of the nurse highlighted the need for Arabic classes.

Conclusion: This study highlights the need for the toolkit to improve the language barriers. Most of the nurses have suggested Arabic classes, access to electronic devices and need for interpreters to overcome the language barrier. The toolkit is important and is to be made available in all areas of the organization.

Keywords: Language; Tool kit; Patient; Arabic; Nurses

Introduction

Communication is considered as an important patient safety goal [1]. The Joint Commission for Accreditation of Health Care Organizations reported that communication barriers are responsible for almost 85% of sentinel events in hospitals [2]. High quality, patient centered care depends on good communication between health care providers and the patient [3]. In multicultural and multilingual environment, language barriers impose an important challenge to health care providers and patients. This language barrier raises question about the holistic care and collaborative decision making among the patients and health care providers [4]. Studies have highlighted that health care provider-patient communication barrier leads to a decrease in patient satisfaction, potentially poor clinical decision making, increased chances of medical errors, longer hospital stays and poor patient outcomes [1]. However, this risk can be reduced by introducing an interpreter and communicating with patients in their preferred language [5]. Nurses are considered as the primary health care provider for the patient. Patients spend more time with the nurses as compared to other health care professionals. Therefore, it is essential for the nurses that they understand the language of their patients, care for them and competently solve their problems. In intensive care setting, patients are critical and rely solely on nurse's care. Therefore, language is considered as an important means of communication among patient, family and health care providers. It may pose a challenge for non-Arabic speaking nurses to overcome the language barriers, ensure high quality care is provided to the patient and maintain high patient satisfaction.

Background of the Study

The mission of the King Faisal Hospital and Research Center (KFSH&RC) is to provide safe and effective care to patients and their families (King Faisal Specialist Hospital and Research Centre Website). Being accredited by the Joint Commission International Accreditation and Magnet designated, communication is considered as an important area for patient safety [2]. The patients admitted in this hospital communicate in Arabic language. Health care workers are employed from close to 67 different nationalities. Nurses mainly spend majority of their time with the patient. KFSH&RC is a tertiary facility providing highly specialized medical treatments to predominantly Saudi nationals. The hospital has 1549 bed capacity and 10,009 employees. There are 3126 employees working under the Nursing Affairs umbrella; this includes registered nurses, clinical educators, care assistants, patient care assistants and ward clerks (King Faisal Specialist Hospital and Research Centre Website).

In the intensive care unit, when the new nurses arrive, interpreters or the family members are utilized to establish appropriate care plans for the patient. This practice does not maintain the patient's confidentiality or privacy.

Study Purpose

The purpose of this study is to focus on the importance of implementing a communication toolkit to enhance the communication between the nurse and the patient. Moreover, this study attempted to evaluate the efficacy of this communication tool prepared for non-Arabic health care providers.

In particular, this study was designed to answer the following questions:

1. What is the efficacy of this communication tool kit?
2. What was the nurses' level of comfort before and after utilizing this tool kit?
3. What other sources can be used to overcome the language barrier?

Literature Search

A systematic and comprehensive search was done in January, 2014, to access research studies on overcoming language barriers among health care professionals and patients. Various words and phrases were used to guide the search that included: communication, language barriers, language conflict, overcoming language barriers and strategies to reduce language barriers. Data bases such as CINAHL, PubMed, Sage and Science Direct were used to guide the search. The search ranged from 2003 to 2014. A total of 230 articles appeared to be relevant, further reading narrowed down the articles to fifteen that met the study purpose.

Study gap

Literature search highlighted that most of the studies were conducted in the western region and very few in the Middle-eastern region [3,6]. In addition, most of the studies have explored the perceptions and feelings of the health care professionals including expatriates nurses and doctors about caring for patients communicating in different language [7]. Studies have emphasized the use of interpreters [6] but none of the studies focus on the interventions such as communication tool kit to overcome the language barriers. Few studies have focused on using communication boards in ICU [4,8]. Therefore, our study is of the highest important as this will focus on utilizing communication tool kit to reduce this language barrier.

Communication Tool Kit

Communication tool kit was designed and created by the direct care staff nurses who encountered daily communication difficulties while providing care to Arabic patients. The team of staff nurses collaborated with the multidisciplinary team to address the language difficulties. Baseline assessment was conducted which highlighted the common words, phrases that were frequently encountered and highlighted by the patients and their relatives. Based on this feedback, draft of the communication tool kit was created, and was enhanced on regular basis (Figure 1). In addition, Arabic speaking staff was involved in the development of this toolkit to ensure that the terminologies and phrases used in this toolkit are culturally appropriate. This communication tool kit addresses the following areas (greetings, pain, personal hygiene, vital signs, intervention, body movements, food, emotions, procedures, staff members, day time and prayer time) with English and Arabic translation along with its pronunciation.

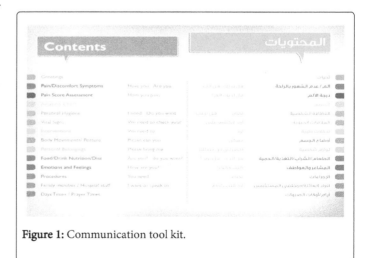

Figure 1: Communication tool kit.

Research Methodology

Descriptive quantitative pre and post-test study design was used in this study.

Study Population and Setting

This study included all adult Intensive Care Units (surgical, medical, chronic and cardiac) and non-Arabic staff nurses after obtaining the RAC approval, the duration of the study was three months.

Inclusion criteria

1. Nurses who are non-Arabic were included in the study.

Exclusion criteria

1. Nurses who do not give voluntary consent were excluded.
2. Arabic speaking staff were excluded.

Data Collection Strategies

1. Briefings about the proposed study and its purpose.
2. Recruitment of the participants was done on the basis of voluntarily participation by the participants.
3. Pre-test questionnaire was distributed to the participants who give voluntarily verbal consent to take part in this study.
4. Communication tool kit was distributed and explanations about the tool kit were given to the targeted audience.
5. Participants to use the toolkit for duration of 3 months.
6. Follow up was done by the researchers within the assessment time to reinforce the participants to utilize this tool kit.
7. The participants ID was coded and kept safe with the principle investigator until the publication is done.
8. Post-test questionnaire was redistributed to the participants after three month from the time specified.

Sample Size

Adult ICU nurses who met the inclusion criteria and agreed to participate in the study. In this study, all adult ICU non-Arabic speaking nurses who gave voluntary verbal consent were the part of this study. On the basis of sample size formula with 95% level of confidence, 73 participants were recruited.

Data Analysis

Statistics analysis of data was done by Statistical Package for Social Scientist (SPSS) version 20. Descriptive statistics were obtained for the quality questionnaires and the demographic data and individual questions on the communication toolkit were analyzed.

Ethical Consideration

The principles of confidentiality and respect for human dignity were followed in this study. The study was conducted after obtaining an approval from the Research Advisory Council and according to the ethical principles of the declaration of Helsinki and the Good Clinical Practice Guidelines. To ensure the right of self-determination, the participants were informed that their participation in the research is voluntary and that they had the right to leave the study at any time. They were also assured that refusal to participate would not have any impact on their job status or benefits. However, voluntary participation of the health care professionals, through an informed verbal consent was taken before the data collection.

Results and Discussion

This part presents an analysis of the findings of the study. This includes details about the questionnaire status, the participants profile, demographics, their level of comfort while speaking Arabic, and their answers regarding the need and applicability of the communication tool kit.

Questionnaire status

A total of 73 participants were enrolled in the study. Only one participant left the study. 72 nurses filled the pre and post questionnaires.

Demographic data

Majority (32%) of the participants enrolled were from Surgical ICU, 19.4 percent from medical ICU, chronic ICU (12.5%) and 35% from cardiac ICU. 89 percent of the nurses recruited were female. Participants' age varied from 25 to 60 years. Most of the participants (62%) were around 26 to 40 years of age. Their education level was diploma and bachelors. 68% of nurses with bachelor's degree were part of this study. Contrary in Al-Harasis [6], 37.9 percent were having bachelor degree in nursing and 3.2% with master's degree in nursing. None of the participants were from gulf region. All of the participants were outside Gulf region. Majority of the nurses were from Asian countries and few were from Western countries (Table 1). This finding is concurrent with other study finding [3] which highlighted that most nurses are from India, Philippines, Malaysia, Australia, America, United Kingdom, South Africa and other Middle Eastern countries with different cultural backgrounds. Almutairi and McCarthy [9] stated that 67.7% of nurses in Saudi Arabia are expatriates.

Nurses nationality	
Country	**Percent**
United States	4.9
Canada	11.8
Pakistan	11.8
India	14.6
Malaysia	18.1
South Africa	2.1
United Kingdom	4.9
Philippines	22.2
Portugal	2.8
Ireland	1.4
Czech republic	3.5
New Zealand	1.4
Total	100

Table 1: Nurses nationality.

Level of comfortability while speaking Arabic

As shown in Table 2, only 39 percent were comfortable while caring for Arabic patient and 38 percent ranked their fluency as poor, 41 percent as fair and 15 percent as good. Similarly in Al-Harasis [6], forty nine percent of the nurses stated difficulty in dealing with patient due to the language barrier.

Eighty one percent of the participants were using interpreters and colleagues to overcome their language barriers while caring for Arabic patients and this finding is similar with Al-Harasis [6]. 6 percent were attending Arabic classes to overcome the language barrier. Contradictory, 90 percent of the nurses in Al-Harasis [6] suggested attending an Arabic course especially during the orientation phase. 2 participants highlighted the use of non-verbal communication and 1 shared the use of internet sites for translation. Similarly in Helmsley et al. [10] study, majority of the nurses were using low technology equipment such as boards, pen and paper which is different from our study. In our study, 10 percent were using booklets prepared by the unit for translating commonly used words. Interestingly, 73 percent nurses in Al-Harasis [6] preferred to use the dictionary for quick reference for commonly used words.

	Frequency	Percent	Valid Percent
Excellent	6	4.2	4.2
Good	55	38.2	38.2
Fair	83	57.6	57.6
Total	144	100	100

Table 2: Levels of compatibility.

In pre-study questionnaire, 94 percent viewed that this communication tool kit will benefit them to overcome the language barrier. 61 percent participants responded it will support them moderately to overcome the language barrier.

Average hours spent using the tool kit

38 percent of the participants used this tool kit twice per week, seventeen percent used it once per week and 7 percent never used the tool kit. 22 percent of the nurses used this tool kit on daily basis or as needed. According to the post questionnaire analysis, 83 percent rated this tool kit as moderate as compared to 13 percent who rated this toolkit as an excellent mode of communication.

Support required and suggestions to overcome this language barrier

Fifty five nurses responded to this question. Majority 50 percent of the nurses highlighted the need for Arabic classes. 2 percent requested electronic devices are made available and accessible to patients. 16.3 percent expressed the need for interpreters. 11 percent identified the need for more communication tool kit accessibility in the units. 4 percent highlighted the need for appreciation. In addition, nurses in the current study raised the matter on who should be the interpreter which is concurrent with Al-Harasis [6] and Timmins [11] study. Timmins [11] suggested hiring trained professional interpreters from the community.

Conclusion

This study has provided information about the need to identify the strategies to overcome the language barrier. In addition, it identifies the nurses' level of comfort speaking Arabic and caring for Arabic patients. Moreover, it highlighted the efficacy and feasibility of this communication tool kit while caring with Arabic patients.

Recommendations

In view of the study findings, following recommendations include importance of:

1. Suitable advertisement and flexible time schedule for Arabic classes.
2. Unit specific communication tool kit with pictures is made available.
3. Practice and commitment is required from the nurses to improve their communication.
4. Tool kit is prepared for beginners, intermediate and advance level including sentences.
5. Flip chart may be created and made accessible to patients that include pictures, words in Arabic and English language.
6. Communication tool kit is portable and pocket size.
7. Online translation tool or laptop is available in every patient room.
8. Employee more Arabic speaking staff

Limitations

This communication tool kit was advantageous for chronic patients who are alert and orientated. In the ICU the patients were sedated and the toolkit was not utilized. The images and written words in English and Arabic assisted the nurses to communicate with the sedated patient's family members. This study did not test the patients' vital signs and emotional parameters. In future, research focus can be a randomized control trial, evaluate patient responses and see the efficacy of this tool kit on sedated patients. In addition, the plan is to test this communication tool kit in the pediatric population and outpatients.

References

1. Gregg J, Saha S (2007) Communicative competence: A framework for understanding language barriers in health care. J Gen Intern Med 22: 368-370.
2. Joint Commission on Accreditation of Healthcare Organizations. (2006) Sentinel Event Statistics
3. Almutairi KM (2015) Culture and language differences as a barrier to provision of quality care by the health workforce in Saudi Arabia. Saudi Med J 36: 425-431.
4. Grossbach I, Stranberg S, Chlan L (2011) Promoting effective communication for patients receiving mechanical ventilation. Crit Care Nurse 31: 46-60.
5. Diamond LC, Jacobs EA (2009) Lets not contribute to disparities: The best method for teaching clinicians how to overcome language barriers to health care. J Gen Intern Med 25: 189-193.
6. Al-Harasis S (2013) Impact of language barrier on quality of nursing care at Armed Forces Hospital, Taif, Saudi Arabia. Middle East Journal of Nursing 7: 12-24.

7. Hudelson P, Vilpert S (2009) Overcoming language barriers with foreign-language speaking patients: A survey to investigate intra-hospital variation in attitudes and practices. BMC Health Serv Res 9: 187.

8. Patak L, Gawlinski A, Fung NI (2006) Communication boards in critical care: Patients' views. Appl Nurs Res 19: 182-90.

9. Almutairi AF, McCarthy A (2012) A multicultural workforce and cultural perspectives in Saudi Arabia: An overview. Health 3: 71-74.

10. Helmsley B, Sigafoos J, Balandin S, Forbes R, Taylor C, et al. (2001) Nursing the patient with severe communication impairment. J Adv Nurs 35: 827-835.

11. Timmins CL (2002) The impact of language barriers on the health care of Latinos in the United States: A review of the literature and guidelines for practice. J Midwifery Womens Health 47: 80-90.

31

Care Management: Perspectives from Managers, Professionals and Users of a Specialized Service Facility Focused on Human Immunodeficiency Virus/Acquired Immune Deficiency Syndrome

Betina Hörner Schlindwein Meirelles*, Samara Eliane Rabelo Suplici, Veridiana Tavares Costa, Aline Daiane Colaço, Bárbara Aparecida Oliveira Forgearini and Valdete Meurer Kuehlkamp

Universidade Federal de Santa Catarina, Florianópolis, Santa Catarina, Brazil

*Corresponding author: Meirelles BHS, Professor of the Department of Nursing and Postgraduate Program in Nursing, Universidade Federal de Santa Catarina Rua Delfino Conti Florianópolis, Santa Catarina 88040-370, Brazil, E-mail: betina.hsm@ufsc.br

Abstract

Background: Complex practices used for care management are developed to include the perspectives of professionals, healthcare organizations and patients. Therefore, to implement strategies to provide quality care, identifying gaps in these practices is crucial. This study seeks to gain a better understanding of the management of health care for people living with Human Immunodeficiency Virus/Acquired Immune Deficiency Syndrome by considering the perspective of health professionals, managers and patients of a specialized service facility in South Brazil that focuses on contagious diseases.

Methods: This qualitative, dialogic, reflexive and interpretative study involved 16 participants. The data were derived from semi-structured interviews conducted during 2013 and 2014. Ethnograph® software was used to provide a descriptive and interpretative data analysis.

Results: The results show that care management multidimensionality requires continuous attention to the way professionals think as well as reorganization of labor processes and the network of services provided. Thus emerged three categories: interdisciplinarity in care management; continuous training in care management; and strengthening of health care networks.

Conclusion: From the perspective of individuals involved in managing and promoting the care and health of people living with Human Immunodeficiency Virus/Acquired Immune Deficiency Syndrome, changes are needed to improve the care of people living with Human Immunodeficiency Virus/Acquired Immune Deficiency Syndrome in terms of the three dimensions of care management.

Keywords: Care management; HIV; Nursing; Health administration; Infectious diseases

Abbreviations AIDS: Acquired Immune Deficiency Syndrome; HIV: Human Immunodeficiency Virus; ART: Antiretroviral Therapy; PLWHA: People Living with HIV/AIDS; CNS: National Health Council; CESPH/UFSC: Human Research Ethics Committee of the Federal University of Santa Catarina; UNAIDS: Joint United Nations Programme on HIV/AIDS

Background

In the more than three decades since Acquired Immune Deficiency Syndrome (AIDS) emerged and grew into a global epidemic, numerous scientific advances have been made to treat AIDS, including identification of Human Immunodeficiency Virus (HIV) disease mechanisms and the introduction of Antiretroviral Therapy (ART). These scientific discoveries resulted in better care and increased the longevity of infected people. Moreover, government and non-government agencies, health professionals and people living with HIV/AIDS (PLWHA) have joined forces to establish a qualified health care model [1].

In terms of care management of PLWHA, HIV infection is no longer considered to be an acute illness, but rather a chronic condition [2]. This re-categorization presents new challenges for health managers and professionals who provide care to PLWHA.

Thus, a new self-management model is needed wherein PLWHA take an active and informed role in decisions about health care practices. This new model requires changes in behavior and social relations, because managing chronic health conditions involves life changes in the biopsychosocial dimension and the adoption of therapeutic treatments [3,4].

Care management can be categorized into three dimensions: professional, organizational and systemic. Professional care management is observed within a professional responsibility, i.e., in establishing a professional-patient relationship that includes ethical, technical-scientific and relational (personal ties) elements. In the organizational dimension, health practices undergo institutionalization, where technical and social issues concerning the division of labor emerge that result in management responsibility and a dynamic conformation of the team and relationships between team members. Finally, the systemic dimension is configured by a set of health care services that have different functions and levels of technological incorporation, as well as various integrations between services that establish a network to offer comprehensive care to patients [4].

Health practices involve complex care that includes dialogue, understanding of human behavior, qualified listening, respect, knowledge, organization of health services and social policy [5]. Therefore, care management of PLWHA becomes relevant and prominent, because effective case management promotes understanding of multidimensional processes and actions with which PLWHA live and also their experience of being ill and feeling healthy.

By investigating the perspectives of managers, health professionals and patients, it is possible to identify gaps in care processes delivered to PLWHA and implement strategies to strengthen actions that enhance care quality.

Thus, the objective of this study was to understand health care management for PLWHA from the perspective of patients and health care professionals at a specialized service facility in southern Brazil that focuses on infectious diseases.

Complex thinking was the theoretical framework for this research that considers the dynamics of reality and is more appropriate for recognizing the multiple facets and diversity of issues related to health and its management.

Method

Design

The research presented here adopted qualitative, dialogical, reflective and interpretative approaches. The study was conducted in the southern Brazilian state of Santa Catarina at a hospital that specializes in treating infectious diseases. According to the classification of the Ministry of Health, this facility provides conventional hospitalization services, day hospital services and a Specialized Care Service for HIV/AIDS.

Procedures

The data from this study were collected through semi-structured interviews conducted by five collectors, all female.

Interviewers number 1 (PhD in nursing and health researcher) and number 2 (master of nursing) work as nursing professors having extensive experience in research and qualitative data collection. This experience is similar to interviewer number 3 (professor in nursing) who work as a clinical nurse. Interviewers number 3 and 4 (nursing students), in turn, were trained to conduct the meetings and the approach of the participants.

Interviewers and participants of this study did not have any direct relationship prior to the survey, however, some managers and health professionals who composed the study sample had references about the curriculum and professional features of number 1 interviewer, because she is a prominent researcher in the HIV/AIDS area.

Research participants

Study participants included managers, health professionals and patients who would enable a comprehensive understanding of care management related to HIV/AIDS, forming a intentional sample

Patients enrolled in the study were >18 years old, were diagnosed with HIV one or more years earlier and were registered and regularly

attending service for treatment and/or monitoring. Professionals and managers in the study must have been directly caring for PLWHA for more than one year. These criteria ensured that the collected data reflected accumulated participant experiences.

The research participants were personally addressed in a hospital that specializes in treating infectious diseases. Of the total addressed people, two refused to participate in the study citing fear of break of confidentiality.

In this qualitative approach, there was no preset number of participants, and the priority was on the theoretical deepening of approaches so that data collection was independent of the number of participants. The study included a total of 8 health professionals, including 2 doctors, 3 nurses, 1 administrator and 2 nursing technicians. Of these, three held management positions. In addition, 8 PLWHA who were patients of the specialized service facility were selected to complete the 16 study enrolees.

The number of participants was determined by theoretical saturation or when the data collection reached a point where no new elements were presented to support the desired theorization [6].

The data collection involved semi-structured interviews composed of questions regarding the professional and organizational dimensions of care management that was created by the authors. The one-to-one meetings were previously scheduled and addressed values, attitudes, beliefs and individual experiences that were relevant to the research.

The meetings occurred in a private room of the hospital, where they were present only an interviewer and the participant. These individual interviews were conducted in only one meeting during on average 30 min and were audio recorded and later transcribed in full without use of field notes. The data collection period was divided into two phases. The first phase was carried out between March and December 2013 and the second phase was done in August 2014. The second phase was included because during collection, transcription and coding of the data for the first phase, the need arose for further exploration of the data in terms of the perspective of PLWHA towards care management.

The interviews were transcribed by hand by all the authors of this study, concomitantly data collection, being in possession of the same until the end of the survey, without returning to the participants.

Data analysis

Qualitative content analysis of the transcripts of interviews was performed by the authors this article using the interactive software Ethnograph®, which assists qualitative researchers in gathering, organizing and analyzing qualitative data [7]. For data analysis, a descriptive and interpretive strategy was adopted.

In structuring analysis and interpretation processes, the first step was an initial and comprehensive reading of the entire text of the interview transcripts, followed by the deconstruction and unitization of the corpus. The aim with this fragmentation or corpus deconstruction, was to highlight the meanings of the text to the limits of its details, with the understanding that this limit is never fully achieved [8].

After rereading and deconstructing, the content relevant and pertinent to the research – termed meaning units – was selected. The second step of the analysis was the categorization of units of analysis where was delimited three main categories. Categorization is a process of constant comparison between the units defined in the initial analysis process, leading to group similar elements. The sets of similar elements form the categories [8].

The research participants were not contacted in order to do that feedback from the search results.

Ethical aspects

To comply with ethical standards, the recommendations of Resolution no. 196/96 of the National Health Council (CNS) of Brazil and its complementary recommendations updated by resolution 466/12, CNS were followed [9]. After receiving authorization from the hosting institution, the assent of the Human Research Ethics Committee of the Federal University of Santa Catarina (CESPH/UFSC) was obtained under Opinion no. 167 681 on December 10, 2012.

The participants were informed of the study objectives and research methods, and were assured of their rights regarding access to data, preservation of anonymity and the possibility to withdraw from the study at any point. All patients signed an Informed Consent Form.

In order to maintain the confidentiality of the research participants, their testimonials were identified with a letter that refers to the sequential sample group followed by a number according to the interview sequence: managers (G1, G2, G3), health professionals (PR1, PR2, ...) and people with HIV/AIDS (PA1, PA2, ...).

Results

The management research participants were all female with a mean age of 41.66 years and average time performance of 16.5 years. Health professionals, in turn, were characterized mostly by women (80%) with operating time in service an average of 14.8 years, and mean age of 39.8 years. Already the PLWHA were mostly male (75%), single (62.5%) and white (87.5%) with mean age of 40.87 years, with a mean time of diagnosis of 11.5 years.

The results of the data analysis process revealed three categories: interdisciplinarity as interface in care management; continuous training in the context of care management; and strengthening of healthcare networks.

Regarding interdisciplinarity, the results showed that both managers and users recognize that interdisciplinarity is required in delivering health services for PLWHA, especially for a perspective that focuses on the quality of care.

The interdisciplinary perspective points to the relevance of comprehensive care to the individual's needs. The quotes below illustrate that fragmenting the work of a multi-professional team complicates the systematization of interdisciplinary and intersectorial relationships as well as interaction practices:

"The team works the multi-professional dimension but do not work the interdisciplinary, you know? Many professionals such as psychiatrists, pharmacists, nurses, doctors, nutritionists [...] they do not exchange experiences [...] people have to get over it and come back to talk about this issue." (G3)

"But when there are health professionals working together with you, understanding your situation, assessing the best options available... this gives you direction... this is important...you have more desire to really come back, to follow the treatment better" (PA4)

However, the perceptions of participants and everyday working practices reinforce a fragmented type of work, where each professional individually fulfills their function, and the interrelationship between them that is so critical for interdisciplinarity gradually disappears. This loss of interdisciplinarity is reflected in a fragmented perception of the patient and the health-disease process instead of a comprehensive view, and may be a consequence of the current model of care management applied in practice.

From the perspective of PLWHA, joint efforts of professionals expand recognition of their care needs and promote more effective participation and commitment. For interdisciplinarity to occur, different disciplines must engage in a dialogue, which may be affected by professional barriers that managers must recognize.

What is needed to ensure long-term and comprehensive care is highlighted by the following participant:

"There is a limitation of each profession, that is why I say they are multiprofessional but do not work the interdisciplinary dimension" (G3)

Thus, continuous training in the context of care management could improve relationships between professionals, and especially between professionals and patients.

This research also identified the need to understand the patient as a person who has complex needs that arise from various determinants of life and health conditions, particularly the challenges of living with HIV/AIDS. This need for a better understanding of the patient as a person is mirrored in the need for professional training to conduct and manage these situations every day as evidenced by this statement:

"I think that continuous training is beyond the technical part. I think it should have something different. There is a human being behind all this. The person arrives here and they have a background, prejudices". (PR4)

However, in the context of this study it was impossible to identify aspects that involve other dimensions of care beyond the technical-scientific, such as interpersonal and institutional relations or conflicts between values and principles.

In addition, on several occasions the interviews highlighted issues such as the importance of continuous training as a tool to enhance the user-professional-user relationship as well as the relationship between professionals. Such training tools should emphasize communicative practices and relational activities that characterize a humanized and welcoming care environment:

"We are discussing some things on continuous training, to make a survey of what the training needs are thinking of the care provided to the patient profile that we meet here. Now my concern is how to bring, how to reformulate a continuous training service thinking of a new model for people to feel responsible for a process of change as well." (G1)

"In daily life I think that the personal relationships are enhanced with continuous training. I think they are two parallel things: fighting with managers to make things work and training, because training is everything! To enhance this I think training is fundamental." (PR4).

In this sense, care could be improved through training processes that include planning and coordination of interactions between knowledge bases and between various professionals.

Finally, the strength of health care networks highlights the need to reorganize network services to provide comprehensive care to PLWHA with the intention of improving care management.

In the testimonials from the professionals participating in this study, difficulties in conducting long-term care are evident and shared among various health facilities:

"There is a lack of an organization of the service as a whole. I think there should be more communication between administrations." (PR1)

Also in terms of care management and creating stronger care networks, interviewees discussed their experiences with overcoming weaknesses of this process. These experiences directly affect the quality of services and satisfaction of professionals and users, as shown by these statements:

"There is a lot of negligence, nobody takes responsibility. I am not satisfied." (PA5)

"One sends the patient from one place to another and the person gets confused. There comes a time that the person is tired! [...] Many drop out of treatment because of that." (PR1)

Thus, the interviews explicitly show dissatisfaction of professionals and users with the lack of coordination between health care services, absence of care lines and no clearly defined referral and counter referral system.

The above statement by PA5, shows that the user perceives negligence by professionals and establishments, i.e., low accountability for the provision of healthcare service.

Another aspect that was highlighted as being important for care management was the decentralization of health services that is intended to facilitate user access and improve the effectiveness in referral processes:

"I think if it was more decentralized, not all patients should come here. Because the biggest problem is the patient who travels a long way to come here." (PR1)

"Because the person goes to the Center (Healthcare Center), then the Center refers them to the specialist. By the time they get an appointment, the person is dead." (PR3)

The professionals are aware of the proposal by the Ministry of Health in Brazil, which intends to decentralize care throughout the health care network, and demonstrates the need to manage the reorganization of services.

Discussion

Given the analysis and results, a limitation of this research is the fact that it was conducted in a specialized service facility, which may affect the data because the participating managers, professionals and PLWHA at the site have better preparation and more experience. However, the data may not reflect the reality of most care services for PLWHA, to whom the multidimensionality of care management does not have as much relevance as it does in a specialized facility.

The interdisciplinarity that is seen as a perspective for care management of PLWHA requires its own team that goes beyond a multi-professional team with fragmented practices. Thus, interdisciplinarity demands a reconnecting of knowledge, since the complexity of life involves both interrelation and interaction between life issues [10].

To achieve interdisciplinarity, efforts must be made to break the hegemony of knowledge in health care and reconnect disciplinary knowledge. Knowledge and experiences of professionals need to be shared so that there is no dominance of one discipline over others or of one professional over others. In doing so, it becomes possible to provide expanded care according to the needs of users, while respecting and accepting the singularities both among health workers and between them and patients [11].

Of note is that continuous training in the context of healthcare management is built from the practice of the teams. Thus, demands for training cannot be solely defined or updated according to a list of needs for individual professionals or by guidelines issued by central management.

The constant professional education that is required in health care guarantees that the professional has knowledge of the best and most effective practices of nursing and medicine. Such attentive, serious and competent care that results from knowledge of best practices can alleviate suffering and even prevent unnecessary deaths. Moreover, professionals must understand that the patient is entitled to accurate diagnosis as well as effective treatment and communication, among other services. Furthermore, they should never be offered care as a favor, but rather as a quality service [12].

The core of continuous training is aimed at reconstructing professional identities and coordinating different areas of knowledge and practices. The training also provides a proactive role for professionals, wherein they are empowered to identify their own strengths and weaknesses, as well as transform the reality, of which they are part, that begins by making a commitment to quality patient care [12].

Another important point highlighted from the perspective of care management for PLWHA refers to the strengthening of healthcare networks, with defined care lines that work to implement a new model of health. Notably, the implementation of health programs that focus on chronic conditions is one of the mandates of the Joint United Nations Program on HIV/AIDS to ensure universal access for PLWHA to programs that prevent and treat their disease as well as provide care and support [13,14].

Maintaining fragmentary healthcare models may be directly related to the failure to achieve goals that are related to controlling chronic disease and the complications that accompany these diseases. Thus, the obsolescence and inadequacy of this compartmentalized organization clearly indicates the need for a new model of care that addresses the needs of people living with a chronic condition [15].

This new model should develop a consolidated, organizational approach to health care that addresses fragmented views of health-disease processes and of the individual patient. In this respect, organization of services in care networks has proven to be a more efficient and effective alternative for professionals, users and managers of health systems [15]. The need for decentralization in HIV/AIDS programs worldwide is reaffirmed by UNAIDS and calls for improved mechanisms through which the population can access services. These mechanisms should include primary care as a protagonist of disease treatment programs [13,14,16].

Although governments and institutions working in the area recognize the importance of committing to reorganized services, this practice is still new to Brazil. In early 2014 the Brazilian government proposed reform measures to consolidate the network of service and technical support to primary healthcare institutions to incorporate the therapeutic management of citizens infected with HIV/AIDS [17].

This reorganization is justified primarily by the promising results reported in the literature for PLWHA who are monitored in a primary care setting [18] and by evidence that centralization of HIV/AIDS services and minimizing the distance between the homes of PLWHA and health facilities are factors that affect the likelihood that PLWHA will follow treatment protocols [19-21].

Conclusion

From the perspective of individuals involved in managing and promoting the care and health of PLWHA, changes are needed to improve the care of PLWHA in terms of the three dimensions of care management (interface interdisciplinarity, training and network strength). Implementing these changes will require continual efforts to address the way in which professionals regard health care and organize their labor in various areas, as well as how services such as continuous training programs and care networks can be re-organized to promote effective patient care.

The research presented in this paper aims to contribute to reflections on the care management practices in nursing and highlight perspectives that can be used for improving activities and services provided to PLWHA at all levels of care.

The various participants involved in this study, whether they were people with HIV/AIDS, or managers and/or professionals, point out the importance of comprehension in health care, and the need to minimize prejudices about uniqueness and diversity. A horizontal perspective of the actions and services is also highlighted, and considers the importance of relationships and interactions that take place around the complex issue of what it means to live with a chronic condition as well as the need for connection and continuous care.

Because this reorganization of services is a process that is still under construction, there will be new long-term challenges to be faced by health professionals and managers who care for PLWHA. Due to the multi-dimensional nature of chronic diseases such as HIV/AIDS, interdisciplinarity, continuous training and the strengthening of health care networks are among the top considerations for care management of PLWHA.

References

1. Mbuagbaw L, Mursleen S, Lytvyn L (2015) Mobile phone text messaging interventions for HIV and other chronic diseases: an overview of systematic reviews and framework for evidence transfer. BMC Health Serv Res 15: 33.

2. Tu D, Belda P, Littlejohn D, Pedersen JS, Valle-Rivera J, et al. (2013) Adoption of the chronic care model to improve HIV care: In a marginalized, largely aboriginal population. Can Fam Physician 59: 650-657.

3. Swendeman D, Ingram BL, Rotheram-Borus MJ (2009) Common elements in self-management of HIV and other chronic illnesses: An integrative framework. AIDS Care 21: 1321-1334.

4. Mosack KE, Petroll A (2009) Patients' perspectives on informal caregiver involvement in HIV health care appointments. AIDS Patient Care STDS 23: 1043-1051.

5. Cecilio LCO (2009) The death of Ivan Ilyich, by Leo Tolstoy: Points to be considered regarding the multiple dimensions of healthcare management. Interface comunicação saúde educação 13: 545-555.

6. Fontanella BJ, Luchesi BM, Saidel MG, Ricas J, Turato ER, et al. (2011) Sampling in qualitative research: A proposal for procedures to detect theoretical saturation. Cad Saude Publica 27: 388-394.

7. Cassiani SHDB, Zago MMF. (1997) Analysis of qualitative data: experiencing the use of The Ethnograph. Acta paul. enferm 10: 100-106.

8. Moraes R (2003) A storm of light: Comprehension made possible by discursive textual analysis. Ciênc educ 9: 191-211.

9. Novoa PC (2014) What changes in research ethics in Brazil: resolution no. 466/12 of the National Health Council. Einstein (Sao Paulo) of the National Health Council. Einstein 12: 7-10.

10. Falcón GS, Erdmann AL, Meirelles, BHS (2006) Complexity in the education of professionals for the health care. Texto Contexto Enferm 15: 343-351.

11. Santos SS, Hammerschmidt KS (2012) Complexity and the reconnection of interdisciplinary knowledge: Contribution of Edgar Morin's thoughts. Rev Bras Enferm 65: 561-565.

12. Silva GM, Seiffert OM (2009) Continuing education in nursing: A methodological proposal. Rev Bras Enferm 62: 362-366.

13. United Nations (2011) Political declaration on HIV/AIDS: Intensifying our efforts.

14. Uebel K, Guise A, Georgeu D, Colvin C, Lewin S (2013) Integrating HIV care into nurse-led primary health care services in South Africa: A synthesis of three linked qualitative studies. BMC Health Serv Res 13: 171.

15. Mendes EV (2010) Health care networks. Cien Saude Colet 15: 2297-2305.

16. Fujita M, Poudel KC, Green K, Wi T, Abeyewickreme I, et al. (2015) HIV service delivery models towards 'Zero AIDS-related Deaths': a collaborative case study of 6 Asia and Pacific countries. BMC Health Serv Res 15: 176.

17. Brazil. Steps for implementation do management of hair infection HIV in primary.

18. Pfeiffer J, Montoya P, Baptista AJ, Karagianis M, Pugas Mde M, et al. (2010) Integration of HIV/AIDS services into African primary health care: Lessons learned for health system strengthening in Mozambique - a case study. J Int AIDS Soc 13: 3.

19. Geng EH, Nash D, Kambugu A, Zhang Y, Braitstein P, et al. (2010) Retention in care among HIV-infected patients in resource-limited settings: Emerging insights and new directions. Curr HIV/AIDS Rep 7: 234-244.

20. Siedner MJ, Lankowski A, Tsai AC, Muzoora C, Martin JN, et al. (2013) GPS-measured distance to clinic, but not self-reported transportation factors, are associated with missed HIV clinic visits in rural Uganda. AIDS 27: 1503-1508.

21. Higa DH, Marks G, Crepaz N, Liau A, Lyles CM (2012) Interventions to improve retention in HIV primary care: a systematic review of U.S. studies. Curr HIV/AIDS Rep 9: 313-325.

32

Assessment of Nursing Care Experience and Associated Factors Among Adult Inpatients in Black-Lion Hospital, Addis Ababa, Ethiopia: An Institution-Based Cross-Sectional Study

Mulugeta Molla[1*], Aster Berhe[2], Ashenafi Shumey[3] and Yohannes Adama[3]

[1]Department of Nursing, College of Health Sciences, Mekelle University, Ethiopia

[2]School of Nursing, College of Medicine and Health Science, Addis Ababa University, Ethiopia

[3]Department of Public Health, College of health sciences, Mekelle University, Ethiopia

*Corresponding author: Mulugeta Molla, Department of Nursing, College of Health Sciences, Mekelle University, Ethiopia, muler.warso@gmail.com

Abstract

Introduction: Patient experience has been used as an indicator to measure the quality of health care provided by nurses. However, this information is rarely available in countries like Ethiopia without which improving the quality of service and demonstrating the benefits of changes in nursing practice is usually difficult. The aim of this study was to assess nursing care experience and associated factors among adult inpatients in Black-Lion hospital, Addis Ababa, Ethiopia from March to April 2012.

Method: An institution-based cross-sectional study was employed among 374 adult patients admitted to Medical, Surgical and Gynecologic wards in Black-Lion hospital, Addis Ababa. Patients admitted during the study period was considered and convenient sampling was used. A modified<Newcastle Experience with Nursing Scales (NENSs) was used as data collection tool. Data were entered with Epi Info version 3.5.1 and cleaning and analysis was done by using SPSS version 16. Frequencies distribution, binary and multiple logistic regressions were done. Odds Ratio and 95% confidence interval was computed.

Result: A total of 374 adult patients from medical, surgical and gynecological wards were approached from the study hospital with 100% response rate. About 90% of patients had rated the experience above the mean. Number of nights the patient spent in the ward (AOR: 0.26) and occupation (AOR: 2.90) were found to be significant predictors of patients' better nursing experience.

Conclusion and Recommendation: Nine out of ten patients had rated nursing experience above the mean which is relatively higher magnitude. Patients who should stay longer have to be given insight to better boost the nursing experience.

Keywords: Patients' experience; Nursing care; Inpatients; Ethiopia

Introduction

Something that satisfies will adequately fulfill expectations, needs or desires and, by giving what is required, leaves no room for complaint [1]. Patient satisfaction with nursing care is the degree of convergence between the expectations patients have of ideal care and their perception of the care they really get [2,3]. And it has a vital role in the effectiveness of care, in increasing patient compliance with medication, advice and in making patients more likely to return for their follow up appointments [4,5]. Though patient satisfaction is a patient's judgment on the quality of care in all aspects, but the interpersonal process, the patient experience, is the major concern. Patient experience is related to technical and interpersonal behavior, partnership building, immediate and positive non-verbal behavior, more social observation, courtesy, consideration, clear communication and information, respectful treatment, frequency of contact, length of consultation, service availability and waiting time [6].

Patient experience has been, therefore, used as an indicator to measure the quality of health care provided by nurses. However, this information is rarely available in countries like Ethiopia without which improving the quality of service and demonstrating the benefits of changes in nursing practice is usually difficult.

The aim of this study was therefore i) to determine nursing care experience among adult inpatients in Black-Lion Hospital, Addis Ababa, Ethiopia from March to April 2012. ii) To identify associated factors among adult inpatients in Black-Lion hospital, Addis Ababa, Ethiopia from March to April 2012.

Materials and Methods

Study area and period

The study was conducted in Addis Ababa, the capital city of Ethiopia and seat of African Union & United Nations World Economic Commission for Africa. Addis Ababa has a population size of over 3 million. Its average elevation is 2,500 m above sea level, and hence has a fairly favorable climate and moderate weather conditions.

The city has 48 hospitals. Thirteen are public hospitals of which, 5 are under Addis Ababa Regional Health Bureau (AARHB) and 5 are specialized referral (central) hospitals. And this study was conducted in Black lion specialized referral teaching hospital which is under Addis Ababa University. The hospital has about 500 beds, seven X-ray, nine surgical and two laboratory diagnostic rooms.

The hospital is providing medical services in the internal medicine, gynecological & obstetrics, Surgical, pediatrics & emergency departments. In addition, the hospital has special units (Referral clinics): Chest, Renal, Neurology, Cardiology, Dermatology & S.T.D, Gastro intestine, Infectious diseases, Orthopedics, General surgical, gynecologic & obstetrics, Diabetic, Hematology, Medical ICU, Surgical ICU Units. The study was conducted from March 25, 2012 to April 28, 2012

Study design, population and sampling

An institution-based cross-sectional study was used to assess patient experience of nursing care among adult patients admitted in medical, surgical and Gynaecology wards, for more than two days, in Black Lion Hospital. Patients who were admitted in ICU, Emergency, Paediatrics, oncology units and those in patients who had cognitive problem and unable to communicate during data collection time were excluded in the study.

The sample size for the study was calculated using single population proportion formula using the assumption that the proportion of patient satisfaction to be 67%, 95% CI, 5% marginal error, and 10% none response rate, a total of 374 inpatients were required for the study.

Number of patients needed from each ward was proportional allocated based on the number of beds there was in medical, surgical and gynaecology ward. Then, convenient sampling was used to select study participants and collect data. Patients who were admitted during data collection were included in the study and new patients who were admitted after we initiated data collection were interviewed after two days of admission. Finally 87,111 and 66 patients were interviewed from gynaecologic, medical and surgical wards, respectively.

Data collection tool

The data were collected according to the Newcastle Experience with Nursing Care Scales (NENSs) users' manual. Questionnaires were translated in to Amharic and back to English to check for consistency. For each ward, one literate non health professional was recruited as data collector to avoid bias and one professional supervisor. Face to face interview was used to collect data. The NENS were developed by Thomas et al. [7] by measuring patients' experiences, based on their perspective. The scales are incorporated into an interview questionnaire, which comprises two sections: (I) experiences of nursing care scale, and (II) demographic information section. The questionnaires were both open and close-ended questions. The scores were categorized into the following levels and this is adopted from the research done in Jordan in 2009 [8].

Criteria for classification of experience score

- Good level and Above good level of experience >60%(those who answer 16 and above)
- Below good level of experience ≤ 60%(those who answer 15 and less)

Data quality control

Training was given to data collectors. The data collectors interviewed the inpatient without wearing gown in order to reduce the social desirability bias and then the quality, clarity and consistency of the questionnaire. The translated questionnaire was pre-tested in 20 patients in St. Paul.

Data analysis, presentation and interpretation

Data were entered using EPI info version 3.5.1 statistical software and cleaning and analysis was made using SPSS version 16. Cleaning was made using frequencies. The open ended questions were coded before entry. Univariate was done to describe dependent and independent variables; percentages, frequency distributions and measures of central tendency and measures of dispersion were used for describing data. Then binary logistic regression was made to see the crude significant relation of each variable with dependant variables. Finally, independent variables found significant were entered to multivariate logistic regressions to control the effect of confounding. Stepwise backward LR was used for multiple logistic regressions. Odds ratio with 95% confidence interval to ascertain association between independent and dependent variable was used.

Ethical considerations

Ethical clearance was obtained from institutional review board of Addis Ababa University. Informed consent was sought from all the study participants and they were reassured that they would be anonymous. Names or any personal identifiers were not recorded. Respondents were clearly told about the study and the variety of information needed from them. They were given the chance to ask anything about the study and made free to refuse or stop the interview at any moment they want if that was their choice.

Results

Socio demographic characteristics

A total of 374 adult inpatients' who had spent two or more days in black lion hospital were included in this study with 100% response rate. The mean age of participants was 40.3(SD=1.55) and the minimum age was 18 and the maximum age was 86 (Table 1).

Variable	Category	Frequency	Percent (%)
Age M(SD)	<=50 years	275	73.5%
	>50 years	99	26.5%
	40.3 (SD=1.55)		
Sex	M	174	46.5%
	F	200	53.5%
Educational Status	Illiterate	72	19.3%
	Literate	302	80.7%
Religion	Orthodox	246	65.8%
	Muslim	85	22.7%
	Others	43	11.5%

Marital Status	Living together	95	25.4%
	Never married	279	74.6%
Nights in the ward M(SD)	0-10	235	62.8%
	11-21	97	25.9%
	>=22	42	11.2%
	13.56 (SD=19.92)		
History of previous Admission	Yes	99	26.5%
	No	275	73.5%
Occupation	Employed	48	12.8%
	Not Employed	326	87.2%

Ethnicity	Amhara	157	42.0
	Tigrie	39	10.4
	Gurage	103	27.5
	Oromo	45	12.0
	Others	30	8.0

Table 1: Participants' characteristics who had been admitted in Black lion Hospital April to March, 2012

The median length of stay was 7 days. Among all respondents, 48.7% of inpatients rated nursing care they receive in the ward very good but 1.1% rate, as it was dreadful (Figure 1).

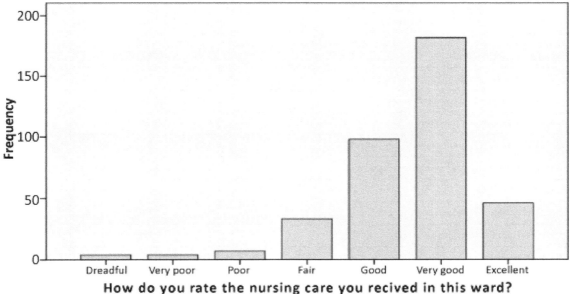

Figure 1: Rate of nursing care received in Surgical, Medical, and Gyn/Obs wards Black Lion Hospital April-March, 2012.

Majority of the respondents, 357 (95.5%), said nurses had good communication and interpersonal skill and 354 (94.7%) inpatients would recommend this hospital to the people they know who might seek medical care in the future.

Patient experience

About 91% (340/374, 95% CI: 87.67%, 93.52%) of the respondents rated their nursing care experience good and above.

Women admitted in Gyn/Obs ward (94.28%) had the highest proportion of "Good and Above Good" scores compared to other wards (surgical (91.48%) and medical (87.38%)).

The mean of experience with nursing care for the total sample was 3.64 (SD=1.43). Participants in Surgical wards had a better experience with nursing care (mean=3.72; SD=1.45) when compared with participants in medical and Gyn/Obs ward (Table 2).

Item	Medical	Gyn/OBs	Surgical

	Mean	SD	Mean	SD	Mean	SD
It was easy to have a laugh with the nurses	5.57	1.39	5.93	1.08	5.89	1.18
#2. Nurses favored some patients over others	1.29	1.19	1.18	0.77	1.22	0.98
#3. Nurses did not tell me enough about my treatment	2.45	2.16	1.38	1.13	1.71	1.61
#4. Nurses were too easy going and laid back	1.52	1.48	1.31	1.03	1.49	1.36
#5. Nurses took a long time when the they were called	2.22	1.92	1.51	1.13	1.83	1.68
Nurses gave me information just when I needed it	5.27	1.46	5.48	1.50	5.80	1.19
#7. Nurses did not seem to know what I was going through	1.74	1.59	1.37	1.05	1.62	1.60
#8. Nurses turned the lights off too late at night	2.46	2.49	2.09	2.32	1.49	1.53
#9. Nurses made me do things before I was ready	1.11	0.65	1.17	0.89	1.37	1.29
No matter how busy nurses were, they made time for me	5.10	1.60	5.51	1.18	5.28	1.50
I saw the nurses as friends	5.01	1.58	5.47	1.33	5.53	1.41
Nurses spent time comforting patients who were upset	5.25	1.47	5.52	1.29	5.65	1.41
Nurses checked regularly to make sure I was okay	5.29	1.51	5.82	1.18	5.90	1.07
# 14. Nurses let things get on top of Them	1.32	1.04	1.32	1.08	1.38	1.04
#15. Nurses took no interest in me as a person	1.74	1.78	1.41	1.35	1.88	1.98
Nurses explained what was wrong with me	4.86	1.82	5.23	1.72	5.43	1.71
Nurses explained what they were going to do to me before they did it	4.84	1.80	5.47	1.41	5.43	1.59
Nurses told the next shift what was happening with my care	3.69	2.45	3.76	2.50	4.09	2.47
Nurses knew what to do without relying on doctors	4.32	2.16	4.07	2.33	4.47	2.40
#20. Nurses used to go away and forget what patients had asked for	1.90	1.69	1.64	1.55	1.91	1.89
Nurses made sure that patients had privacy when they needed it	6.13	1.50	6.29	1.21	6.28	1.23
Nurses had time to sit and talk to me	1.37	1.10	1.80	1.62	1.38	1.09
Doctors and nurses worked well together as a team	5.33	1.50	6.01	0.79	6.06	1.12
#24. Nurses did not seem to know what each other was doing	1.43	1.22	1.18	0.67	1.38	1.24
Nurses knew what to do for the Best	5.63	0.93	6.03	1.17	6.15	0.96
There was a happy atmosphere in the ward, thanks to the nurses	5.90	1.41	6.43	1.10	6.16	1.18
Average 3.57 1.53 3.63 1.32 3.72 1.45						

Table 2: Mean and Standard deviations for patient's Experience of nursing care in Black-Lion hospital, Addis Ababa, Ethiopia from March-April 2012.

#All these negative items were reversed during analysis to be positive items

Factors found associated with inpatients' nursing care experience

After applying bivariate and multiple logistic regressions two variables were found to be significantly associated with inpatients nursing care experience in Black-Lion hospital, Addis Ababa. These were the number of nights they spent in the ward (95%CI, AOR: 0.26(0.12, 0.57)) and occupation of the inpatients (95%CI, AOR: 2.90(1.10, 7.62)). People who spent 10-22 days are less likely to have a good and above good level of experience than those patients who spent <10 days. People who were not employed had a better experience than those who were employed (Table 3).

Variable	Category	Experience of patient with Nursing		COR (95% CI)	AOR (95% CI)
		Below good level of experience	Good & above level of experience		
Sex	Male	21	153	1.00	1.00
	Female	13	187	1.97(0.96,4.07)	1.99(0.79,5.02)
Age	<=50 years	22	253	1.00	1.00
	>50 years	12	87	0.63(0.30,1.33)	0.50(0.20,1.21)
Ward	Surgical	15	161	1.00	1.00
	Medical	14	97	0.65 (0.30,1.40)	0.61(0.26,1.44)
	Gynecology	5	82	1.53 (0.54,4.35)	0.70(0.18,2.74)
Nights in ward	2-10	14	221	1.00	1.00
	11-21	18	79	0.28(0.13,0.59)	0.26(0.12,0.57)*
	>=22	2	40	1.27(0.28,5.79)	1.34(0.28,6.40)
Religion	Orthodox	21	225	1.00	1.00
	Muslim	12	73	0.59(0.27,1.21)	0.46(0.20,1.06)
	Others	1	42	3.92(0.51,29.4)	3.19(0.40,25.18)
Occupation	Employed	8	40	1.00	1.00
	Not employed	26	300	2.31(0.98,5.44)	2.90(1.10,7.62)*

Table 3: Factors affecting experiences of patients' with nursing care in BLH April to March 2012

*Significantly associated (p<0.05, **highly significantly associated (P<0.001)

Discussion

The result of our study revealed that the proportion of patients who experienced good or above nursing care was 91%. Number of nights the patient spent and occupation of the patients were found to be the independent predictors of nursing care experience among the adult inpatients.

The 91% good and above experience of nursing care among inpatients was high in magnitude when compared with other studies conducted in Jordan and Japan [9,10]. This might be related with the low awareness of the people on how should be nursing care and the recent movement of Ethiopian Ministry of Health to ameliorate the nursing care.

In this study participants had above the mean level of experiences in different measurements such as Doctors and nurses worked well together as a team, nurses knew what to do for the best, it was easy to laugh with nurses and nurses didn't forget what the patients' had asked for. These findings were consistent with the finding in Newcastle and Jordan [6,9]. Such results indicate the important collaborative role and patients' relationship with nurses and doctors.

Participants of this study had lower experience of nursing care with aspects such as nurses told the next shift what was happening with my care, nurses did not made me do things before I was ready, nurses did not favored some patients over others and nurses did not tell me

enough about my treatment when compared with findings from Jordan and New castle [6,9]. The reason for this might be high workload and lack of knowledge, attitude and practice to those particular issues.

In this study number of nights spent in the ward had a significant relationships with patients' experience of nursing care which was similar with the findings in Japan and Turkey [10,11]. This might be because as the patients stayed for a long period of time it might be related with poor prognosis of their problems and their expectation and frustration might be increased or the nurses might be faded up with low prognosis of patients.

In this study occupation also had an association with patients' experience which contrasts the findings of Jordan, Japan, and Turkey studies [8,9,11]. Those who were not employed had better experience than those who were employed. This might be because those who were employed had better overall health related awareness and might not need the same care as unemployed/poorer people.

This study found that gender, age, ward and religion seemed to have no effect on their experience with nursing care, which was consistent with the findings in Turkey [11].

Conclusion

In this research, the overall patient experiences were 91% and this implied that the nursing care service that provided in Black lion hospital was better. The number of nights spent in the ward and occupation were found to affect patient experience with nursing care.

Acknowledgement

We would like to thank the NSNS team at the University of Newcastle up on Tyne for their permission to use the NSNS standardized questionnaire in this study particularly Professor Elaine McColl. And we thank Addis Ababa University for financial support. We would also like to give our special gratitude to Federal Ministry of Health Quality management team, especially Mohammedamin Adem, officer, Medical Services Directorate for providing Ethiopian Hospital Reform Implementation guidelines.

We want to spread out our gratefulness to our study participants for their willingness to participate in our study and data collectors are also acknowledged.

References

1. Crow R, Gage H, Hampson S, Hart J, Kimber A, et al. (2002) The measurement of satisfaction with healthcare: implications for practice from a systematic review of the literature. Health Technol Assess 6: 1-244.

2. Risser NL (1975) Development of an instrument to measure patient satisfaction with nurses and nursing care in primary care settings. Nurs Res 24: 45-52.

3. Merkouris A, Ifantopoulos J, Lanara V, Lemonidou C (1999) Patient satisfaction: a key concept for evaluating and improving nursing services. J Nurs Manag 7: 19-28.

4. Bond S, Thomas LH (1992) Measuring patients' satisfaction with nursing care. J Adv Nurs 17: 52-63.

5. Yilmaz M Saglik bakim kalitesinin bir olcutu: hasta memnuniyeti (2001) [Patient satisfaction: an indicator for quality of health care]. Cumhuriyet Universitesi Hemsirelik Yuksekokulu Dergisi 5: 69–74. Issues in clinical nursing Newcastle Satisfaction with Nursing Care Scale.

6. Westaway MS, Rheeder P, Van Zyl DG, Seager JR (2003) Interpersonal and organizational dimensions of patient satisfaction: the moderating effects of health status. Int J Qual Health Care 15: 337-344.

7. Thomas LH, McColl E, Priest J, Bond S, Boys RJ (1996) Newcastle satisfaction with nursing scales: an instrument for quality assessments of nursing care. Qual Health Care 5: 67-72.

8. Alhusban MA, Abualrub RF (2009) Patient satisfaction with nursing care in Jordan. J Nurs Manag 17: 749-758.

9. Ahmad MM, Alasad JA (2004) Predictors of patients' experiences of nursing care in medical-surgical wards. Int J Nurs Pract 10: 235-241.

10. Tokunaga J, Imanaka Y, Nobutomo K (2002) Influence of length of stay on patient satisfaction with hospital care in Japan. International Journal for Quality in Health Care 12 (5) : 395-401.

11. Findik UY, Unsar S, Sut N (2010) Patient satisfaction with nursing care and its relationship with patient characteristics. Nurs Health Sci 12: 162-169.

Permissions

All chapters in this book were first published in JNC, by OMICS International; hereby published with permission under the Creative Commons Attribution License or equivalent. Every chapter published in this book has been scrutinized by our experts. Their significance has been extensively debated. The topics covered herein carry significant findings which will fuel the growth of the discipline. They may even be implemented as practical applications or may be referred to as a beginning point for another development.

The contributors of this book come from diverse backgrounds, making this book a truly international effort. This book will bring forth new frontiers with its revolutionizing research information and detailed analysis of the nascent developments around the world.

We would like to thank all the contributing authors for lending their expertise to make the book truly unique. They have played a crucial role in the development of this book. Without their invaluable contributions this book wouldn't have been possible. They have made vital efforts to compile up to date information on the varied aspects of this subject to make this book a valuable addition to the collection of many professionals and students.

This book was conceptualized with the vision of imparting up-to-date information and advanced data in this field. To ensure the same, a matchless editorial board was set up. Every individual on the board went through rigorous rounds of assessment to prove their worth. After which they invested a large part of their time researching and compiling the most relevant data for our readers.

The editorial board has been involved in producing this book since its inception. They have spent rigorous hours researching and exploring the diverse topics which have resulted in the successful publishing of this book. They have passed on their knowledge of decades through this book. To expedite this challenging task, the publisher supported the team at every step. A small team of assistant editors was also appointed to further simplify the editing procedure and attain best results for the readers.

Apart from the editorial board, the designing team has also invested a significant amount of their time in understanding the subject and creating the most relevant covers. They scrutinized every image to scout for the most suitable representation of the subject and create an appropriate cover for the book.

The publishing team has been an ardent support to the editorial, designing and production team. Their endless efforts to recruit the best for this project, has resulted in the accomplishment of this book. They are a veteran in the field of academics and their pool of knowledge is as vast as their experience in printing. Their expertise and guidance has proved useful at every step. Their uncompromising quality standards have made this book an exceptional effort. Their encouragement from time to time has been an inspiration for everyone.

The publisher and the editorial board hope that this book will prove to be a valuable piece of knowledge for researchers, students, practitioners and scholars across the globe.

List of Contributors

Mulugeta Aseratie
Department of Nursing, College of Health Science, Addis Ababa Science and Technology University, Addis Ababa Ethiopia

Rajalakshmi Murugan
School of Nursing, College of Health Science, Addis Ababa University, Addis Ababa, Ethiopia

Mulugeta Molla, Ashenafi Shumey and Yohannes Adama
Department of Nursing, College of Health Science, Mekelle University, Mekelle, Ethiopia

Cheryl Ann Alexander
Department of Nursing, University of Phoenix, USA

Lidong Wang
Department of Engineering Technology, Mississippi Valley State University, USA

Geofery Luntsi, Aishatu Babagana Ajikolo, Nkubli Bobuin Flaviuos, Chigozie Nwobi, Jamila Muhammed Hassan and Fati Adamu Malgwi
Department of Medical Radiography, College of Medical Sciences, University of Maiduguri, Borno State, Nigeria

Lola Nelson
Department of Nursing Sciences, College of Medical Sciences, University of Maiduguri, Borno State, Nigeria

Mafumo JL, Netshandama VO and Netshikweta L
Department of Advanced Nursing Science, University of Venda, South Africa

Zakaria A Mani and Mohammed Abutaleb
Ministry of Health, Nursing Education, Saudi Arabia

Tim Henwood
The University of Queensland, University of Queensland/ Blue Care Research and Practice Development Centre, School of Nursing, Midwifery and Social Work, Brisbane, Australia

Anthony Tuckett
The University of Queensland, School of Nursing, Midwifery and Social Work, Brisbane, Australia

Nadja E –Bagadi
School of Nursing and Midwifery, Freiburg University, Freiburg, Germany

John Oliffe
School of Nursing, University of British Columbia, Vancouver, Canada

Bi Lian Chen
Department of Nursing, Taichung Veterans General Hospital, Taiwan

David O Ajeigbe
Alumni University of California School of Nursing, Nurse Manage Ambulatory Managed Care Service, Inland Empire Health Plan, Rancho Cucamonga, California, USA

Donna McNeese-Smith
Emerita University of California School of Nursing, Los Angeles, CA, USA

Linda R Phillips
Sectional Chair, Acute and Chronic Health Services, University of California School of Nursing, Los Angeles, CA, USA

Linda Searle Leach
University of California School of Nursing, Los Angeles, CA, USA

Naglaa Abd El- Aziz El Seesy and Faten El Sebaey
Alexandria University, Department of Nursing Administration, Faculty of Nursing, Alexandria, Egypt

Ragusa
Heath Technology Assessment Committee, University Hospital, Italy
Committee against nosocomial infection, University Hospital "G. Rodolico" Catania, Italy
Direzione Medica di Presidio, University Hospital "G. Rodolico" Catania, Italy

Lombardo
Heath Technology Assessment Committee, University Hospital, Italy
Committee against nosocomial infection, University Hospital "G. Rodolico" Catania, Italy
Nursing for the Control of Hospital Infections, University Hospital "G. Rodolico" Catania, Italy

Bruno A
Nursing for the Control of Hospital Infections, University Hospital "G. Rodolico" Catania, Italy

Sciacca A
Committee against nosocomial infection, University Hospital "G. Rodolico" Catania, Italy
Department of Biomedical and Biotechnological Sciences, University of Catania, Italy

Lupo L
Heath Technology Assessment Committee, University Hospital, Italy
Department of Medical and Surgical Sciences and advanced technologies, University of Catania, Italy

Vasanthrie Naidoo
School of Nursing, Department of Medical and Surgical Nursing, Life College of Learning-KZN, South Africa

Sibiya MN
School of Nursing, Faculty of Health Sciences, Durban University of Technology, South Africa

Nurdan Gezer
Medical Surgical Nursing Department, Nursing Faculty, Adnan Menderes University, Aydın, Turkey

Belgin Yildirim
Health Nursing Department, Nursing Faculty, Adnan Menderes University, Aydın, Turkey

Esma Özaydın
Adnan Menderes University Hospital Intensive Care Unit, Aydın, Turkey

Do Thi Ha and Khanitta Nuntaboot
Faculty of Nursing, Khon Kaen University, Vietnam

Tereza Cristina Guimaraes Felippe
Coordinator of the Heart Failure and Cardiac Transplantation of the National Institute of Cardiology / Rio de Janeiro, Brazil

Deyse Conceicao Santoro
Department of Medical Surgical EEAN / UFRJ, Brazil

Maria Jirwe and Azita Emami
Department of Neurobiology, Care Sciences and Society, Division of Nursing, Karolinska Institutet, Sweden

Kate Gerrish
School of Nursing and Midwifery, University of Sheffield, UK

Aysun Ünal
Department of Pediatric Surgery, Dokuz Eylul University, Izmir, Turkey

Seyda Seren
Department of Nursing Management, Dokuz Eylul University, Izmir, Turkey

Jemal Beker and Tesafa Bamlie
Department of Nursing, College of Public Health and Medical Sciences, Jimma University, Ethiopia

Anette C Ekstrom, Lena Nilsson and Lena B Martensson
School of Health and Education, University of Skovde, SE-54128 Skovde, Sweden

Caroline Apell
The Municipality of Alingsas, SE-44181 Alingsas, Sweden

David Palmius
Skaraborg Hospital Skovde, SE-54182 Skovde, Sweden

Adriana Lima Pimenta, Maria de Lourdes de Souza and Flavia Regina de Souza Ramos
Federal University of Santa, Brazil

Donna M. Glynn, Kelsey W. ILL, Margaret Taylor, Athena Lynch and Jodi DeLibertis
Simmons College, School of Nursing and Health Sciences, USA.

Ji Young Noh
Severance Hospital, Yonsei University, Korea

Eui Geum Oh, Won Hee Lee and Mona Choi
College of Nursing, Yonsei University, Korea

Marica Guevarra Estrada and Crestita Tan
The Graduate School University of Santo Tomas, Philippines
University of Santo Tomas College of Nursing, Philippines

Zeljko Vlaisavljević and Ivan Rankovic
University of Mississippi Clinical Centre of Serbia, Clinic for Gastroenterolgy and Hepatology, Street of Dr Koste Todorovica 2, 11 000 Belgrade, Serbia

Anita Afua Davies
School of Nursing, University of Cape coast, Cape Coast, Ghana

Christiana Buxton
Department of Mathematics and Science Education, University of Cape Coast, Ghana

Ya-Lie Ku
Fooyin University, Kaohsiung, Taiwan

Donna J. Plonczynski
Northern Illinois University, USA

Donna Kruse
Clinical Educator/Magnet Program Director, Advocate Sherman Hospital, USA

Nurilign Abebe and Habtamu Abera
Nursing Department, Medicine and Health Sciences College, Debre Markos University, Debre Markos, Ethiopia

Mulatu Ayana
Public Health Department, Medicine and Health Sciences College, Debre Markos University, Debre Markos, Ethiopia

Mikiko Natsume
Department of Nursing College of Life and Health Sciences, Chubu University, Japan

Katusmasa OTA
Nagoya University Graduate School of Medicine Doctor of Medical Sciences, Japan

Líscia Divana Carvalho Silva and Marli Villela Mamede
Universidade Federal do Maranhão. São Luís, MA, Brazil

Shirin Badruddin and Shazia Arif
King Faisal Specialist Hospital and Research Center, Surgical Intensive Care Unit, Riyadh, Saudi Arabia

Betina Hörner Schlindwein Meirelles, Samara Eliane Rabelo Suplici, Veridiana Tavares Costa, Aline Daiane Colaço, Bárbara Aparecida Oliveira Forgearini and Valdete Meurer Kuehlkamp
Universidade Federal de Santa Catarina, Florianópolis, Santa Catarina, Brazil

Aster Berhe
School of Nursing, College of Medicine and Health Science, Addis Ababa University, Ethiopia

Index

CPSIA information can be obtained
at www.ICGtesting.com
Printed in the USA
BVHW090936120619
550807BV00003B/100/P

9 781632 425850